The Acquisition of Motor Behavior
in Vertebrates

The Acquisition of Motor Behavior in Vertebrates

edited by James R. Bloedel, Timothy J. Ebner, and Steven P. Wise

A Bradford Book
The MIT Press
Cambridge, Massachusetts
London, England

This book was set in Palatino by Asco Trade Typesetting Ltd., Hong Kong and was printed and bound in the United States of America.

Library of Congress Cataloging-in-Publication Data
Acquisition of motor behavior in vertebrates / edited by James R.
 Bloedel, Timothy J. Ebner, and Steven P. Wise.
      p.   cm.
  "The proceedings of a satellite meeting held at the fifth annual
 Neural Control of Movement meeting in Key West, Florida from April
 23 to April 25, 1995"—Pref.
 "A Bradford book".
 Includes bibliographical references and index.
 ISBN 0-262-02404-7 (hc : alk. paper)
  1. Motor learning—Congresses. 2. Efferent pathways—Congresses.
 I. Bloedel, James R. II. Ebner, Timothy J. III. Wise, Steven P.
 QP303.A66   1996
 599'.01852—dc20   95-46159
                                                            CIP

Contents

Preface

Practice makes perfect or at least predicates perfect performance. It does so both because experience promotes the learning of how and when to do something and because learning *to do* virtually anything requires the nervous system to acquire new (and modify old) motor behaviors. In athletics, dance, music, and even in countless daily chores, our motor learning capabilities determine how we work and play. Our ability to master movements and to synthesize them into seamless sequences forms a natural limit to our athletic and artistic talents, both individually and as a species. As for other animals, even those most well-endowed in flesh and bone have much to learn from experience, be it practice or play.

In this volume are the proceedings of a satellite seminar held at the fifth annual Neural Control of Movement meeting in Key West, Florida from April 23 to April 25, 1995. These chapters explore motor learning and some of the mechanisms underlying the acquisition of motor behavior in vertebrates. Though we made no effort to construct a comprehensive compendium on motor learning, we did seek to develop a broad survey that would convey the character of much contemporary investigation into the subject. The diverse disciplines represented here include physiology, psychology, evolutionary biology, neurology, and computational modeling. It is our belief that such diversity promotes a more thorough understanding of motor learning than would concentration on any one of the traditional academic disciplines alone.

We hope this book will lend itself to the needs of those undergraduate and graduate students interested in advanced topics in neurobiology or other interdisciplinary fields of inquiry. Of course, we also expect that experts in the traditional fields of physiology and psychology, in exercise and sports science, and in clinical neurology will find topics of interest among the present chapters. Researchers in the burgeoning fields of human brain imaging and computational modeling should find analyses and approaches that will prove to be highly pertinent to their investigations as well.

Acquisition of Motor Behavior in Vertebrates

1 Introduction

James R. Bloedel, Timothy J. Ebner, and
Steven P. Wise

The acquisition of a motor behavior implies that motor learning has taken place, even though the meaning of the phrase *motor learning* remains subject to debate. Although several of the contributors to this volume (e.g., Harvey and Welsh, Hallett et al., Ebner et al., Stelmach, and Donoghue et al.) attempt useful definitions of one sort or another, we find ourselves in accord with Medawar and Medawar (1993, p. 66) in recognizing that although "a principal purpose of definition is to bring peace of mind...[s]ometimes...it is too dearly bought." Accordingly, we have embraced no single definition of motor learning and have elected from the outset to include a diversity of relevant topics. We trust that a useful perspective can be obtained by inclusion of research areas apart from the traditional approaches to motor learning (e.g., Pew, 1974; Summers, 1981, 1992; Schmidt, 1988, 1991; Adams, 1987; Rosenbaum, 1991), including the study of nonassociative reflexes, conditioned reflexes, and learning the context for the performance of already learned movements.

From a biological perspective, the function of the central nervous system (CNS) is to acquire a behavioral repertoire and to select from it those actions most likely to enhance an individual's fitness. As demonstrated in chapter 3, this information storage can accrue over generations and be expressed epigenetically, or it might occur in one or a few instances of an individual's experience. Adaptation of reflexes, such as changes in vestibuloocular and postural reflexes, forms one aspect of motor learning that has been subject to intense scrutiny. The first part of this book is devoted to that topic. The second part addresses the controversial area of associative, conditioned reflexes, which modify behavior through linking different sources of information. Complex patterns of actions, including movement sequences, and the visual guidance of movement, all require practice for their modification. These topics comprise the subsequent two parts. In the final part, several broader perspectives on motor learning are offered.

Notwithstanding our intent to include a broad consideration of motor learning, practical limitations required exclusions. At the outset, we limited the meeting and volume to the acquisition of motor behavior in vertebrates, without implying that motor learning in invertebrates holds less intrinsic interest. Further, despite the occasional reference to molecular biology (e.g., see chapter 7), readers primarily interested in the molecular basis of motor learning should examine other sources (e.g., Dudai, 1989). In formulating the meeting's content, we chose to concentrate instead on the emergent properties of relatively intact biological systems. As for computational neuroscience, we included a selection of models (see chapters 2, 4, and 20) but recognized that comprehensive coverage of this area in its own right would have required volumes. An encyclopedia of the subject, *The Handbook of Brain Theory and Neural Networks*, is available from the MIT Press (Arbib, 1995).

On the general topics that we did include, many additional specific studies are worthy of equal attention. We point specifically to *Models of Information Processing in the Basal Ganglia*, also published by the MIT Press (Houk, Davis, and Beiser, 1995b). That volume includes several chapters on motor learning primarily in relation to the basal ganglia (Arbib and Dominey, 1995; Barto, 1995; Gabrielli, 1995; Graybiel and Kimura, 1995; Houk, Adams, and Barto, 1995a; Schultz, Apicella, Romo, and Scarnati, 1995; Schultz, Romo, Ljünberg, Mirenowicz, Hollerman, and Dickinson, 1995). We expect that future treatments of motor learning will explore further the relative contributions of basal ganglia, cerebellum, cerebral cortex, and brainstem to various aspects of motor learning.

Finally, we expect that a substantial proportion of future research into motor learning will make use of positron emission tomography and functional magnetic resonance imaging. These topics are briefly summarized here (see chapters 11 and 13), but are not particularly emphasized. Despite its promise, such research remains in its infancy. Future works on motor learning will contain many contributions from—and perhaps be dominated by—those new and developing technologies. It is our hope that the present volume summarizes research that will motivate and provide a firm foundation for such studies.

ACKNOWLEDGMENTS

We would like to thank Barry Peterson and Peter Strick for sharing the resources and administrative support of the Neural Control of Movement meeting. Anna and Ken Taylor were the conference organizers. We wish to acknowledge the generous financial support of the Barrow Neurological Institute of St. Joseph's Hospital and Medical Center and the Department of Neurosurgery of the University of Minnesota. We are indebted to Fiona Stevens of MIT Press for her efforts on behalf of this volume and to both Jan Carey and Susan Mann for providing secretarial support. We are especially grateful to the many authors who expedited production of this volume by observing, with due respect, the much-abused "deadline."

REFERENCES

Adams JA (1987). Historical review and appraisal of research on the learning, retention and transfer of human motor skills. Psych Bull 101:41−74.

Arbib MA (1995). The Handbook of Brain Theory and Neural Networks. Cambridge: MIT Press.

Arbib MA, Dominey PF (1995). Modeling the roles of basal ganglia in timing and sequencing saccadic eye movements. In JC Houk, JL Davis, DG Beiser (eds), Models of Information Processing in the Basal Ganglia. Cambridge: MIT Press, pp 149−162.

Barto AG (1995). Adaptive critics and the basal ganglia. In JC Houk, JL Davis, DG Beiser (eds), Models of Information Processing in the Basal Ganglia. Cambridge: MIT Press, pp 215−232.

Dudai Y (1989). The Neurobiology of Memory: Concepts, Findings, Trends. Oxford: Oxford University Press.

Gabrielli J (1995). Contribution of the basal ganglia to skill learning and working memory in humans. In JC Houk, JL Davis, DG Beiser (eds), Models of Information Processing in the Basal Ganglia. Cambridge: MIT Press, pp 277−294.

Graybiel AM, Kimura M (1995). Adaptive neural networks in the basal ganglia. In JC Houk, JL Davis, DG Beiser (eds), Models of Information Processing in the Basal Ganglia. Cambridge: MIT Press, pp 103−116.

Houk JC, Adams JL, Barto AG (1995a). A model of how the basal ganglia generate and use neural signals that predict reinforcement. In JC Houk, JL Davis, DG Beiser (eds), Models of Information Processing in the Basal Ganglia. Cambridge: MIT Press, pp 249−270.

Houk JC, Davis JL, Beiser DG (1995b). Models of Information Processing in the Basal Ganglia. Cambridge: MIT Press.

Medawar P, Medawar J (1983). Aristotle to Zoos. A Philosophical Dictionary of Biology. Oxford: Oxford University Press.

Pew RW (1974). Levels of analysis in motor control. Brain Res 71:393−400.

Rosenbaum DA (1991). Human Motor Control. San Diego: Academic Press.

Schmidt RA (1988). Motor Control and Learning. Champaign: Human Kinetics Books.

Schmidt, RA (1991). Motor Learning and Performance: From Principles to Practice. Champaign, IL: Human Kinetics Books.

Schultz W, Apicella P, Romo R, Scarnati E (1995). Context-dependent activity in primate striatum reflecting past and future behavioral events. In JC Houk, JL Davis, DG Beiser (eds), Models of Information Processing in the Basal Ganglia. Cambridge: MIT Press, pp 11−28.

Schultz W, Romo R, Ljüngberg T, Mirenowicz J, Hollerman JR, Dickinson A (1995). Reward-related signals carried by dopamine neurons. In JC Houk, JL Davis, DG Beiser (eds), Models of Information Processing in the Basal Ganglia. Cambridge: MIT Press, pp 233−248.

Summers JJ (1981). Motor programs. In D Holding (ed), Human Skills. New York: Wiley, pp 41−64.

Summers JJ (1992). Approaches to the Study of Motor Control and Learning. Amsterdam: Elsevier.

I   Reflex Adaptation

2 Learning and Memory in the Vestibuloocular Reflex

Stephen G. Lisberger

In 1972, Ito first proposed the vestibuloocular reflex (VOR) as a model system for investigating the general question of the function of the cerebellum and its role in motor learning. His proposal was based on the theories of Marr (1969) and Albus (1971), both of which postulated that the cerebellar cortex was a site at which changes in the strength of synaptic transmission would cause changes in the motor response to a given combination of sensory stimuli. According to these general theories of cerebellar function and learning, the climbing fiber inputs to the cerebellar cortex carried "teaching" signals that guide learning; the synapse between parallel fibers and Purkinje cells would be the site of the changes (see also chapters 10 and 11, this volume). Conjuctive activity of the climbing-fiber input to a given Purkinje cell and a set of its parallel fiber inputs would cause changes in the strength of transmission from the active parallel fibers to the Purkinje cell.

Ito's proposal was based on two discoveries. First, a number of laboratories had discovered the physiological substrate for cerebellar participation in the VOR (Fukuda, Highstein, and Ito, 1972; Baker, Precht, and Llinas, 1972; Highstein, 1973). A part of the cerebellum called the *flocculus* sends inhibitory inputs directly to brainstem neurons that are interposed between vestibular primary afferents and extraocular motoneurons, thus forming interneurons in the most direct of the brainstem VOR pathways. Second, Gonshor and Melvill Jones (1976) had discovered that the VOR is subject to long-term adaptive modifications if a human subject wears prisms that cause left-right reversal of vision. Normally, the VOR compensates well for head turns so that angular head rotation in one direction causes smooth eye rotation in the opposite direction at close to the same speed as that of the head rotation. As a result, visual acuity remains excellent during head motion because normally the eyes are nearly stabilized in space, and images from the stationary surroundings remain stable with respect to the eyeball and the retina. Gonshor and Melvill Jones demonstrated that the gain of the VOR, defined as eye speed divided by head speed during angular head turns in darkness, gradually becomes lower if humans wear left-right-reversing prisms for several days. If measured during mental arithmetic, the gain of the VOR declined from a normal value of 0.7 to values as low as 0.2.[1] It is now known that motor learning in the VOR is a form of experience-dependent adaptation that normally occurs when visual image motion is persistently paired with head turns.

Based on the behavioral evidence of learning in the VOR, the electrophysiological demonstration of a direction project from cerebellar Purkinje cells to the brainstem VOR pathways, and the theories of Marr and Albus, Ito (1972) proposed that the function of the flocculus was to modulate transmission through the brainstem VOR pathways. He suggested that *long-term* modulation would occur through changes in the strength of synaptic transmission of vestibular input signals from parallel fibers to Purkinje cells. According to Ito's hypothesis, the visual signals that guide motor learning in the VOR would be provided by the climbing fiber inputs to the flocculus and the conjunction of visual climbing fiber and vestibular parallel fiber inputs to a given Purkinje cell would alter the strength of transmission of vestibular inputs provided by parallel fibers. The organization of the anatomical pathways dictates the relationship between the gain of the VOR and the strength of transmission in the vestibular pathways to Purkinje cells. The brainstem targets of floccular Purkinje cells (called *floccular target neurons* or *FTNs* by Lisberger, Pavelko, and Broussard, 1994a) receive vestibular signals over an excitatory pathway from the vestibular primary afferents and an inhibitory pathway from the flocculus. During a head turn, both inputs are present and their effects on the responses of FTNs are antagonistic: If learning causes an increase in the size of the vestibular response of Purkinje cells with no change in the strength of the input from the vestibular afferents, then the responses of FTNs to a given head turn will decrease. Thus, increases in the strength of the vestibular input to Purkinje cells will cause decreases in the gain of the VOR, and vice versa.

In this chapter, we want to emphasize the agreement of available data on motor learning in the VOR, even though in the 24 years since Ito's original hypothesis, considerable disagreement and controversy have arisen about the function of the cerebellum in general and its role in motor learning in the VOR. Although many important issues remain unresolved, we believe that the data support a single unified hypothesis for motor learning in the VOR. Our goal will be to show the general agreement among experiments on different species and in different laboratories. At the same time, we will highlight areas where further experiments are needed and point out assumptions that are critical to the single unified hypothesis that we propose.

EFFECT OF CEREBELLAR ABLATIONS ON LEARNING AND MEMORY IN THE VOR

It is important to distinguish between the dynamic events that cause changes in the gain of the VOR and their expression as the VOR that is evoked by head turns in the dark at any given moment. We will adopt the terminology of du Lac, Raymond, Sejnowski, and Lisberger, (1995), in which *learning* refers to the dynamic process by which combined image motion and head turns modify the VOR and *memory* refers to changes that are retained and measured during head turns in darkness.

Lesion studies generally agree that the cerebellum is essential for learning in the VOR, although the exact details of the results have differed slightly among species. One kind of experiment has ablated parts of the cerebellum when the gain of the VOR was normal and has discovered which parts of the cerebellum are necessary to allow learning. In cats, complete cerebellectomy prevents learning (Robinson, 1976), whereas in rabbits and goldfish, ablations reportedly restricted to the flocculus are sufficient to prevent learning (Schairer and Bennett, 1981; Nagao, 1983; Pastor, de la Cruz, and Baker, 1994). In primates, the situation is more complex (Lisberger, Miles, and Zee, 1984). Data from two animals have been reported. In one monkey, complete ablation of the flocculus, the associated ventral paraflocculus, and the surrounding dorsal paraflocculus completely prevented learning. In a second monkey, the same structures were ablated except that several of the most rostral folia of the ventral paraflocculus were spared. Learning in the VOR was slowed but not completely prevented.

A second kind of experiment, to date done only in nonprimate species, has investigated the role of the cerebellum in remembering a modified VOR. In goldfish, much but not all of the modified VOR was retained if the flocculus was ablated bilaterally after the VOR had been modified (Michnovicz and Bennett, 1987; Pastor et al., 1994). Exactly the same ablations reportedly prevented any further learning in the VOR, so that stimulation with combined visual and vestibular stimulation was not able to drive the VOR back to normal gains. In cats, simple-spike activity in the flocculus was ablated reversibly by stimulating the climbing fiber inputs electrically at a frequency of 7 Hz (Luebke and Robinson, 1988). If the "ablation" was applied during head rotation in darkness, preexisting motor learning in the VOR was remembered, and the gain of the VOR was the same as that during head rotation in darkness without stimulation. If the "ablation" continued as the animal was exposed to head rotation in stationary surroundings, the gain of the VOR did not return to normal.

These data demonstrate that the flocculus plays an important role in learning, but that it is not the only site of memory for an altered VOR and, at least in cats, may not be a site of memory at all. However, the exact identity of the relevant cerebellar structures has been a matter of controversy, especially in primates. The flocculus exists clearly in both primate and nonprimate species and, in primates, consists of four folia. In primates, the ventral paraflocculus is much more developed than in nonprimate species and consists of six or seven folia. All published reports agree that the flocculus and ventral flocculus have similar input connections from the vestibular nuclei, the nucleus prepositus, and the inferior olive, and similar output connections to the vestibular nuclei. The two stuctures differ primarily in the source of their visual mossy fiber inputs which arise in the dorsolateral pontine nuclei for the ventral paraflocculus and in the nucleus reticulari tegmenti pontis for the flocculus (Gerrits and Voogd, 1989). Our view (see Lisberger, Pavelko, Bronte-Stewart, and Stone, 1994c) has been that the flocculus and ventral paraflocculus have similar functions, whereas Nagao (1992) has suggested that the flocculus participates in the VOR and the ventral paraflocculus only in pursuit. Nagao's single-unit recordings completely fail to substantiate his position. Our data (reviewed later) argue that a group of Purkinje cells found in large numbers in the ventral paraflocculus plays an important role in learning in the VOR. At the same time, our data provide only a small amount of information about the primate flocculus, and new experiments are needed to resolve this issue. In the meantime, we will refer to the flocculus and ventral paraflocculus together as the *floccular lobe*.

BEHAVIORAL ANALYSIS OF MODIFIED AND UNMODIFIED COMPONENTS OF THE VOR

Recordings of the eye movements evoked by natural and electrical stimulation of the vestibular apparatus have placed a number of important constraints on sites of memory for the VOR. We (Lisberger, 1984), for example, demonstrated that changes in the gain of the VOR did not affect the first 5 ms of the eye velocity evoked by these "rapid changes in head velocity." The VOR had a latency of 14 ms, but the earliest expression of learning did not occur until 19 ms after the onset of the head-velocity stimulus. These data imply that the VOR has separate modified and unmodified components and raise the possibility that the two components are mediated by separate neural pathways. It is tempting to interpret the difference in the latency of the modified and unmodified components of the VOR as evidence that the sites of memory for the VOR are not in the disynaptic VOR pathways, but two more recent articles disagree with this reasoning. Using a much more rapid head acceleration than we used, Khater et al. (1993) reported that changes in the gain of the VOR are expressed at the onset of the VOR.[2] Broussard et al. (1992) demonstrated that changes in the gain of the VOR altered the earliest part of the eye velocities evoked by electrical stimulation of the vestibular apparatus with single pulses. The fact that changes in the gain of the VOR can be expressed in the shortest latency part of the response demonstrates that the cerebellar cortex cannot be the only site of memory in the VOR. Only a site of memory in the disynaptic, brainstem VOR pathways could support such short latency expression of changes in the gain of the VOR.

We think that the different latencies of the modified component of the VOR in different experiments are entirely compatible and that they can be understood if (1) there are separate modified and unmodified VOR pathways, (2) the modified and unmodified pathways both include disynaptic VOR pathways, and (3) the modified and unmodified pathways receive inputs from different vestibular primary afferents. These assumptions imply that the minimum conduction time through the modified and unmodified pathways should be the same and that any difference in the latencies of the modified components of the VOR should arise from the latency of vestibular primary afferents. Available data are consistent with this interpretation. We (Lisberger and Pavelko, 1986) recorded the responses of primary afferents to the rapid changes in head velocity that we had previously used (Lisberger, 1984). We found that the latency from the onset of head velocity to the onset of primary afferent responses ranged from 5 to 14 ms. If the afferents with the shortest latencies project into unmodified VOR pathways and only the afferents with latencies in excess of 10 ms project into the modified pathways, then the first 5 ms of the VOR would not be modified, even if the modified pathway includes a disynaptic component.[3] We recorded (Bronte-Stewart and Lisberger, 1994) the responses of primary afferents to electrical stimulation of the vestibular apparatus with single pulses and found that the latencies ranged from 0.6 to 1.5 ms. Because of the small range of latencies in the afferent responses, it would not be possible to distinguish the modified and unmodified components of the eye movements evoked by electrical stimulation. If both the minimum and range of latencies of primary afferent responses decrease as a function of head acceleration, the head accelerations used by Khater et al. (1993) may have been high enough so that the latencies were similar for afferents projecting into the modified and unmodified pathways: The modified and unmodified components of the VOR should have the same latency for such a stimulus.

LEARNING-RELATED CHANGES IN THE DYNAMICS OF THE VOR

A number of results have shown that the dynamics of the VOR are modified in association with motor learning, arguing that it is probably incorrect to think of the mechanism of motor learning as a simple volume control. In one approach, a number of laboratories have demonstrated that motor learning in the VOR is frequency specific (e.g., Collewijn and Grootendorst, 1979; Lisberger, 1988). If the VOR is adapted by sinusoidal oscillation at a single sinusoidal frequency, the gain of the VOR shows the greatest changes when tested at the adapting frequency and smaller or no change at testing frequencies above and below the adapting frequency. Because the vestibular afferents themselves do not show frequency-tuned responses, frequency selectivity must be a property of the VOR pathways. Further, the site of memory must be within or downstream from the part of the system that generates the frequency selectivity. Although frequency-selective adaptation of the VOR has been modeled successfully, no plausible biological explanation exists.

In a second approach, we found (Lisberger and Pavelko, 1986) that adaptation with natural head turns also caused changes in the dynamics of the VOR. When the vestibular testing stimulus was a rapid change in head velocity, the eye velocity evoked in darkness showed impressive transient overshoot when the gain of the VOR was low and no transient overshoot at all when the gain of the VOR was high. Our original explanation (Lisberger and Pavelko,

1986) for this change in dynamics—that the modified VOR pathways transmitted inputs selectively from primary afferents with little transient overshoot in firing rate—is almost certainly wrong. Recent computer simulations have suggested that the VOR dynamics may depend critically on properties of the neural network mediating the VOR and not on the dynamics of the afferents that project into the modified or unmodified pathways. For example, we discovered (Lisberger and Sejnowski, 1992) that the effect of motor learning on the gain *and* dynamics of the VOR can be reproduced if the memory is in the vestibular pathways through the cerebellum and if the mechanism is a change in the *time-course* rather than in the gain of transmission through these pathways. We showed (1994) that changes in the time course of transmission of vestibular signal through the floccular lobe allowed a VOR model with realistic "anatomy" to reproduce the effect of changes in the VOR gain on the time courses of both eye movements and unit responses during brief head turns. However, it remains to be determined whether a change in the time constant of transmission of vestibular signals is "realistic" physiology.

NEURAL EXPRESSION OF MOTOR LEARNING IN THE VOR

All available data now agree about the effects of changes in the gain of the VOR on the responses of neurons in the VOR pathways (figure 2.1). Single-unit recordings have now evaluated the effect of motor learning on the responses to Purkinje cells in the floccular lobe, in FTNs in the vestibular nuclei, in "position-vestibular-pause" (PVP) cells in the vestibular nucleus, and in abducens neurons.

Purkinje Cells in the Floccular Lobe

The greatest controversy about the effect of motor learning on neuronal responses has concerned the activity of Purkinje cells in the floccular lobe, and most readers who have followed this line of research over the years will be astonished to read our assertion that the available data from all laboratories and all species are in good qualitative agreement.

If recordings are made during the VOR in the dark, the simple-spike responses of Purkinje cells show changes that are in the direction originally postulated by Ito (1972), (i.e., the correct direction to support the associated changes in the gain of the VOR). This result has been obtained in rabbits and in monkeys by members of Ito's laboratory (Dufosse, Ito, Jastreboff, and Miyaskita, 1978; Watanabe, 1984) and in monkeys by Miles, Fuller, Braitman, and Dow (1980) and Lisberger et al. (1994c). The same result was obtained both when following individual Purkinje cells during small changes in the VOR gain over an hour of adaptation (Dufosse et al., 1978; Watanabe, 1984) and when recording large samples of Purkinje cells before and after large increases or decreases in the VOR gain (Miles et al., 1980; Lisberger et al., 1994c). The same result was obtained in Purkinje cells identified as "horizontal-

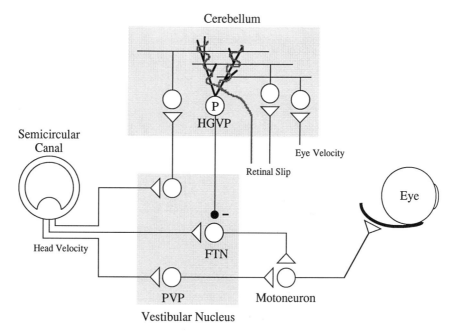

Figure 2.1 Simplified circuit diagram of the brainstem and cerebellar circuitry for the VOR. Vestibular inputs arise in the semicircular canals at the left of the diagram. Two disynaptic pathways transmit the vestibular information to ocular motoneurons via interneurons in the vestibular nucleus. One interneuron in the diagram is called *FTN* or floccular target neuron because it represents a group of cells that are inhibited with monosynaptic latencies by stimulation of the floccular lobe with single electrical pulses (Lisberger et al., 1994a). The second interneuron represents PVP cells, which are not inhibited by stimulation in the floccular lobe. Horizontal-gaze-velocity Purkinje (HGVP) cells in the floccular lobe of the cerebellum receive parallel converging fiber inputs related to vestibular stimulation, eye velocity, and retinal image slip. They also receive visual information about image slip over the climbing fiber pathway. No attempt to represent the bilateral nature of the VOR pathways or midline crossings is made in this simplified diagram.

gaze-velocity Purkinje" (HGVP) cells by studying their responses during smooth-tracking eye movements as well as during the VOR (after Lisberger and Fuchs, 1978a) and in Purkinje cells that were not identified according to their other response properties.

If recordings are made while the monkey tracks a target that moves exactly with it during passive head rotation, the HGVP cells' response is modified in association with learning, but the change in the strength of the vestibular inputs to HGVP cells is in the wrong direction to cause the associated changes in the VOR gain. The use of this tracking paradigm, called *cancellation of the VOR*, provides a direct estimate of the strength of the vestibular input to HGVP cells, independent of other inputs such as those related to eye velocity. When Miles et al. (1980) first made this observation, they concluded that their data were incompatible with the hypothesis that the site of memory for the VOR was in the vestibular pathways through the cerebellar cortex.

Still, these authors did reveal learning in the vestibular pathways through HGVP cells, even if the purpose of the learning was not to change the gain of the VOR. We now realize that these measurements, made in 1980 and confirmed by Lisberger et al. (1994c), reveal only the steady-state strength of vestibular transmission through HGVP cells. It remains plausible that there are changes in a transient component of vestibular sensitivity that are in the correct direction to cause the associated changes in the VOR gain, and our models show that such a change would be one way to account for available data on learning in the VOR. Unfortunately, it is not clear how to design an experiment to evaluate the transient behavior of vestibular inputs to HGVP cells.

From these experiments, we conclude that the output of the floccular lobe in the primate supports changes in the gain of the VOR. If it were possible to ablate the floccular lobe bilaterally in primates after learning in the VOR, we would expect that some but not all of the memory would be lost, as reported in the goldfish by Pastor et al. (1994). At the same time, the responses of HGVP cells during cancellation of the VOR reveal wrong-way changes in the strength of vestibular transmission through the floccular lobe, making it impossible to conclude at this time that changes in the VOR gain are caused by a site of memory in the vestibular pathways through the floccular lobe.

Floccular Target Neurons in the Vestibular Nucleus

Two studies have used quite different approaches to demonstrate what appear to be the same learning-related changes in the responses of FTNs in the vestibular nucleus and the dorsal Y-group. We studied three samples of FTNs for horizontal eye movements when the VOR gain was normal or after a week or more of learning had caused the gain of the VOR to become asymptotically low or high (Lisberger, Pavelko, and Broussard, 1994b). Partsalis, Zhang, and Highstein (1995) followed individual FTNs for vertical eye movements during approximately an hour of learning. Their data agree that FTN firing during the VOR is modified in a direction that is appropriate to cause the changes in the VOR gain. The only difference between the two studies is in the baseline responses of the FTNs during the VOR in the dark. The vertical FTNs in the squirrel monkey show little modulation of firing rate during the VOR in the dark when the VOR gain is normal and become modulated with increases in firing for pitch up or down when the VOR gain is increased or decreased, respectively. The horizontal FTNs in the rhesus monkey show strong modulation of firing rate during the VOR in the dark when the VOR gain is normal, and the depth of modulation either increases when the VOR gain is high or decreases and ultimately reverses direction when the VOR gain is low. Thus, the learning-related changes in firing are the same in the two studies, even if the baseline responses during the normal VOR in the dark differ quantitatively. The effect of motor learning on the responses of FTNs in the monkey may account for the findings in an earlier study in the cat (Keller and Precht, 1979). These authors recorded all vestibular neurons that showed modulation of firing rate during the VOR in the dark and did not identify FTNs by stimulation in the floccular lobe. Decreases in the VOR gain were associated with a failure to record (and apparent loss of) vestibular responses with a specific quantitative relationship to head velocity; this change in the sample of vestibular responses is in agreement with the changes now known to occur in the responses of FTNs when the gain of the VOR is low.

Position-Vestibular-Pause Neurons in the Vestibular Nucleus

There is no evidence for learning-related changes in vestibular transmission to PVP cells (Lisberger et al., 1994b). Under the same conditions that caused large changes in the responses of FTNs during the VOR in the dark, PVP cells showed only a small expression of learning and that only for head rotations away from the side of recording. Because there was no associated change in the vestibular responses of PVP cells during cancellation of the VOR, we attribute these small changes to feedback of eye velocity signals that cause the firing of PVP cells to modulate in relation to eye position and velocity.

Abducens Neurons

Because abducens neurons drive eye movements, it is not surprising that changes in the gain of the VOR are associated with changes in the relationship between abducens neuron firing and head velocity (SG Lisberger, DM Broussard, C DeCharms, and EJ Morris, unpublished observations). However, the relationship between the firing rate of abducens neurons and the parameters of eye movement appears to be unaffected by changes in the gain of the VOR (Broussard, de Charms, and Lisberger, 1995).

TIMING OF LEARNING-RELATED CHANGES IN NEURONAL RESPONSES

For a rapid-change head velocity with a mean acceleration of $600°/s^2$, that the latency of the VOR is 14 ms and the latency of the modified component of the VOR is 19 ms (Lisberger, 1984). Recordings from PVP cells, FTNs, and HGVP cells have now demonstrated the correspondence between the latency of neuronal responses and the latencies of the modified and unmodified components of the VOR. PVP cells respond to the same rapid change in head velocity after latencies of 7 ms, FTNs respond with a range of latencies tightly grouped around 13 ms, and HGVP cells response with a broad range of latencies distributed around a mean of 23 ms. Because both PVP cells and FTNs project directly to abducens neurons, a change in the firing rate of each will affect eye movement 7 ms later. Thus, responses that begin in PVP cells and FTNs at 7 and 13 ms after the onset of head velocity will affect eye movement at 14 and 20 ms after the onset of head movement. These latencies correspond well to the latencies of the unmodified and modified components of the VOR. The relatively long latency of HGVP cells during the VOR evoked by rapid changes in head velocity implies that the earliest change in the responses of FTNs cannot be driven by the postulated connection from HGVP cells to FTNs. We conclude that the disynaptic pathway through PVP cells contributes to the unmodified component of the VOR, the FTNs are interneurons in pathways that drive the modified component of the VOR, and one excellent candidate for a site of memory is the synapse between primary vestibular afferents and FTNs.[4]

BEHAVIORAL ANALYSIS OF SITES OF MEMORY

Because much of the circuitry illustrated in figure 2.1 is shared with other kinds of eye movements, information about possible sites of memory can be gained by analyzing whether changes in the gain of the VOR generalize to other kinds of eye movements. We demonstrated (Lisberger, Miles, Optican, and Eighmy, 1981) that learning in the VOR generalizes extremely well to the long time-constant component of the optokinetic response but not to the rapid, early component of the response. The changes in the long time-constant component of optokinetic nystagmus (OKN)—expressed as a long-lasting optokinetic afternystagmus called *OKAN*—would be expected because the control signals for OKAN masquerade as vestibular signals and are present on all secondary vestibular neurons (Henn et al., 1974). It follows that other central vestibular neurons, specifically HGVP cells, should respond the same way during the OKAN as they do during the VOR, and this expectation has been verified by Buttner and Waespe (1984). The effect on OKAN of changing the VOR gain has one important implication for the site of memory in the VOR. Because the signals that drive OKAN are not seen in the firing of vestibular primary afferents (Buttner and Waespe, 1981; JM Goldberg, SG Lisberger, and FA Miles, unpublished observations), modifications restricted to the synapse from primary vestibular afferents to FTNs would alter the gain of the VOR but would not alter OKAN. This finding makes it unlikely that this first central synapse is the only site of memory, and points out the likely importance of changes in the cellular operation of FTNs or sites of memory elsewhere in the central pathways that mediate the VOR.

We showed that changes in the VOR gain have little or no effect on either the initiation or maintenance of smooth-pursuit eye movements for a small moving target, or on the eye movements evoked by electrical stimulation of the floccular lobe with single pulses or trains of pulses (Lisberger, 1994). In contrast, changes in the gain of the VOR caused pronounced changes in the eye movements evoked by electrical stimulation of the vestibular apparatus with trains of pulses (Broussard, Bronte-Stewart, and Lisberger, 1992; Bronte-

Stewart and Lisberger, 1994) and small but measurable changes in the eye movements evoked by single pulses (Broussard et al., 1992).

The eye velocity positive-feedback pathway in figure 2.1 is an essential component of the interpretation of these data. The following reasoning suggests the existence of this positive feedback of the motor commands for pursuit. First, in the floccular lobe, HGVP cells respond as strongly during smooth pursuit with the head stationary as they do during head rotation with cancellation of the VOR. These data demonstrate that HGVP cells are important for pursuit as well as for the VOR. Second, analysis of the responses of HGVP cells during pursuit has revealed that the modulation of simple-spike firing during pursuit is related to smooth eye velocity per se, not to visual imputs; the modulation persists when the tracking target is stabilized on the fovea during ongoing pursuit. Third, many of the input elements and non-Purkinje cells recorded in the floccular lobe respond to eye movements during both pursuit and the VOR. These inputs may arise from the nucleus prepositus (Baker, Gresty, and Berthoz, 1975; McFarland and Fuchs, 1992), which projects abundantly to the floccular lobe (Alley, Baker, and Simpson, 1975; Langer, Fuchs, Chubb, Scudder, and Lisberger, 1985) and contains neurons with discharge patterns similar to those recorded in the floccular lobe by Lisberger and Fuchs, 1978b. Fourth, the nucleus prepositus receives disynaptic vestibular inputs relayed through the vestibular nucleus (Baker and Berthoz, 1975). Direct anatomic and physiologic demonstration of a positive-feedback loop is still needed, but available evidence suggests that the anatomic pathway could be from HGVP cells to FTNs to the nucleus prepositus and back to the floccular lobe.

If the positive feedback pathway has a gain close to one, it would operate as a velocity-memory system, remembering the eye velocity at one moment and using it as a major part of the command for eye velocity at the next moment. This organization of the pursuit system was first suggested by Young, Forster, and Van Houtte (1968) and Robinson (1971), and it has major advantages for providing accurate tracking and stability at the same time. In addition, a velocity memory system would account for our finding that pursuit continues at its current speed if the target is stabilized on the fovea during ongoing tracking at constant speed (Morris and Lisberger, 1987).

We think that the absence of any changes in pursuit eye movements with even large changes in the VOR gain preclude a site of memory in pathways that are shared by pursuit and the VOR. Specifically, we do not think that memory resides in the eye velocity positive-feedback loop or in its outputs to the extraocular motoneurons. Computer models show that it is possible to modify both the gain and dynamics of the VOR by altering either the gain or time course of transmission through the positive feedback pathway, but that this change has effects on pursuit eye movements that are large enough to measure. Further, our finding that changes in the gain of the VOR do not alter the eye movements evoked by electrical stimulation of the floccular lobe suggests that the VOR memory site cannot be in the pathway from HGVP cells to FTNs to extraocular motoneurons. However, these conclusions could be wrong. It is now clear that pursuit eye movements are subject to adaptive modification (Optican, Zee, and Chu, 1985; Kahlon and Lisberger, 1994). With this in mind, our data are also consistent with the possibility that the VOR memory site is in pathways that are shared with pursuit and that changes in the gain of the VOR do alter pursuit eye movements, but that motor learning in pursuit corrects those changes and restores pursuit performance so that it appears to be independent of the VOR gain.

USE OF COMPUTER SIMULATION TO FORM HYPOTHESES ABOUT SITES OF MEMORY

We wish to know the sites of memory, but our research tools have allowed us to measure only the neural and behavioral expressions of memory. Because of the feedback loops in the neural network that generates the VOR, we must rely on quantitative theories to make the connection from what we can measure to what we wish to know. In our research, computer simulations and analytical treatments have led to a hypothesis of the sites of memory that allows models to reproduce the effects of changes in the VOR gain on the time courses of both the evoked eye movements and the responses of relevant neurons, including HGVP cells, FTNs, PVP cells, and abducens motoneurons.

Figure 2.2 shows the structure of the model we have simulated. The details of the model can be found in our recent publications (Lisberger and Sejnowski, 1992; Lisberger, 1994). Briefly, the model was selected to mimic the anatomy implied by the schematic circuit diagram of figure 2.1. It includes nodes that represent HGVP cells, FTNs, and PVP cells, and it performs simulations of head velocity, eye velocity, and neural firing as a function of time on a millisecond time scale. Figure 2.3 shows that appropriate changes in the parameters of the model allow in to reproduce the effects of increases and decreases in the gain of the VOR on the time course of eye velocity and of the firing rates of HGVP cells and FTNs. To decrease the model's VOR gain, we decreased the strength of vestibular transmission to HGVP cells and FTNs in parallel and by the same amount, and we decreased the time constant of filtering in the vestibular inputs to HGVP cells. To increase the gain of the VOR, we made the opposite modifications. All of these parameter changes were necessary to obtain the simulations illustrated on the left side of figure 2.3 without altering the performance of the model during pursuit.

1. Changes in the strength of vestibular transmission to HGVP cells were required to account for the effect of changes in the gain of the VOR on the responses of HGVP cells during cancellation of the VOR. The size of these changes was restricted by the size of the changes recorded by Miles et al. (1980) and Lisberger, Pavelko, Bronte-Stewart, and Stone (1994c).

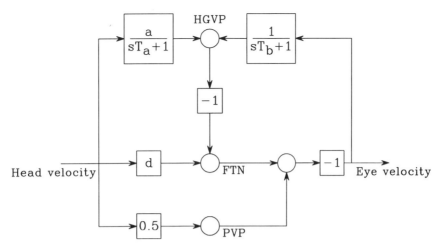

Figure 2.2 Simplified mathematical model of the VOR pathways, showing nodes that represent HGVP cells in the floccular lobe as well as PVP cells and FTNs in the vestibular nucleus. Vestibular inputs related to head velocity enter the pathways at the left side of the model and motor outputs related to eye velocity emerge at the right side of the model. Parameters a and d represent gains that control the strength of transmission of vestibular signals, whereas T_a and T_b are time-constants that control the time-course of responses to changes in input signals. The circular nodes operate as summing junctions that add their various inputs.

2. Changes in the strength of vestibular transmission to FTNs had to be made to cause changes in the gain of the VOR and had to be the same magnitude as the changes in vestibular transmission to HGVP cells to maintain stability of the system.

3. Changes in the time course of vestibular transmission to HGVP cells was required to obtain a large enough change in the gain of the VOR and, given the existence of the eye-velocity feedback pathway to HGVP cells, allowed the model to reproduce the effect of changes in the gain of the VOR on the responses of HGVP cells during the VOR in the dark. Contrary to our earlier intuition (Lisberger, 1988), changes in only the strength of vestibular transmission to FTNs and HGVP cells did not allow the model to reproduce this general finding.

The strength of the model in figure 2.2 is its ability to reproduce available data from multiple laboratories and species. The weakness of the model is that its predictions are strongly dependent on some of its assumptions. For example, if the eye velocity responses of HGVP cells are not due to a positive-feedback pathway, then other combinations of parameter changes may be able to reproduce available data.

ERROR SIGNALS THAT GUIDE LEARNING

Now that putative sites of memory have been identified, we can ask whether those sites receive signals that are appropriate to guide learning. The model

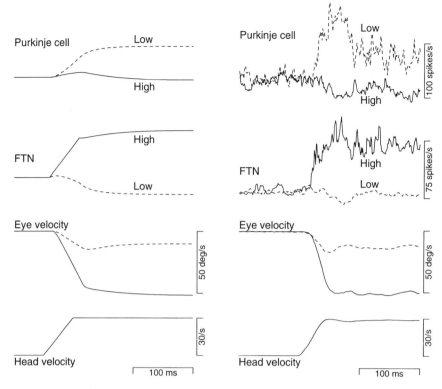

Figure 2.3 (Left) Comparison of the effect of changes in the gain of the VOR on the responses of the model in figure 2.2 and the eye movements. (Right) Neuronal firing rates measured in monkeys. Each pair of traces compares responses when the gain of the VOR was high (solid lines) or low (dashed lines). In all cases, neuronal responses are shown for head turns toward the side of the recording. The data for neuronal responses were selected to represent the typical response across the population of neurons. The database for this selection can be found in other publications (Lisberger et al., 1994b,c).

suggests that there is learning in the vestibular inputs to HGVP cells. Though some or all of this learning could occur in the brainstem pathways that relay vestibular inputs to the floccular lobe, it is plausible to assume that the site of learning is in parallel fiber transmission to Purkinje cells. Cerebellar long-term depression (LTD) provides a workable mechanism of learning in Purkinje cells (Ito, 1989), and the requisite input signals to guide learning in the VOR are available in the cerebellar cortex of the floccular lobe. Vestibular inputs arise over mossy fibers, and visual information about image motion is transmitted by climbing fibers in all species that have been studied (rabbit: Simpson and Alley, 1974; cat: Simpson, Precht, and Llinás, 1974; monkey: Stone and Lisberger, 1990b; chicken: M Vetter and SG Lisberger, unpublished data). At the same time, analysis in a more functional context of LTD as a possible mechanism of learning revealed many issues of specificity and timing of LTD that need to be resolved (du Lac et al., 1995). Given what is known about the adequate stimuli for climbing-fiber responses, for example, LTD would be in the correct direction to cause the changes in transient vestibular sensitivity of HGVP cells postulated by our model but would be in the wrong direction to cause the changes in steady-state vestibular sensitivity of HGVP cells actually recorded during cancellation of the VOR (Miles et al., 1980).

Visual signals are also available to guide learning in the vestibular inputs to FTNs. Direct brainstem visual pathways to FTNs have not been documented but may exist. Some HGVP cells respond directly to visual image motion (Stone and Lisberger, 1990a) and would provide useful information that could guide learning in FTNs. In addition, the simple-spike firing of all HGVP cells would provide FTNs with clear direction about whether the gain of the VOR should increase or decrease, at least for vestibular stimulation with low-frequency sine waves (Lisberger and Fuchs, 1978a). However, the simple-spike discharge of HGVP cells cannot function alone to guide changes in FTNs, because the firing of HGVP cells is modulated during the VOR in the dark after learning and would cause further inappropriate changes in the gain of the VOR without any visual inputs. To us, it seems plausible to think that HGVP cells play an important role in setting the firing rate of FTNs at levels that are suitable for learning, but some other, visual, influence is needed to enable changes in the strength of vestibular transmission through FTNs.

FROM EXISTING MODELS TO BIOLOGICAL REALISM

One of the current challenges in research on the VOR is to make the transition to biologically realistic models from our current models (which view the VOR as a lumped system and implement the mechanisms of motor learning as lumped changes in internal gain, such as volume controls, or as changes in time-constants). Electrical stimulation of the vestibular apparatus, used either to activate vestibular afferents synchronously or to ablate specific subpopulations of vestibular afferents reversibly, has begun this transition. In our laboratory, electrical stimulation of the vestibular apparatus has suggested that only a subset of vestibular afferents provides inputs to the VOR and yet another subset of those projects into pathways that are modified in association with learning (Bronte-Stewart and Lisberger, 1994). For example, electrical stimulation at low currents activates all afferents with highly irregular spontaneous discharge but does not evoke any measurable eye movement. The absence of an eye movement cannot result from a failure to bring central neurons to threshold because almost all neurons in the VOR pathways are spontaneously active with the head stationary and the eyes at straightahead gaze. Experiments with reversible ablation of these "irregular" afferents (Minor and Goldberg, 1992) agree with our conclusion that these afferents do not contribute to the VOR. There is a similar dissociation between the evoked eye movements and the thresholds for afferents at high currents. Beyond a certain level, increasing the stimulation current continues to recruit the vestibular afferents with the most regular spontaneous discharge but does not evoke any further increase in the amplitude of the evoked eye movement.

This finding may represent saturation in the central vestibular pathways if all secondary vestibular neurons are emitting one spike, but it may also reflect a failure of the most "regular" afferents to contribute to the VOR.

A similar approach using trains of electrical stimuli has revealed that some afferents contribute to the VOR but do not project into pathways the are modified in association with learning (Bronte-Stewart and Lisberger, 1994). Over the first third of the range of stimulation currents that evokes an eye movement, the eye movements evoked by trains of stimuli are not modified in association with learning. At higher currents, the eye movements evoked by trains of electrical stimuli undergo large changes in association with learning. This kind of observation emphasizes the fact that the VOR pathways are highly distributed. There are multiple parallel VOR pathways with different functions, and vestibular primary afferents with different physiological properties project differentially into these VOR pathways. Similar conclusions have been reached based on physiologic studies of the input profile of different central neurons (Highstein et al., 1987), although our data on the eye movements of monkeys revealed much more order than was apparent in the distribution to individual cells of afferents with different thresholds for electrical stimulation.

Comparison of the eye movements evoked by single electrical pulses with those evoked by trains of pulses emphasizes the flaws in regarding the motor learning mechanisms in the VOR as a volume control, presumably implemented as a change in the strength of transmission across certain synapses. Although quantitative analysis was able to reveal that changes in the gain of the VOR affected the eye movements evoked by stimulation of the vestibular apparatus with single electrical pulses, the effects were small (Broussard et al., 1992). This was true even when we used stimulation currents for which changes in the gain of the VOR caused large changes in the eye movements evoked by trains of stimuli. If the VOR motor learning mechanism were a large change in the strength of synaptic transmission, such as has been demonstrated for long-term potentiation (LTP) in the hippocampus, we would have expected changes in the VOR gain to cause large changes in the eye movements evoked by single electrical pulses.

There are two general explanations that could account for the profound difference in the effect of changes in the gain of the VOR on the eye movements evoked by single pulses versus trains of electrical stimuli: First, the mechanism of learning may indeed be a small change in the strength of synaptic transmission. When probed with a single electrical pulse, the small change in synaptic transmission would be expressed as a small change in the evoked eye movement. When probed with a train of electrical pulses or a head turn, the small change in cellular function may be amplified by feedback loops in the VOR pathways so that it quickly grows and is expressed as a large change in the evoked eye movements. Second, the mechanism of learning may be in a cellular function that determines the temporal dynamics of cellular activity (e.g., the ionic currents that determine the relationship between input current and firing rate). A single electrical pulse would not probe this kind of modification very effectively, and there would be little or no change in the evoked eye movement. However, a train of pulses or a natural stimulus would much more effectively probe cellular mechanisms that generate firing rate, and motor learning would be expressed much more prominently in the eye movements evoked by these stimuli. In our opinion, available data offer obstacles to each of these alternatives, although the obstacles could be removed by suitable albeit difficult experimental approaches.

CONCLUSIONS

We have argued that a single interpretation can be applied to all available data on the effect of changes in the gain of the VOR on eye movements and neuronal responses. It is possible to reproduce the data from all laboratories and species by a model in which there are multiple sites of memory. One site is a change in the strength of transmission in the brainstem vestibular pathways to FTNs. A second site involves a change in both the strength and time-course of vestibular input transmission to Purkinje cells in the floccular lobe of the cerebellum. This model accounts for extensive disagreements about the interpretation of the effect of motor learning on the responses of Purkinje cells in the floccular lobe. However, models are made to be broken and perhaps we should view the model proposed here as a starting point for research that, while refining and possibly replacing the model, will lead to an understanding of motor learning in the VOR at a systems level. In so doing, we hope that we can put the cerebellum in its appropriate place, as an important part of a greater neuronal system that mediates the VOR and motor learning thereof.

NOTES

1. In humans, the gain of the VOR depends on the instructions given to the subject. At least for sinusoidal head rotation at low frequencies, the gain is near 1 if the subject is instructed to imagine a target fixed to the wall, and is near 0 if the subject is instructed to imagine a target rotating exactly with the head (Barr, Schultheis, and Robinson, 1976). Gauthier and Robinson (1975) have shown that this "parametric" modulation of the VOR gain is different from long-term adaptation and that magnifying and miniaturizing spectacles cause changes in the gain of the VOR that are expressed consistently whether the subject is instructed to do mental arithmetic or to imagine a target either fixed to the wall or moving with the head.

2. In these experiments, the VOR was adapted by subjecting cats to vertical oscillation of the visual stimulus during horizontal vestibular oscillation at low frequencies.

3. We disagree with Minor and Goldberg (1992), who argue that their data disprove the contribution of afferents with short latencies to the unmodified component of the VOR. They found that the VOR was not altered by reversible ablations of all primary afferents with irregular spontaneous firing rate and some of the afferents with intermediate spontaneous firing rate. Because some of the afferents with short latency responses during rapid changes in head velocity also have irregular or intermediate spontaneous discharge, Minor and Goldberg

concluded that afferents with short latency responses could not contribute to the VOR. Their logic overlooks that fact that many of the afferents with short latency responses to natural stimuli also had regular spontaneous discharge and therefore remained candidates to contribute to the unmodified component of the VOR as outlined here.

4. The rather long (19-ms) latency of the modified component of the VOR can be consistent with a site of memory in the monosynaptic vestibular inputs to FTNs, as long as our hypothesis is correct that the longer latencies of the modified component of the VOR result primarily from longer latencies in the vestibular primary afferents that project into the modified pathways.

REFERENCES

Albus JS (1971). A theory of cerebellar function. Math Biosci 10:25−61.

Alley K, Baker R, Simpson JI (1975). Afferents to the vestibulo-cerebellum and the origin of visual climbing fibers in the rabbit. Brain Res 98:582−589.

Baker R, Berthoz A (1975). Is the prepositus hypoglossi nucleus the source of another vestibulo-ocular pathway? Brain Res 86:121−127.

Baker R, Gresty M, Berthoz A (1975). Neuronal activity in the prepositus hypoglossi nucleus correlated with vertical and horizontal eye movement in the cat. Brain Res 101:366−371.

Baker R, Precht W, Llinas R (1972). Cerebellar modulatory action on the vestibulotrochlear pathway in the cat. Exp Brain Res 15:364−385.

Barr CC, Schultheis LW, Robinson DA (1976). Voluntary, non-visual control of the human vestibulo-ocular reflex. Acta Otolaryngol 81:365−75.

Bronte-Stewart HM, Lisberger SG (1994). Physiological properties of vestibular primary afferents that mediate motor learning and normal performance of the vestibuloocular reflex in monkeys. J Neurosci 14:1290−1308.

Broussard DM, Bronte-Stewart HM, Lisberger SG (1992). Expression of motor learning in the response of the primate vestibuloocular pathway to electrical stimulation. J Neurophysiol 67:1493−1508.

Broussard DM, de Charms RC, Lisberger SG (1995). Inputs from the ipsilateral and contralateral vestibular apparatus to behaviorally-characterized abducens neurons in rhesus monkeys. J Neurophysiol 74:2449−2459

Buttner U, Waespe W (1984). Purkinje cell activity in the primate flocculus during optokinetic stimulation, smooth pursuit eye movements and VOR-suppression. Exp Brain Res 55:97−104.

Buttner U, Waespe W (1981). Vestibular nerve activity in the alert monkey during vestibular and optokinetic nystagmus. Exp Brain Res 41:310−315.

Collewijn, H, Grootendorst AF (1979). Adaptation of optoknetic and vestibulo-ocular reflexes to modified visual input in the rabbit. In R Granit, O Pompeiano (eds), Reflex Control of Posture and Movement. Amsterdam: Elsevier pp 772−781.

Dufosse M, Ito M, Jastreboff PJ, Miyashita Y (1978). A neuronal correlate in rabbit's cerebellum to adaptive modification of the vestibulo-ocular reflex. Brain Res 150:611−616.

du Lac S, Raymond JL, Sejnowski TJ, Lisberger SG (1995). Learning and memory in the vestibulo-ocular reflex. Annu Rev Neurosci 18:409−41.

Fukuda J, Highstein SM, Ito M (1972). Cerebellar inhibitory control of the vestibuloocular reflex investigated in rabbit IIIrd nucleus. Exp Brain Res 14:511−526.

Gauthier GM, Robinson DA (1975). Adaptation of the human vestibuloocular reflex to magnifying lenses. Brain Res 92:331–5.

Gerrits NM, Voogd J (1989). The topographical organization of climbing and mossy fiber afferents in the flocculus and the ventral paraflocculus in rabbit, cat, and monkey. Exp Brain Res Suppl 17:26–29.

Gonshor A, Melvill Jones G (1976). Extreme vestibulo-ocular adaptation induced by prolonged optical reversal of vision. J Physiol (Lond) 256:381–414.

Henn V, Young LR, Finley C (1974). Vestibular nucleus units in alert monkeys are also influenced by moving visual fields. Brain Res 71:144–149.

Highstein SM (1973). Synaptic linkage in the vestibulo-ocular and cerebello-vestibular pathways to the VIth nucleus in the rabbit. Exp Brain Res 17:301–314.

Highstein SM, Goldberg JM, Moschovakis AK, Fernandez C (1987). Inputs from regularly and irregularly discharging vestibular nerve afferents to secondary neurons in the vestibular nuclei of the squirrel monkey: II. Correlation with output pathways of secondary neurons. J Neurophysiol 58:719–738.

Ito M (1972). Neural design of the cerebellar motor control system. Brain Res 40:80–84.

Ito M (1989). Long term depression. Annu Rev Neurosci 12:85–102.

Kahlon M, Lisberger SG (1994). Adaptation of open-loop smooth pursuit responses in the rhesus monkey. Soc Neurosci Abstr 20:1193.

Keller EL, Precht W (1979). Adaptive modification of central vestibular neurons in response to visual stimulation through reversing prisms. J Neurophysiol 42:896–911.

Khater TT, Quinn KJ, Pena J, Baker JF, Peterson BW (1993). The latency of the cat vestibulo-ocular reflex before and after short- and long-term adaptation. Exp Brain Res 94:16–32.

Langer R, Fuchs AF, Chubb MC, Scudder CA, Lisberger SG (1985). Floccular efferents in the rhesus macaque as revealed by autoradiography and horseradish peroxidase. J Comp Neurol 235:26–37.

Lisberger SG (1988). The neural basis for motor learning in the vestibulo-ocular reflex in monkeys. Trends Neurosci 11:147–152.

Lisberger SG (1994). Neural basis for motor learning in the vestibulo-ocular reflex in primates: III. Behavioral and computational analysis of the sites of learning. J Neurophysiol 72:954–973.

Lisberger SG, Fuchs AF (1978a). Role of primate flocculus during rapid behavioral modification of vestibuloocular reflex: I. Purkinje cell activity during visually guided horizontal smooth-pursuit eye movements and passive head rotation. J Neurophysiol 41:733–763.

Lisberger SG, Fuchs AF (1978b). Role of primate flocculus during rapid behavioral modification of vestibuloocular reflex: II. Mossy fiber firing patterns during horizontal head rotation and eye movement. J Neurophysiol 41:764–777.

Lisberger SG, Miles FA, Zee DS (1984). Signals used to compute errors in monkey vestibulo-ocular reflex: possible role of flocculus. J Neurophysiol 52:1140–1153.

Lisberger SG, Miles FA, Optican LM, Eighmy BB (1981). Optokinetic response in monkey: Underlying mechanisms and their sensitivity to long-term adaptive changes in vestibulo-ocular reflex. J. Neurophysiol. 45:869–890.

Lisberger SG, Pavelko TA (1986). Vestibular signals carried by pathways subserving plasticity of the vestibulo-ocular reflex in monkeys. J Neurosci 6:346–354.

Lisberger SG, Pavelko TA, Bronte-Stewart HM, Stone LS (1994c). Neural basis for motor learning in the vestibulo-ocular reflex in primates: II. Changes in the responses of Purkinje cells in the cerebellar flocculus and ventral paraflocculus. J Neurophysiol 72:974–998.

Lisberger SG, Pavelko TA, Broussard DM (1994a). Responses during eye movement of brainstem neurons that receive monosynaptic inhibition from the flocculus and ventral paraflocculus in monkeys. J Neurophysiol 72:909–927.

Lisberger SG, Pavelko TA, Broussard DM (1994b). Neural basis for motor learning in the vestibulo-ocular reflex of primates: I. Changes in the responses of brainstem neurons. J Neurophysiol 72:928–953.

Lisberger SG, Sejnowski TJ (1992). A novel mechanism of motor learning in a recurrent network model based on the vestibulo-ocular reflex. Nature 360:159–161.

Luebke AE, Robinson DA (1988). Transition dynamics between pursuit and fixation suggest different systems. Vision Res 28:941–946.

Marr D (1969). A theory of cerebellar cortex. J Physiol (Lond) 202:437–470.

McFarland JL, Fuchs AF (1992). Discharge patterns in nucleus prepositus hypoglossi and adjacent medial vestibular nucleus during horizontal eye movement in behaving macaques. J Neurophysiol 68:319–332.

Michnovicz JJ, Bennett MVL (1987). Effects of rapid cerebellectomy on adaptive gain control of the vestibulo-ocular reflex in alert goldfish. Exp Brain Res 66:287–294.

Miles FA, Fuller JH, Braitman DJ, Dow BM (1980). Long-term adaptive changes in primate vestibulo-ocular reflex: III. Electrophysiological observations in flocculus of normal monkey. J Neurophysiol 43:1437–1476.

Minor LB, Goldberg JM (1992). Vestibular-nerve inputs to the vestibulo-ocular reflex: A functional-ablation study in the squirrel monkey. J Neurosci 11:1636–1648.

Morris EJ, Lisberger SG (1987). Different responses to small visual errors during initiation and maintenance of smooth-pursuit eye movements in monkeys. J Neurophysiol 58:1351–1369.

Nagao S (1983). Effects of vestibulocerebellar lesions upon dynamic characteristics and adaptation of vestibulo-ocular and optokinetic responses in pigmented rabbits. Exp Brain Res 53:36–46.

Nagao S (1992). Different roles of flocculus and ventral paraflocculus for oculomotor control in the primate. Neuroreport 3:13–16.

Optican LM, Zee DS, Chu FC (1985). Adaptive response to ocular muscle weakness in human pursuit and saccadic eye movements. J Neurophysiol 54:110–122.

Partsalis AM, Zhang Y, Highstein SM (1995). Dorsal Y group in the squirrel monkey. I. Neuronal responses during rapid and long-term modifications of the vertical VOR. J Neurophysiol 73.615–650.

Pastor AM, de la Cruz RR, Baker R (1994). Cerebellar role in adaptation of the goldfish vestibuloocular reflex. J Neurophysiol 72:1383–94.

Robinson DA (1976). Models of oculomotor neural organizations. In P. Bach-y-Rita, CC Collins (eds), The Control of Eye Movements. New York: Academic, p 519.

Schairer JO, Bennett MVL (1981). Cerebellectomy in goldfish prevents adaptive gain control of the VOR without affecting the optokinetic system. In G Gaultierotti (ed), Vestibular Function and Morphology. S Berlin: Springer-Verlag, pp 463–477.

Schultheis LW, Robinson DA (1981). Directional plasticity of the vestibulo-ocular reflex in the cat. Ann N Y Acad Sci 374:504–512.

Simpson JI, Alley KE (1974). Visual climbing-fiber input to rabbit vestibulo-cerebellum: A source of direction-specific information. Brain Res 82:302–308.

Simpson JI, Precht W, and Llinás R (1974). Sensory separation in climbing and mossy fiber inputs to cat vestibulocerebellum. Pflügers Arch 351:183–193.

Stone LS, Lisberger SG (1990a). Visual responses of Purkinje cells in the cerebellar flocculus during smooth-pursuit eye movements in monkeys: I. Simple spikes. J Neurophysiol 63: 1241–1261.

Stone LS, Lisberger SG (1990b). Visual responses of Purkinje cells in the cerebellar flocculus during smooth-pursuit eye movements in monkeys: II. Complex spikes. J Neurophysiol 63: 1262–1275.

Watanabe E (1984). Neuronal events correlated with long-term adaptation of the horizontal vestibulo-ocular reflex in the primate flocculus. Brain Res 297:169–174.

Young LR, Forster JD, Van Houtte N (1968). A revised stochastic sampled data model for eye tracking movements. Fourth Annual NASA—University Conference on Manual Control. Ann Arbor: University of Michigan.

3 The Evolution of Hindbrain Visual and Vestibular Innovations Responsible for Oculomotor Function

Robert Baker and Edwin Gilland

"...the ancient and original function of the eye muscles was not really to move the eye but rather to hold it still with respect to the environment..."
—Walls, 1962

In his classic, contemplative introduction to the evolutionary history of eye movements, Walls (1962) correctly identified the *raison d'etre* of oculomotor existence in our Paleozoic ancestors. The argument, however, did not focus exclusively on the need to maintain retinal constancy of objects in the environment but also on the ability to perceive an object as changing its egocentric direction (i.e., as moving in external space in respect to the viewer). The key concept stated that "something about the eye movement keeps equal and opposite retinal-image movement from connoting object movement" (Walls, 1962). That "something" implies, in essence, that whether objects or their retinal locations are either stationary or moving, "What makes the difference is the matter of whether the eyes themselves are moving or not." This essay argues that from the onset of vertebrate evolution, the need to determine egocentric direction was the major biological force responsible for neuronal innovations underlying sensorimotor function, particularly in the oculomotor system. Consequently, the "ancient, original task" for this part of the central nervous system (CNS) was to produce neural signals proportional to eye motion that could hold the eyes still with respect to the environment, under all conditions of movement, especially independent of object motion. We propose that this type of neuronal processing was achieved effectively more than 450 million years ago by early evolutionary innovations in the hindbrain developing in parallel with cerebellar circuitry. Subsequently, this oculomotor blueprint was used to attain sophisticated visual tracking that truly could acquire and sustain object motion. We ascribe the origin of the visual and vestibular premotor nuclei, including related cerebellar pathways, to alar plate and rhombic lip derivatives originating from discrete locations in hindbrain rhombomeric segments (rhs) 1 to 8. We propose that all hindbrain neurons with eye-motion-related signals may have originated from a special group of migratory precursor cells originating largely, perhaps exclusively, from rhs 7 and 8. Specification of this visuooculomotor circuitry is hypothesized to represent a unique neuroepithelial founder event that became locked throughout vertebrate phylogeny by a dedicated regulator-gene interaction.

TACKLING THE PRIMITIVE OCULOMOTOR PLAN

Because fossilized vertebrate visuooculomotor and vestibulooculomotor circuits do not exist, their evolution must be deduced by comparison of extant taxa. Fortunately, recent evidence suggests much greater conservation than previously suspected, not only in the central circuitry underlying oculomotor behavior but also in the genetic information and developmental interactions responsible for building this circuitry. Comparison of behavior, neuronal organization and physiological signals in extant species shows that oculomotor traits are phylogenetically well-preserved. The distribution of oculomotor features across taxa provides valuable information about brain evolution, including the basis for reconstructing aspects of neuronal function in our fossilized ancestors (Northcutt, 1985; Baker, 1991). Nonetheless, the idea that motor circuits in a living CNS might either substitute for or allow a reconstruction of oculomotor evolution is generally met with skepticism. However, we suggest that early, highly conserved, embryonic gene expression patterns presage adult oculomotor organization rather well and may provide independent criteria outlining oculomotor history.

The striking conservation of genetic material and developmental interactions, both within vertebrates and throughout metazoans in general, are among the prominent features leading to specific neuronal characteristics (Ruddle, Bentley, Murtha, and Risch, 1994; Carroll, 1995). In particular, evidence from comparative molecular studies has begun to provide an initial blueprint of genes and protein products correlated with both the early development and later phenotypic characterization of hindbrain sensorimotor organization (Holland, 1992; Krumlauf, 1992; McGinnis and Krumlauf, 1992; Krumlauf, Marshall, Studer, Nonchev, Sham, and Lumsden, 1993). If, as recently proposed, specific gene products became identified with unique developmental processes during evolution (Holland, 1992; Manak and Scott, 1994), it seems probable that these in turn also may have become linked to identified physiologic processes. We will argue that circumstantial evidence exists for these linkages, and that, for example, Hox genes—especially the *deformed* gene homologues—may be essential for establishing the neuroepithelial sites for rhythmic motor behavior. More specifically, it appears that particular paired-box and wnt gene products may be involved in specifying the visuomotor pathways (McGinnis and Krumlauf, 1992; Stoykova and Gruss, 1994).

ORIGIN OF VISUAL AND VESTIBULAR MOTOR PATHWAYS IN THE HINDBRAIN

A previous essay elaborated a set of hypotheses concerning the production of rhythmic motor behavior by neurons derived from hindbrain rhs 7 and 8

(Bass and Baker, 1996). The initial hypothesis was based on identifying essential motor behaviors, largely cardio-respiratory, that became specified in rhs 7 and 8 at the protochordate-vertebrate transition. The evolution of particular subsets of pacemaker and pattern-generating neurons arising from rhs 7 and 8 were described in relationship to motoneurons and occipital muscles associated with vocal behavior (Bass and Baker, 1996).

A corollary hypothesis proposed that the brainstem premotor circuitry responsible for other rhythmic motor behaviors such as electromotor, oculomotor, locomotor, and masticatory, also were derived largely from rhs 7 and 8 (Bass and Baker, 1996). In contrast to the sonic motor system, the behaviors in each of these cases were produced by motoneurons originating from other rhombomeres, innervating muscles derived from the head somitomeres, not from the classical occipital somites. In the oculomotor system, for example, neurons associated with rhythmic bursting behavior and others with higher-level neuronal processing, such as eye velocity and position integration, were suggested to originate from rhs 7 and 8 (Gilland and Baker, 1994; Pastor et al., 1994b). Current observations suggest that cerebellar pathways are necessary for attaining autonomous, adaptive visuomotor (optokinetic) and vestibuloocular reflexes (OKR and VOR, respectively) (Lisberger, Pavelko, Bronte-Stewart, and Stone, 1994; Marsh, Pastor, and Baker, 1994; Pastor et al., 1994a). Image and eye motion signals were found to be mediated by hindbrain mossy and inferior olivary climbing fibers (Stone and Lisberger, 1990; Simpson, 1984) originating from neurons arising in rhs 7 and 8 (Altman and Bayer, 1987a; Sotelo and Wassef, 1991; Boss and Baker, 1996). Evidence presented in the previous essay also suggested that the inferior olive, particularly in respect to oscillation and pacemaker properties, might represent the highest-order hindbrain pattern-generating circuit, because of its essential role in providing a timing signal for a variety of rhythmic vertebrate behaviors (Llinas and Yarom, 1986; Llinas and Pare, 1994). Thus, it may be argued that the cerebellum is essential for bringing into existence specific evolutionary changes in oculomotor circuit design.

Determining which of the oculomotor traits evolved first—vestibular or visual—and whether their relationship to eye motion evolved in coordination or independently, are important issues to resolve before one or the other can be labeled as either "primitive" or "advanced" (Collewijn, 1989). This essay attempts to address these issues by deriving a framework for distinguishing cellular details of particular taxa from the general principles of visuooculomotor and vestibulooculomotor organization. In time, certain experimental models (e.g., cypriniformes [zebrafish] and mammals [mice]) that allow for true genetic analysis of neurons and circuits will eventually specify the neurophysiological profiles and pathways relevant to all species (Kimmel, 1989; Solnica-Krezel Schier, and Driever, 1994). By integrating development, evolution, and genetics, it may be possible to build a hypothetical primitive oculomotor plan that can be evaluated within the context of established physiological signals and neuron types (Keller, 1991; Scudder and Fuchs, 1992). Therefore, we propose that a genetic-based phylogenetic analysis of relevant neurons and circuits provides the best approach for assessing all oculomotor organization.

HYPOTHESES REGARDING THE EVOLUTION OF OCULOMOTOR FUNCTION

Five hypotheses are presented that outline the pattern of behavioral and neuronal innovations transpiring over 550 million years of vertebrate oculomotor evolution. The inferred evolutionary changes shown in the cladogram of figure 3.1 lead to the supposition that the processing of visual signals, while playing a subordinate role to inertial responses in the first 50 million years of vertebrate evolution, provided the major biological determinant guiding the selection of more sophisticated brainstem and cerebellar circuits generating eye movements during the ensuing 100 million years.

Hypothesis 1 The protochordate-vertebrate transition was characterized by elaboration of light-sensitive forebrain areas and statoreceptors whose signals we propose converged onto pacemaker neurons in caudal hindbrain rhombomeres to induce rhythmic locomotion. Hence, sensory signals appropriate for eye movements predated the entire oculomotor system and were available to be coopted by neurons specifically related to "eye" locomotion. We suggest that this "primitive" visual and vestibular convergence was largely forged in hindbrain compartments distinguished as rhombomeric segments 7 and 8.

Hypothesis 2 The early visuo-vestibulo-cerebellooculomotor template appears to have originated from neuroepithelial columns extending throughout the dorsal alar derivatives of rhs 2 to 8 in the common ancestors of lamprey and gnathostomes. The anterior-intermediate vestibuloocular neurons (rhs 2–5) were designed to respond to ipsilateral head rotation, roll, and forward tilt, and likely were regulated directly by the primitive vestibulocerebellum (rhs 1 and 2). For reasons still not clear, the ipsilateral posterior vestibular neurons (rhs 6 and 7) projecting to the contralateral abducens nucleus appear to have been only indirectly regulated through vestibulo- and visuocerebellar pathways. We suggest the latter connections originated from a hindbrain visuomotor center (rhs 7 and 8) that, in addition, projected directly to the abducens nuclei. This neuronal plan has remained intimately linked with horizontal oculomotor function throughout phylogeny and may have provided the biological impetus for contriving abducens internuclear neurons (rhs 5 and 6), thus attaining true conjugate horizontal eye movements.

Hypothesis 3 In gnathostomes, we hypothesize that convergence of specific vertical axis–related visual and vestibular motion signals was responsible for the diversification and accumulation of neurons in rhs 7 and 8 capable of generating directionally specific signals for eye and head motion, including

Vertebrate Oculomotor Innovations

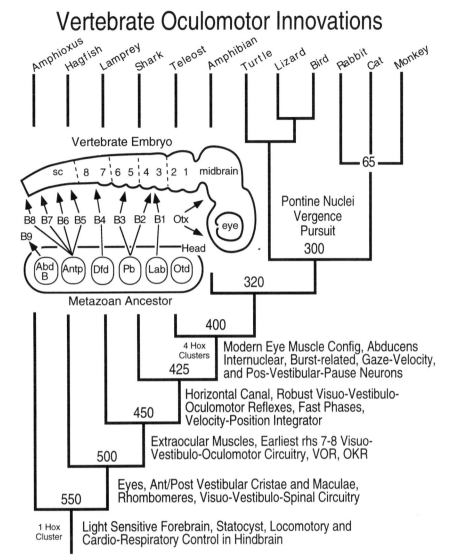

Figure 3.1 Diagram illustrating the sequence of appearance of vertebrate oculomotor innovations, including the theoretical evolution of vertebrate Hox gene clusters from an ancestral metazoan Hox cluster. An informal scheme depicts the relationships of some representative species with approximate times of their divergence indicated at the nodes in millions of years. The oculomotor features indicated to the right suggest these features to be present at origination of the descendant species. The evolution of pontine nuclei and associated vergence-pursuit behaviors are illustrated as occurring within the tetrapods; however, the distribution of these traits and their common or independent origins are unknown. The Hox B gene cluster is illustrated for hindbrain segments with continuation into the spinal cord. The primordial Hox cluster in the metazoan ancestor are shown with *Drosophila* nomenclature as summarized in the recent literature (Holland, 1992; Krumlauf, 1992). One Hox cluster is present in protochordates, while four are known from zebrafish and tetrapods. At least three clusters are present in lampreys, and the number is unknown in sharks and hagfish. Abd B, abdominal B; Antp, antennepedia; Dfd, deformed; Pb, proboscipedia; Lab, labial; Otd, orthodenticle; B1–B9, vertebrate Hox genes; 1–8, rhombomeres; sc, spinal cord.

eye position. In addition, burst-related neurons evolved to generate rapid eye velocity and reset eye position as well as to allow object motion to be attended by saccadic eye movements. We suggest that all these unique vestibulo- and visuomotor neurons and pathways originated in the earliest jawed vertebrates some 450 million years ago. As a result, the evolving oculomotor system had by then virtually accomplished Wall's goal of "holding the eye still with respect to the environment."

Hypothesis 4 Signals conveying image motion, initially arising from the pretectum and later the cortex, converged onto the evolving pontine nuclei of tetrapods to allow object motion to be tracked about rotational and translational axes, with either parallel or independent eye movement. We hypothesize that the unique pontocerebellar pathways responsible for visual pursuit originated from iteration and migration of neurons located within the pre-existing rhs 7 and 8 brainstem neuroepithelial template. As a result, we propose that the mechanisms for converting image slip to eye velocity were implemented in earlier vertebrates by rhs 7 and 8 dorsal column derivatives and then transferred to the pontine nuclei by neuronal migration. Accordingly, the primary visuomotor role of forwarding eye motion signals to the cerebellum by rhs 7 and 8 neurons was largely coopted to serve higher-order visual processing. The oculomotor innovations underlying pursuit therefore may represent the elaboration and refinement of existent visuomotor signal-processing capabilities as opposed to the acquisition of new ones. In this evolutionary scenario, the pontine nuclei have emerged as part of the consummate visuo-vestibulo-cerebellooculomotor circuit, because both pursuit and ocular following (OKR) are mediated directly through VOR interneuronal pathways.

Hypothesis 5 The history of oculomotor function is chronicled largely in the development and structure of the vertebrate hindbrain rhombic lip derivatives. If the prepositus and pontine nuclei, including the olivo-cerebellar pathways, are found to arise in rhs 7 and 8, then the genetic basis for visuomotor behavior in the brainstem may be concluded to originate from a specific segmented origin. Therefore, we suggest that interaction between multiple gene products, many already identified, may be viewed as a neuroepithelial founder event specifying unique neuronal phenotypes (Scott, 1994). As a result, we postulate that dedicated regulator-gene interactions have become linked to particular oculomotor roles throughout phylogeny. This hypothesis appears to be testable through manipulation and characterization of the physiological profiles in identified brainstem and cerebellar neurons of extant vertebrates.

STRUCTURAL AND GENETIC PATTERNING OF THE HINDBRAIN

In the late nineteenth century, researchers established the concept that the early vertebrate hindbrain is organized into segments known as *rhombomeres*:

(Neal, 1898; Vaage, 1969). These segments give rise to particular neuronal types in stereotypical patterns and are overlain by axial and dorsoventral expression patterns of numerous developmentally regulated genes (see figure 3.1). Experimental rhombomere transplants (Guthrie, Muchamore, Kuroiwa, Marshall, Krumlauf, and Lumsden, 1992) and perturbation of gene expression patterns indicate an autonomous genetic pattern for hindbrain compartmentalization and neuronal specification (McGinnis and Krumlauf, 1992). Because cranial motor nuclei of nerves III-XII share a conserved relationship with embryonic hindbrain compartments (Lumsden and Keynes, 1989; Gilland and Baker, 1993; Keynes and Krumlauf, 1994), gene expression patterns may provide useful criteria for identifying motoneurons, and presumably interneurons, throughout phylogeny. The conserved segmental origin of homologous reticulospinal neurons indicates that the correlative gene expression patterns specifying interneurons related to oculomotor function are also likely to have been established early in vertebrate hindbrain evolution (Metcalfe, Mendelson, and Kimmel, 1986; Hanneman, Trevarrow, Metcalfe, Kimmel, and Westerfield, 1988; Gilland and Baker, 1995). As a result, we believe that the principal features of an archetypical vertebrate "sensorimotor bauplan" originated in early jawless fishes much nearer to the onset of vertebrate evolution 500 million years ago than to the radiation of modern mammals, the usual experimental benchmark, 60 million years ago.

Recent work in both jawless (lamprey) and jawed (teleost) fish indicates that many segmentally organized features initiated in early embryogenesis persist through larval and adult periods (Gilland and Baker, 1994, 1995; Pastor et al., 1994b; Lee, Eaton, and Zottoli, 1993). Therefore, rhombomeres can be viewed as not only providing an initial blueprint for neurogenesis (lineage) and early circuit development (fate) but also as a permanent framework for sustaining functional neuronal circuitry (Fraser, Keynes, and Lumsden, 1990; Puelles and Rubenstein, 1993; Lumsden, Clarke, Keynes, and Fraser, 1994). If continuity of lineage-determinant mechanisms can be shown to exist from neuronal origin to adult phenotype, as appears likely, then individual genes and their protein products will be helpful for establishing a reliable phylogenetic history of particular neurons and circuits in extant vertebrates. Once "homologous" identity of neurons and circuits between species is better defined, the neuronal basis of visuo- and vestibulooculomotor function can be studied not only on a physiological basis but also within the context of a genetic biography. Insertional mutagenesis of genes (e.g., *deformed, wingless, paired-box, muscle segment*) will make it possible to address directly the developmental mechanisms for neuronal specificity accounting for VOR and OKR circuit design (Malicki, Cianetti, Peschle, and McGinnis, 1992).

Vertebrates possess numerous anatomical and physiological features not seen in their closest living relatives, *Branchiostoma* and the urochordates, for example, amphioxus and tunicates. (Northcutt and Gans, 1983; Forey and Janvier, 1993). Particularly relevant among these features are the appearance of embryonic neural crest and cephalic neuromeres. We believe that the current attempts to derive a vertebrate bauplan from either extant invertebrate taxa or hypothetial ancestral forms, by using developmental regulator genes and comparative developmental biology of extant relatives, are directly relevant to the evolution of brainstem and cerebellar regulation of oculomotor function (Gruss and Kessel, 1991; Holland, Garcia-Fernandez, Williams, and Sidow, 1994). The foremost feature of the bauplan so far revealed is the occurrence in most metazoan species studied (including all vertebrates) of a linear cluster of homeotic selector genes (Hox) encoding sequence-specific transcription factors lying within a cluster that mirrors the order of their overlapping expression domains along the anterior-posterior axis of the embryo (see figure 3.1) (Holland, 1992; Krumlauf, 1992; McGinnis and Krumlauf, 1992). In essence, Hox genes appear always to have organized the primary anterior-posterior axis in the animal kingdom (Slack, Holland, and Graham, 1993). This extraordinary conservation of structure and function emanating from a primary precursor set of four to six Hox genes (Garcia-Fernandez and Holland 1994; Manak and Scott, 1994; Ruddle et al., 1994) and the eventual quadruplication of the original Hox gene cluster in gnathostomes (Holland et al., 1994) (see figure 3.1) suggest to us that gene duplication was probably critical for the neuronal diversification postulated to occur here in hindbrain rhombomeres.

Central to our hypotheses is the apparent contemporaneous appearance of extensive hindbrain neuronal diversity, enhanced oculomotor capability, and additional genetic capacity during early phases of vertebrate evolution. This argument proposes that a suite of neurogenic innovations relevant to oculomotor performance (among other motor capabilities) emerged at different levels (i.e., physiological, behavioral, and genetic) within vertebrate organization and that their acquisition was historically contemporaneous. Comparison of these patterns indicates that the cooccurrence was not just fortuitous but instead might have been based on a common set of genetic and ontogenetic mechanisms. Both the evolutionary origination and subsequent repeated enhancements of oculomotor performance were suggested in hypothesis 4 to result from duplication and divergence of existing neuronal types and their resultant signals. We propose that the underlying ontogenetic system allowing for this neuronal-signal diversification was itself based on genetic regulation within neuroepithelial segments (rhombomeres), whose origin and diversification stemmed from the duplication (twice) of the primordial cluster of iterated Hox genes and their related chromosomal companions (Holland et al., 1994).

The apposite ancestral Hox gene in the case of rhs 7 and 8 is the chordate homologue of *Drosophila* deformed (Wilkinson, Bhatt, Cook, Boncinelli, and Krumlauf, 1989; McGinnis and Krumlauf, 1992). Though only one homologue of deformed appears to be present in amphioxus, at least two and probably three paralogous, deformed-type genes exist in lamprey (Wilkinson et al., 1989; McGinnis and Krumlauf, 1992; Holland et al., 1994); and four copies

(A4, B4, C4, and D4) are likely to be expressed in rhs 7 and 8 of jawed vertebrates. However, causality underlying vestibulo- and visuomotor capability clearly cannot be ascribed either directly or only to Hox gene duplication. Many other genes coding for transcription factors, and a host of genes coding for particular components of signal transduction pathways mediating cellular interactions, are also certainly necessary for downstream determination of distinct neuronal phenotypes within each rhombomere. In the case of vestibulo- and visuomotor interneuronal populations, genes coding for transcriptional factors containing paired-box motifs (e.g., *pax 3–6*) appear likely to be particularly relevant for determining the neuronal derivatives arising near to and from the rhombic lip, as opposed to basal neuroepithelium (Gruss and Walther, 1992; Stoykova and Gruss, 1994). Overall, the evolutionary rationale for the existence of rhombomeres thus appears to be that they provide a cellular spatial framework that allows for coexistence of genetic specificity with combinatorial diversity and neuronal specificity with expansive phenotypic diversity. Unfortunately, this suggestion rests primarily on the phylogenetic conservation and covariation of patterns between neuroepithelial compartments, spatially restricted gene expression, and later-appearing neuronal types. Documentation of cellular detail, let alone circuit composition, has yet to be accomplished in *any* species (Fraser et al., 1990; Clarke and Lumsden, 1993; Gilland and Baker, 1993; Glover, 1993; Lumsden et al., 1994).

The five hypotheses presented here argue that modification of primitive sensorimotor traits is likely carried out by a process of homeotic iteration of common neuroepithelial precursors, implying that diversification of innovative signal processing is compatible with retention of the original neuronal phenotypes. Consequently, if oculomotor innovations in a wide range of vertebrates originate ontogenetically from a segmental scaffold (Gilland and Baker, 1993; Guthrie, 1995) it follows that specific subdivisions of the hindbrain neuroepithelium probably were defined early in vertebrate evolution to generate particular neuronal subtypes and circuits underlying specific types of eye movement. As a result, it should be possible to follow the evolution of constituent neurons in vestibuloocular and optokinetic reflexes to provide a logical basis specifying neurophysiological principles of circuit processing in the brainstem and cerebellum throughout vertebrates.

VISUAL AND VESTIBULAR RELATIONSHIPS IN THE ANCIENT HINDBRAIN

The earliest vertebrates possessed both light- and stato-sensitive neuroepithelial areas regulating locomotion. Some type of phototactic behavior is present in most multicellular and many unicellular animals. It is likely that some components of a common, homologous chordate visuomotor system still exist in vertebrates, though available evidence remains fragmentary. Protochordates and urochordates exhibit phototactic light-avoidance responses and may provide evidence regarding the earliest chordate visuomotor reflexes (Berrill, 1987; Bone, 1987). Phototactic responses also are known from amphioxus, and possible homologues of vertebrate lateral and pineal photoreceptors along with their connections with CNS locomotory centers are being examined in an ongoing series of ultrastructural studies by Lacalli and colleagues (Lacalli, Holland, and West, 1994). In addition to phototactic responses mediated by retinal and pineal systems, larval lampreys exhibit body movements in response to dermal photostimulation and even to illumination of nonretinal encephalic photoreceptors (Young, 1935; Ullen, Orlovsky, Dellagini, and Grillner, 1993). Retinal signals through pretectal nuclei were shown to project bilaterally to the lamprey hindbrain (Fritzsch and Collin, 1990) and are likely to be spatially specific (Deliagina Grillner, Orlovsky, and Ullen, 1993). Although hagfish are generally considered to be blind, they possess retinal photoreceptors and ganglion cells with restricted, yet fairly typical central visual pathways (Holmberg, 1979; Wicht and Northcutt, 1990). All these more or less primitive chordates also locomote using a homologous axial motor system comprised of somite-derived myotomes and centrally located motoneurons. Based on features seen in gnathostomes, Bass and Baker (1996) proposed that an ensemble of neural elements whose properties and connectivity gave rise to rhythmical pattern generation coordinating locomotor and cardiorespiratory mechanisms may have originated from hindbrain rhs 7 and 8. Hence, we suggest in hypothesis 1 that light-sensitive forebrain areas established central connections with comparable pacemaker-like neurons in rhs 7 and 8. As a result, the directionally tuned, visual-avoidance motor responses could be implemented by hindbrain spino-locomotor pathways.

Another major character determinant of early vertebrates was the presence of an inner ear with presumed vestibular sensitivity (Forey and Janvier, 1993). One of the earliest sensory capabilities of vertebrates was probably determination of spatial relations to the earth, namely orientation in respect to a single direction (i.e., gravity) (Graf, 1988). The ubiquitous distribution of hair cells across the body surface underlying both electrical reception and mechanical transduction may will have preceded an inner ear with hair cells specifically designed for either gravity or angular displacement (Boord and Campbell, 1977). As a result, several inertia-independent, environment-specific spatial mechanisms were present long before the labyrinth and eye muscles (Northcutt, 1985). Hence, the earliest brainstem-cerebellar interaction must have been based largely on the use of electro- and mechanoreception for object detection in respect to locomotion and posture (Northcutt and Gans, 1983). A reasonable proposal might be that the early evolving reference frames leading to an integrated inertial and visual coordinate system emerged gradually by refinement of sensorimotor maps from separate but diverse hair cell systems. Their convergence onto autorhythmical premotor centers in hindbrain rhs 7 and 8 provided the first clearly definable visuo- and vestibulo-motor circuitry. Retinal and inertial signals would have been selected for by primitive brainstem-cerebellar circuitry because these senses exhibited an invariant relationship with the environment (i.e., gravity and world motion) (Simpson and Graf, 1985). Hence, the early octavolateral organization, including vestibular nuclei, consisted of neurons conveying spatial information sensing either self-motion (vestibular), that of the environment (lateral-line), or objects therein (electroreception), to central pattern-generating neurons located in rhs 7 and 8 controlling locomotion and the cardiorespiratory pump (Bass and Baker, 1996).

Body orientation is maintained in lampreys with the dorsal side up, and this appears to be a vestibular-driven control system that can be modified by visual input (i.e., dorsal light reflex) (Deliagina et al., 1992). An extensive synaptic interaction between visual and vestibular signals has been described in lamprey reticulospinal neurons that is clearly distinguished from effects occurring directly in octavomotor neurons (Deliagina, Orlovsky, Grillner, and Wallen, 1993). Vestibular influences have been found on the same subset of reticular neurons influencing both body orientation and locomotion (Orlovsky, Deliagina, and Wallen, 1992). Both roll and pitch trigger the spinal locomotor's central pattern generator that modulates neurons in rhs 7 and 8 through, presumably, efferent-copy brainstem signals related to locomotor rhythm. These observations provide evidence that the visual and vestibular mechanisms, including their coordinate axes, are operational before either the eye or extraocular muscles become functional (Rubinson and Cain, 1989).

Living representatives of early agnathan lineages, namely the hagfish and lamprey, both exhibit a labyrinth but with two particularly incomplete canals (Simpson and Graf, 1985). Considerable debate exists about relationships between ancient fishes and early vertebrate sensorimotor history (Forey and Janvier, 1993); however, there are several observations that address the issue of vertebrate oculomotor innovations. First, lampreys and hagfish exhibit long and separate histories related by fossil agnathan groups consisting of osteostracans, anapsids, and heterostracans (Forey and Janvier, 1993). This fossil evidence suggests that closely related taxa were quite different in overall body shape and equally distinct in respect to eye position regarding body axis. For example, eyes in heterostracans (and related hagfish) were located more frontally than in either anaspids (including lampreys) or cephalaspids. The latter were the closest agnathan relatives of gnathostomes and had dorsally positioned eyes with well-developed extrinsic eye muscles. Therefore, long before jawed vertebrates, all eye locations (lateral, frontal, dorsal), both with and without extraocular muscles, had largely been experimented with in the rich diversity of the fossil agnathans.

Not all the relationships between eye morphogenesis, differentiation of the retina, and the presence of eye muscles in early vertebrates are well understood (Fritzsch, 1991). The eye anlage evaginates and forms the optic cup, including formation of the lens placode before species-related appearance of extrinsic extraocular muscles (and therefore a visuo- and vestibulooculomotor system). For instance, a neural retina clearly preceded either intrinsic or extrinsic eye muscles, even at a time when the retina exhibited both afferent and efferent relationships with the CNS (Fritzsch and Collin, 1990). Thus it is likely that the extraocular eye muscles occurred at the transition between, or in the ancestor of, hagfish and lampreys (see figure 3.1). Hence, arguments about the origins of eye muscles revolve around agnathans (both fossil and living) and their relationship to jawed vertebrates. In any case, it can be concluded that the origins of extraocular muscles lie somewhere within the history of the long-extinct jawless fishes represented today as lampreys and hagfishes (Neal, 1918).

If convergence of visual and vestibular afferents onto rhs 7 and 8 pacemaker neurons that produced rhythmic self-motion predated the entire oculomotor system, then the appropriate sensory signals were already present in rhs 7 and 8 to be coopted for innervation of neuroepithelial derivatives specifically related to eye movement (hypothesis 1). Assuming that the absence of extraocular muscles is a primitive feature and is not found in hagfish, it is possible to infer that the visual and vestibular locomotor circuits preceded those of visuo- and vestibulooculomotor circuits described in lampreys (Pombal, Rodicio, and Anadón, 1994). Though lampreys and hagfishes are thought not to form a monophyletic group, interpretation of their phylogeny was determined independent of either visuo- or vestibulomotor traits. Early history was largely established based upon an analysis of nasal and hypophyseal regions (Forey and Janvier, 1993); however, other seemingly unrelated characters such as dermal skeleton, rudimentary vestibular and visual sensory end organs, and paired pectoral fins in cephalaspids, may have some relevance to the issue of the evolution of motor coordination (Bunker and Machin, 1991). These observations suggest that posture served as a significant biological determinant in agnathans, instigating morphogenetic transformations leading to the focus of visuovestibular convergence in hindbrain rhs 7 and 8. We believe that the proximate relationship of amphioxus with early Paleozoic vertebrates (Gee, 1994) and the ability to locate and map homeobox genes in amphioxus neuroepithelium (Holland, Holland, Williams, and Holland, 1992) will allow the expression domains of homologous genes to be correlated with morphological landmarks in the neural plate and the distribution of neuronal phenotypes along the body axis throughout vertebrates (Holland, 1992; Gilland and Baker, 1993; Slack et al., 1993). Such data will provide the basis for constructing a prototypical neuroepithelial scaffold from which it will be possible to infer the exact locations of the earliest visuomotor neurons and circuits, herein hypothesized to be located in rhs 7 and 8.

RHOMBOMERIC ORIGIN OF VISUO- AND VESTIBULOMOTOR INTERNEURONS AND CIRCUITS

Comparison of the extraocular muscles and motoneuronal innervation in lamprey, elasmobranch, and bony fish provides evidence regarding visuo- and vestibulooocular organization in early gnathostomes (Graf and Brunken,

1984; Fritzsch, Sonntag, Dubuc, Ohta, and Grillner, 1990). The origin and insertion of extraocular muscles in the lamprey orbit differing from that of jawed fishes was suggested to occur in response to organizational changes in the inner ear, i.e., a causal correlation with either a two- or three-semicircular-canal arrangement. By contrast, the divergence in extraocular innervation patterns between sharks and bony fish has been explained as retention of the primitive gnathostome pattern by sharks (Graf and Brunken, 1984). These proposals are consistent with the fact that lampreys and hagfish lack a horizontal canal and that sharks appear to exhibit an embryonic pattern of eye muscle development quite different from other vertebrates (Baker, 1991). However, our recent observations on rhombomeres and eye muscle development (Gilland and Baker, 1995) and the ideas introduced by Fritzsch et al. (1990) could be equally well interpreted by assuming that vestibuloocular organization in lampreys is primitive to (i.e., ancestral to) that found in jawed vertebrates. Hence, oculomotor organization in elasmobranchs may be truly divergent from that of other jawed vertebrates and as a result provides an extremely interesting outgroup comparison of visuo- and vestibuloocular pathways.

Based on developmental studies in lamprey and chicken (Larsell, 1967; Glover and Petursdottir, 1991; Pombal et al., 1994; Marín and Puelles, 1995) our second hypothesis proposed that the primitive vestibulooculomotor brainstem template originated from a distinct longitudinal column extending throughout the rhombic lip of rhs 2 to 8 in the common ancestors to lampreys and gnathostomes. The neuronal organization of the ventral octavolateral column in the lamprey hindbrain provides a plausible picture of an early stage in the evolution of VOR interneurons and circuits (Tretjakoff, 1909; Larsell, 1947; Rovainen, 1982; Pombal et al., 1994). This longitudinal region includes the anterior, intermediate, and posterior octavomotor nuclei which have been shown to contain VOR interneurons (Pombal et al., 1994). Based on their relationship to segmentally identified neuronal groups (Gilland and Baker, 1995) these VOR neurons are hypothesized to originate from separate locations in rhs 2 to 7. In summary, these VOR neurons may represent the ancestral, excitatory projections to the contralateral superior rectus (rhs 2 and 3), ipsilateral medial rectus (rhs 4 and 5), and contralateral abducens (rhs 6 and 7) motor pools. VOR interneurons appear to be derived from more medio-ventral neuroepithelial precursor areas than are either the cerebellar nuclei or cortex (Rudeberg, 1961).

The intermediate and posterior octavomotor nuclei described in lamprey are relevant for understanding rotations about the vertical axis and horizontal eye movement. The intermediate nucleus gives rise to ipsilateral rostral projections that enter the medial longitudinal fasciculus (MLF) just prior to the oculomotor nucleus (Pombal et al., 1994). Based on cell location, axonal trajectory, and presumed target (the rostral rectus subnucleus in the oculomotor complex (Fritzsch et al., 1990) these neurons are likely to be homologous to those forming the ascending tract of Deiters and may represent the ancestral condition (Highstein and McCrea, 1988). By contrast, posterior octavomotor neurons innervate the contralateral abducens motor nucleus; however, they also exhibit bifurcating axon collaterals projecting to the spinal cord (Pombal et al., 1994). These VOR interneurons are located near the posterior lateral line entry zone, and the underlying hindbrain topography suggests origination from rhs 6 and 7 (Gilland and Baker, 1995).

The anterior-intermediate vestibuloocular neurons (rhs 2–4) appear to respond to ipsilateral head rotation, roll, and forward tilt (Rovainen, 1976). In gnathostomes, the homologous VOR interneurons are directly inhibited by the vestibulocerebellum (de La Cruz, Pastor, and Baker, 1993). A constitutive brainstem-cerebellar circuit may be an intrinsic attribute of rhs 1 and 2, as both the vestibulocerebellum and subsets of VOR interneurons appear to originate from the same hindbrain rhombomeric compartments. We believe this primitive feature is also significant for the origin of the pontine nuclei in descendant vertebrates (see hypothesis 4). In contrast, although the posterior vestibular neurons (rhs 6 and 7) projecting to the contralateral abducens nucleus are also directly responsive to ipsilateral head rotation, there is no evidence in any vertebrate that these VOR neurons were ever directly regulated by the cerebellum (Ito, 1982). In hypothesis 2, we proposed that these horizontal VOR interneurons are likely connected indirectly with the vestibulocerebellum through the hindbrain visuomotor nucleus originating from rhs 7 and 8. Evidence in bony fishes shows that this visuomotor area projects to both the vestibular and abducens nuclei and that all the eye-motion-related neurons contained therein are directly regulated by the cerebellum (de La Cruz et al., 1993). Confirmation of these UOR and OKR pathways in lampreys would suggest the possibility that a similar organization of three octavomotor nuclei in early agnathans rendered the ancestral basis for one of the most significant transitions in the evolution of oculomotor function, namely from the nearly exclusive reliance on statoreceptors (inertia) to that of photoreceptors (vision).

HOLDING THE EYE STILL WITH RESPECT TO THE ENVIRONMENT THROUGH VISION

The two semicircular canals in lampreys appear sufficient to produce three axes of eye movement (Rovainen, 1976); yet, the evolutionary transition at the origin of jawed fishes was accompanied by elaboration of a separate horizontal canal. However, contrary to suggestions in the literature, this does not demonstrate that newly acquired brainstem signals were either driven by or causally related to the evolution of vestibular function. Arguably, vision was the sensory stimulus bearing the most consequence, and although the terminology *visuomotor evolution* is unsound, it more aptly represents the major evolutionary impetus for the selection and design of gnathostom brainstem eye movement circuitry. Specifically, visual input was exploited to build up the temporal-spatial frequency range, particularly the insufficient vestibular time-constant (Raphan and Cohen, 1985). Moreover, the unceasing need for vestibulooculomotor reflex calibration must have been a critical early evolutionary pressure, because the image-forming retina could view objects, as opposed to just merely noting their motion (Fritzsch, 1991; Miles and Busettini, 1992). As a result, we hypothesize that rapid transformations occurred in the brainstem-cerebellar circuits, in respect to the location and diversity of neuronal phenotypes.

As explicitly set forth in hypothesis 3, the convergence of visual and vestibular motion-related signals in hindbrain rhs 7 and 8 provided the physiological rationale for generating a novel subset of neurons by a process of developmental iteration. In this instance, preexisting vestibular connections were sustained, and new collaterals provided the formative foundation for an entirely new "vertical axis" visuovestibular organization correlated with the horizontal canal. This idea presupposes that separate visuomotor and vestibulomotor pathways existed in the agnathans and that the vestibulovisual interface in hindbrain rhs 7 and 8 developed largely for postural compensation. The necessity of visual signals for parallel, symmetric oculomotor control likely provided the functional rationale for the coevolution of abducens internuclear neurons with motoneurons in rhs 5 and 6 (Baker, 1991). As a result, either visual or vestibular stimuli could produce conjugate movement of the two eyes even though the primitive vestibulo-cerebellomotor circuits were capable of directly regulating only ipsilateral brainstem neurons.

Evidence in ray-finned fishes (e.g., goldfish) suggests that convergence of vertical axis vestibular and visual input to rhs 7 and 8 was responsible for developing neurons capable of generating directionally specific eye motion (i.e., velocity), combined eye-head sensitivity, and eye-position signals (Pastor et al., 1994b). For example, in response to either vertical axis vestibular or visual stimuli, both horizontal eye velocity signals and eye position signals have been observed in separate subsets of neurons located in rhs 7 and 8. Burst-related neurons capable of generating rapid eye velocity to reset eye position and saccadic eye movements were also identified in the same region of the goldfish hindbrain. Hence, it is plausible to hypothesize that neurons generating rapid eye velocity, either for resetting purposes or scanning the environment, would also be selected from the same hindbrain rhs 7 and 8 neuroepithelial precursors.

Several subsets of identifiable saccade-related neurons can be found located medial to, and between, the eye position and velocity integrators in the hindbrain (Pastor et al., 1994b). One unique physiological profile called the *burst driver* was illustrated in a previous essay (Bass and Baker, 1996) because these cells seem to play the role of a hindbrain fast-phase integrator and, like the other oculomotor integrators, lie in the caudal hindbrain. This type of neuron uniquely integrates information from the visuo- and vestibulomotor system to generate resetting fast-phases and responds as well to motor commands from the superior colliculus to attend discrete objects (Sasaki and Shimazu, 1981). Burst-driver neurons project onto immediately adjacent neurons, described as short-lead burst generators (Pastor et al., 1994b), that provide the command-velocity signals directly to the appropriate abducens motoneuron-internuclear neurons, including collaterals to VOR interneurons (Keller, 1991). Based on morphological profiles, transmitters, and early lineage markers, all the saccade-related neurons are likely derived from rhs 7 and 8 (Metcalfe et al., 1986; Hanneman et al., 1988; Spencer, Wenthold, and Baker, 1990).

In summary, all the aforementioned unique vestibulo- and visuomotor neurons and circuits described in hypotheses 2 and 3 appear to have originated some 450 million years ago in the common ancestor to lamprey and gnathostomes. As a result, by then the essence of "holding the eye still with respect to the environment" had been virtually realized. In this respect, our viewpoint on evolution of the oculomotor system differs from that usually argued, because we emphasize that the focus of natural selection switched early, and abruptly, from vestibular to visual signal processing. For instance, we advance the idea that all the oculomotor innovations necessary and sufficient for generating both the slow and fast-phases of vertical axis eye movement in vertebrates were clearly present in the earliest bony fishes. Hence, nearly all the physiological types previously studied in other vertebrates (i.e., mammals) must necessarily have been present in earlier taxa. Consequently, the genetic basis of interactive visuovestibular eye movement, including motor adaptation, also must have existed some 450 million years ago and has been highly conserved since then. Therefore, the question arises: Are any significant oculomotor innovations not included to this point in evolutionary history (i.e., before the origin of tetrapods)? The answer is equally both unambiguous and surprising.

ORIGIN OF THE PONTINE NUCLEI AND THE PURSUIT OF OBJECT MOTION

Image motion signals arising from the pretectum and cortex converge onto pontine nuclei of tetrapods and, through bilateral projections to the cerebellum, allow object motion about any axes to be tracked with symmetrical eye movements (Keller, 1991; Fuchs, Mustari, Robinson, and Kaneko, 1992; Miles and Busettini, 1992). Hypothesis 4 proposed that this trait—called *smooth pursuit*—may have been achieved primarily through developmental iteration of the preexisting brainstem and cerebellar neuronal templates. Most notably, we suggest that the eye motion–related neurons of the dorsolateral pontine nuclei and nucleus reticularis tegmenti pontis were probably exclusively derived from rhs 7 and 8 precursors. During embryogenesis in birds and mammals, pontine neurons from the visuomotor rhombic lip column migrate and form distinct nuclei located in the pons (Marin and Puelles, 1995). Therefore, the insertion of eye motion signal processing into the same hindbrain site from which the vestibulo-, cerebello-, and oculomotor circuits originate (rhs 2 and 4) established the structural basis for ocular pursuit to be directly produced through VOR interneuronal pathways.

Neurons originating from the alar (dorsal) and basal (ventral) neuroepithelial regions can be clearly distinguished in embryonic material (e.g., zebrafish [Metcalfe et al., 1986], mammals [Altman and Bayer, 1987b], and birds [Tan and LeDourarin, 1991]). Although neither cell lineage nor migration from the rhombic lip have been studied in respect to visuovestibular oculomotor function, we believe the available evidence indicates that all motion-related neurons originate dorsally along the entire extent of hindbrain rhombomeres 2 to 8. As noted much earlier by Essick (1912), "the rhombic lip must be regarded as the germ center for the cells which form the olive, pons, and other nuclei of the brainstem" (e.g., prepositus, vestibular, cochlear, and raphé nuclei). At particular stages of development in both birds and mammals, continuous strands of cells exhibiting varying degrees of differentiation extend ventromedially from the caudal medullary rhombic lip (Harkmark, 1954). Vestibular interneurons originate from more medial precursors than do visuomotor neurons, in agreement with the demonstration of separate, direct OKR and VOR connections to the abducens motor complex (Weiser, Marsh, and Baker, 1995). Visuovestibular control of eye movement thus may be regarded as an autonomous trait of a subset of cells derived from the dorsolateral-longitudinal cell columns of rhs 2 to 8, in which vertical-axis optokinetic and pursuit neurons arose largely from rhs 7 and 8, and VOR interneurons from rhs 4 to 7. Included are inferior olivary neurons that convey retinal slip signals to the vestibulocerebellum (Simpson, 1984) and also originate from rhs 7 and 8 rhombic lip precursors (Harkmark, 1954; Sotelo and Wassef, 1991). Hence, nearly all of the cerebellar afferent circuitry (i.e., mossy and climbing fibers) related to retinal slip and eye motion (for both VOR and OKR function) originates from rhs 7 and 8. Assuming that visuovestibular signals converged onto subsets of rhs 7 and 8-derived reticular neurons before the evolution of the visuooculomotor column in gnathostomes, we suggest that recently acquired rhombic lip derivatives arise from juxtaposed neuroepithelial precursors and in all cases have selected migration towards the source of "new" visual signals. Therefore, the adult phenotypic location of the visually related prepositus, olivary, and pontine nuclei (as seen in mammals, for example) is neither enigmatic nor the result of random displacement of nuclei.

The primitive visuomotor role of optokinetic-related neurons arising from rhs 7 and 8, including their cerebellar projections, thus appears to have been coopted largely during the evolution of pontine nuclei in mammals. In effect, the mechanisms for converting image slip to eye velocity were transferred along with the rhs 7 and 8 neuronal migration. In most ray-finned fishes, the brainstem-cerebellar circuits are well designed for independent control and calibration of the VOR and OKR (Pastor, de la Cruz, and Baker, 1992, 1994a). Retinal specializations (including foveation) are present in some species, allowing eye movements that briefly follow object motion (Weiser, Bass,

McElligot, and Baker, 1988). Hence, though some comparable mechanism probably existed in Paleozoic fish and tetrapods to track objects, development of smooth pursuit called for sustained suppression of the optokinetic surround, which required cortical projections to the pretectum along with convergence of image motion signals onto the pontine nuclei with feedforward signal processing through the vestibulocerebellum. Clearly, evolution of the pontine nuclei led to the acquisition of smooth pursuit; however, we suggest that neurons responsible for ocular tracking behavior, irrespective of hindbrain location, have been generated as iterative homologues from rhs 7 and 8 throughout phylogeny.

At some point in early tetrapod evolution, the pontine nuclei appear to have arisen by migration into a brainstem region already determined as a forebrain afferent recipient zone (Harkmark, 1954; Karten, 1991). In early gnathostomes, the development of jaws occurred from branchial arch derivatives innervated from rhs 2 and 3 with the elaboration of both tectal and forebrain signals allowing for prey recognition, acquisition, and mastication. Convergence of diverse sensorimotor systems at a single axial level may have provided a behavioral rationale for the evolution of the cortico- and pontocerebellar loops in motor control, especially for the visual cortex in the case of pursuit (Miles and Busettini, 1992; Fuchs et al., 1992). We suspect that neurons from the rhs 7 and 8 rhombic lip migrated to a more rostral hindbrain location (rhs 2 and 4) at least partly in response to the established rhs 2 vestibulo- and cerebellooculomotor circuits described in hypothesis 2. Hence, we propose that the visuo- and vestibulooculomotor organization in higher vertebrates arose by superimposition of additional neuroepithelial derivatives on the preexisting 450-million-year-old blueprint. If so, oculomotor innovations in advanced tetrapods should be viewed as the elaboration of existent neuronal traits rather than the de novo acquisition of novel neurons and circuits.

The argument forwarded in hypothesis 5 is that all visual motion–related signals involved with oculomotor behavior (both precerebellar and premotoneuronal) are uniquely specified by combinatorial gene transcripts that we propose can eventually be shown to characterize hindbrain rhs 7 and 8 oculomotor derivatives. This genetics-based supposition has important implications in the phylogenetic shift from fish to tetrapods because rhs 7 and 8 derivatives appear to underlie the structural basis of all visuomotor behavior. If the relevant brainstem cerebellooculomotor pathways, including the inferior olive, originate from rhs 7 and 8, we argue that a rational framework exists for interpreting the entire evolution of visual and vestibular oculomotor function. In particular, the major transitions in oculomotor history have largely occurred because of the expansion of neuronal potential in the vertebrate hindbrain rhombic lip. Hence, we suggest that multiple gene products, some of which already have been identified (e.g., deformed, paired-box, wingless, muscle segment), collectively constitute a neuroepithelial founder event (Scott, 1994). Consequently, a particular gene interaction has become linked to the physiological phenotypes underlying a given oculomotor behavior throughout phylogeny. This hypothesis can be tested on the basis of available knowledge regarding signal processing and genetic profiles of identified visuomotor neurons in the hindbrain.

SYNOPSIS OF PHYSIOLOGICAL SIGNALS IN BRAINSTEM AND CEREBELLAR NEURONS

The original 450-million-year-old draft of the VOR and OKR circuitry had a significant and lasting impact on determining the physiologic signals and types of neurons found in the brainstem and cerebellum of all vertebrates. By and large, all types of signal processing described in the brainstem and cerebellum of more derived vertebrates (e.g., mammals) are found in teleosts and thus probably exist in all gnathostomes. We propose that this design arose primarily from the convergence of head and eye motion (i.e., velocity) signals in the cerebellum and the parcellation of Purkinje cell projections onto VOR and OKR interneurons located in the different brainstem subnuclei as outlined in hypotheses 2 and 3. The signals in derived tetrapod pontine neurons actually represent the same type of signal processing described in earlier vertebrates. Because some brainstem targets of the cerebellum, especially the VOR interneurons, appear to have been preserved nearly intact in the transition from fish to tetrapods, our surmise is that nearly all the physiological subtypes described in the mammalian VOR and OKR pathways (Keller, 1991; Scudder and Fuchs, 1992) existed in the primitive hindbrain 450 million years ago. Additional physiological response profiles, however, have arisen from the primitive neuronal substrate to implement oculomotor behaviors capable of combining translational and rotational axes in attending object motion via smooth pursuit and vergence.

Analysis of physiological signal processing in the mammalian vestibular nuclei has revealed a seemingly infinite variety of cell types related to the dynamics of the VOR, OKR, smooth pursuit, and vergence, including saccadic eye movements (Scudder and Fuchs, 1992). Vestibular neurons have been subdivided into classes based on spatial traits related to semicircular canal planes aligned with extraocular muscle action (Simpson and Graf, 1985); coordinate transformations (Robinson, 1992); signal conversions (e.g., velocity and position integration) (Robinson, 1989); and structure-function correlates related to targets (Graf and Ezure, 1986; McCrea, Strassman, May, and Highstein, 1987; Highstein and McCrea, 1988). Most of this work, carried on without benefit of any evolutionary rationale, has supported the belief that indigenous visual signals project directly onto VOR interneurons through prepositus, pontine, or pretectal nuclei rather than indirectly from the same pathways, but through the cerebellum.

An example relevant to vertical axis eye movements concerns the cell type called *position-vestibular-pause* (PVP) but originally named *tonic-vestibular-pause*

(TVP) (Keller, 1991). During VOR and OKR performance, PVP discharge correlates with eye and head velocity but only with the latter during VOR cancellation. These neurons were found to be the major VOR interneuron projecting to the abducens nucleus; however, another subtype called *eye-head velocity* (EHV; also termed *FTN*) was identified as an interneuron in the three-neuron horizontal VOR (Scudder and Fuchs, 1992). These cells are likely cerebellar targets (Lisberger et al., 1994b; see also chapter 2). In addition, similar types have been distinguished in vertical (up-down) eye movements (Zhang, Partsalis, and Highstein, 1995).

Given the diversity of cell types in the vestibular complex (McCrea et al., 1987; Scudder and Fuchs, 1992), it may be possible to shift the relative strengths of head and eye velocity sensitivity between neurons (e.g., by the cerebellum) so that one type—for example, PVP—might be converted to another—for example, EHV. This hypothesis is supported by the demonstration that adaptive mechanisms managing the VOR and OKR can produce sustained changes in the physiological sensitivity of vestibular neurons (Lisberger et al., 1994a). A similar explanation has been advanced for intra- and interspecies differences in vestibular types (Scudder and Fuchs, 1992). The rationale in both cases suggests that during evolution, additional unique phenotypes might have arisen through diversification of common neuronal precursors with closely aligned physiological fate (Kimmel, 1990; Karten, 1991). We believe this sort of developmental mechanism may be analogous to manipulation of physiological signals in vestibular neurons achieved by cerebellar processing. Thus, in the context of eye movements, the proposed developmental hypothesis may be thought of as an example in which the evolution of neurons and circuits have followed, not preceded, already established oculomotor behavior.

CONCLUSIONS

The oculomotor blueprint in the hindbrain was founded on an evolutionary history in which visual and vestibular motor circuits evolved separately with respect to each eye and the direction of movement. Early vestibular and visual premotor nuclei contained largely (maybe only) one type of neuron, PVP. In this arrangement, the cerebellum could, independently and adaptively, regulate eye and head velocity sensitivity in each reflex (Pastor et al., 1992, 1994a, de La Cruz et al., 1993). During the evolution of more sophisticated oculomotor function, phylogenetic history appears to have prevailed because the cerebellum has retained direct relationships to VOR neurons related to the control of ipsilateral brainstem neurons and eye muscles. Particularly, in all vertebrates the VOR projection to the contralateral abducens nucleus is indirectly controlled via the original rhs 7 and 8 neurons constituting the prepositus nucleus. With the addition of pontine eye-motion-related signals operating through cerebellar circuits, the physiological sensitivity of vestibular neurons could be altered, producing, in effect, an evolution of new

VOR phenotypes. This adaptability likely depended on intrinsic properties of neurons permitting pacemakerlike discharge sustaining the positive feed-forward cerebellar pathways (Llinas and Pare, 1994; Bass and Baker, 1996). These hindbrain innovations could produce stable eye velocity for any combination of self or surround movements, including that of tracking objects.

Though the plan for "holding the eyes still" about the vertical axis was complete in early jawed fish, the physiological signals and circuits from rhs 7 and 8 were later coopted during evolution to pursue discrete objects. Although ocular tracking has been considered a unique trait of foveated mammals (Miles and Busettini, 1992), aspects of this behavior also exist in teleost fish (Marsh et al., 1994). Genuine pursuit required more extensive visual motion sensitivity to generate the correct velocity command to move both eyes in the same direction and at the same speed. Hence, the dorsolateral pontine nuclei acquired neurons exhibiting directionally selective receptive fields that either were quite wide (like prepositus) or smaller (several degrees) and highly dependent on speed (Keller, 1991). We have suggested that the appearance of these speed-sensitive signals in the pons resulted from the migration of neurons from rhs 7 and 8. Thus, it is not surprising that similar visual motion and eye velocity sensitivity appears in the mammalian pons and prepositus (Fuchs et al., 1992). Irrespective of the location of visual motion–sensitive neurons, either in rhs 7 and 8 prepositus or the rhs 2 and 3 pontine site, the signals have always converged within the same cerebello- and vestibulo-oculomotor circuitry that existed in early gnathostomes. Evolution appears to have exercised an option to shift the balance of synaptic strength by capitalizing on the extant properties of neuronal subtypes. Therefore, we suggest that while considerable diversification has occurred in vertical axis signal subtypes, the general principles of neuronal processing have changed remarkably little, if at all.

In short, sensorioculomotor circuits were largely "designed" in early evolution to fulfill the goal of holding the eye still with respect to the environment so that visual processing, whatever it may be in any species, could distinguish objects and their movements with respect to the self (Walls, 1962). However, nature tinkered with continuous adaptation of each reflex, the VOR and OKR, leading to a large transformation of the visuomotor blueprint in which both developmental and adaptive modifications became largely interpolated into VOR interneuronal pathways. Thus, in amniotes, refinement of ocular following has occurred through the vestibular nuclei, so that, in contrast to teleosts, VOR modification influences OKR performance (Lisberger, Miles, Optican, and Eighmy, 1981; Marsh et al., 1994). Because visuomotor function was coopted by the pontine motion-sensitive pathways, the only oculomotor processing clearly retained in the rhs 7 and 8 hindbrain of higher vertebrates is that which generates eye velocity signals (i.e., the prepositus nucleus). Significantly, this hindbrain site has remained throughout vertebrates as the critical source for the eye motion signals alluded to "as responsible for the ancient and original function of eye muscles."

REFERENCES

Altman J, Bayer SA (1987a). Development of the precerebellar nuclei in the rat: II. The intramural olivary migratory stream and the neurogenetic organization of the inferior olive. J Comp Neurol 257:490–512.

Altman J, Bayer SA (1987b). Development of the precerebellar nuclei in the rat: IV. The anterior precerebellar extramural migratory stream and the nucleus reticularis tegmenti pontis and the basal pontine gray. J Comp Neurol 257:529–552.

Baker R (1991). A contemporary view of the history of eye muscles and motoneurons. In H. Shimazu, Y. Shinoda (eds), Vestibular and Brainstem Control of Eye, Head, and Body Movements. Tokyo: Springer Verlag and Japan Scientific Society Press, pp 3–19.

Bass AH, Baker R (1996). Phenotypic specification of hindbrain rhomobomeres and the origins of rhythmic circuits in vertebrates. Brain Behav Evol, in press.

Berrill NJ (1987). Early chordate evolution part 2. Amphioxus and ascidians, to settle or not to settle. Int J Invert Reprod Dev 11:15–28.

Bone Q (1987). Tunicates. In MA Ali (ed). Nervous Systems in Invertebrates. New York: Plenum, pp 527–557.

Boord RL, Campbell CBG (1977). Structural and fuctional organization of the lateral line system of sharks. Am Zool 17:431–441.

Bunker SJ, Machin KE (1991). The hydrodynamics of cephalaspids. In JMV Rayner, RJ Wootton, (eds), Biomeohomics in Evolutiron. Cambridge University Press, pp 113–129.

Carroll SB (1995). Homeotic genes and the evolution of arthropods and chordates. Nature 376:479–485.

Clarke JD, Lumsden A (1993). Segmental repetition of neuronal phenotype sets in the chick embryo hindbrain. Development 118:151–162.

Collewijn H (1989). The vestibulo-ocular reflex: An outdated concept? Prog Brain Res 80: 197–209.

De La Cruz RR, Pastor AM, Baker R (1993). Eye and head velocity signals in the vestibulo-cerebellum and brainstem of the goldfish. Soc Neurosci Abstr 19:858.

Deliagina TG, Grillner S, Orlovsky GN, Ullen F (1993). Visual input affects the response to roll in reticulospinal neurons of the lamprey. Exp Brain Res 95:421–428.

Deliagina TG, Orlovsky GN, Grillner S, Wallen P (1992). Vestibular control of swimming in lamprey: II. Characteristics of spatial sensitivity of reticulospinal neurons. Exp Brain Res 90: 489–498.

Essick CR (1912). The development of the nuclei pontis and the nucleus arcuatus in man. Am J Anat 13:25–54.

Forey P, Janvier P (1993). Agnathans and the origin of jawed vertebrates. Nature 361: 129–134.

Fraser SK, Keynes R, Lumsden A (1990). Segmentation in the chick embryo hindbrain is defined by cell lineage restrictions. Nature 344:431–435.

Fritzsch B (1991). Ontogenetic clues to the phylogeny of the visual system. In P Bagnoli, W Hodos (eds). The Changing Visual System. New York: Plenum, pp 33–49.

Fritzsch B, Collin SP (1990). Dendritic distribution of two populations of ganglion cells and the retinopetal fibers in the retina of the silver lamprey (*Ichthyomyzon unicuspis*). Visual Neurosci 4:533–545.

Fritzsch B, Sonntag R, Dubuc R, Ohta Y, Grillner S (1990). Organization of the six motor nuclei innervating the ocular muscles in lamprey. J Comp Neurol 294:491–506.

Fuchs AF, Mustari MJ, Robinson FR, Kaneko CR (1992). Visual signals in the nucleus of the optic tract and their brain stem destinations. In B Cohen, DL Tomko, F Guedry (eds), Sensing and Controlling Motion: Vestibular and Sensorimotor Function. New York: New York Academy of Sciences, pp 266–276.

Garcia-Fernandez J, Holland PW (1994). Archetypal organization of the amphioxus Hox gene cluster. Nature 370:563–566.

Gee H (1994). Return of the amphioxus. Nature 370:504–505.

Gilland E, Baker R (1993). Conservation of neuroepithelial and mesodermal segments in the embryonic vertebrate head. Acta Anat 148:110–123.

Gilland E, Baker R (1994). Phylogenetic diversification within embryonic hindbrain rhombomeres and the neuronal organization underlying postural control. Soc Neurosci Abstr 20: 1274.

Gilland E, Baker R (1995). Organization of rhombomeres and brainstem efferent neuronal populations in larval sea lamprey, Petromyzon marinus. Soc Neurosci Abstr 21:779.

Glover JC (1993). The development of brain stem projections to the spinal cord in the chicken embryo. Brain Res Bull 30:265–271.

Glover JC, Petursdottir G (1991). Regional specificity of developing reticulospinal, vestibulospinal, and vestibulo-ocular projections in the chicken embryo. J Neurobiol 22:353–376.

Graf W (1988). Motion detection in physical space and its peripheral and central representation. Ann N Y Acad Sci 545:154–169.

Graf W, Brunken WJ (1984). Elasmobranch oculomotor organization: Anatomical and theoretical aspects of the phylogenetic development of vestibulo-oculomotor connectivity. J Comp Neurol 227:569–581.

Graf W, Ezure K (1986). Morphology of vertical canal related second order vestibular neurons in the cat. Exp Brain Res 63:35–48.

Gruss P, Kessel M (1991). Axial specification in higher vertebrates. Curr Opin Genet Devel 1:204–210.

Gruss P, Walther C (1992). Pax in development. Cell 69:719–22.

Guthrie S (1995). The status of the neural segment. Trends Neurosci 18:74–79.

Guthrie S, Muchamore I, Kuroiwa A, Marshall H, Krumlauf R, Lumsden A (1992). Neuroectodermal autonomy of Hox-2.9 expression revealed by rhombomere transpositions. Nature 356:157–159.

Hanneman E, Trevarrow B, Metcalfe WK, Kimmel CB, Westerfield M (1988). Segmental pattern of development of the hindbrain and spinal cord of the zebrafish embryo. Development 103:49–58.

Harkmark W (1954). Cell migrations from the rhombic lip to the inferior olive, the nucleus raphe and the pons. A morphological and experimental investigation on chicken embryos. J Comp Neurol 100:115–209.

Highstein SM, McCrea RA (1988). The anatomy of the vestibular nuclei. Rev Oculomot Res 2:177–202.

Holland P (1992). Homeobox genes in vertebrate evolution. Bioessays 14:267–273.

Holland PW, Holland LZ, Williams NA, Holland ND (1992). An amphioxus homeobox gene: Sequence conservation, spatial expression during development and insights into vertebrate evolution. Development 116:653–661.

Holland PWH, Garcia-Fernàndez J, Williams NA, Sidow A (1994). Gene duplications and the origins of vertebrate development. Development (Suppl) 125–133.

Holmberg K (1977). The cyclostome retina. In F Grescitelli (ed), The Visual System in Vertebrates: Handbook of Sensory Physiology, Vol VII/5. Berlin: Springer-Verlag, pp 47–66.

Ito M (1982). Cerebellar control of the vestibulo-ocular reflex around the flocculus hypothesis. Annu Rev Neurosci 5:275–296.

Karten HJ (1991). Homology and evolutionary origins of the 'neocortex'. Brain Behav Evol 38:264–272.

Keller EL (1991). The brainstem. In RHS Carpenter, (ed), Eye Movements. Boca Raton: CRC Press, pp 200–223.

Keynes R, Krumlauf R (1994). Hox genes and regionalization of the nervous system. Annu Rev Neurosci 17:109–132.

Kimmel C (1989). Genetics and early development of zebrafish. Trends Genet 5:283–288.

Kimmel CB (1990). Embryonic origins of segmented nervous systems. In S Roth (ed), Molecular Approaches Toward Supracellular Phenomena. Philadelphia: University of Pennsylvania Press, pp 136–174.

Krumlauf R (1992). Evolution of the vertebrate Hox homeobox genes. Bioessays 14:245–252.

Krumlauf R, Marshall H, Studer M, Nonchev S, Sham MH, Lumsden A (1993). Hox homeobox genes and regionalisation of the nervous system. J Neurobiol 24:1328–1340.

Lacalli TC, Holland ND, West JE (1994). Landmarks in the anterior central nervous system of amphioxus larvae. Philos Trans R Soc Lond [B] 344:165–185.

Larsell O (1947). The cerebellum of myxinoids and petromyzonts including developmental stages in the lamprey. J Comp Neurol 86:395–445.

Larsell O (1967). The Comparative Anatomy and Histology of the Cerebellum from Myxinoids Through Birds. Minneapolis: University of Minnesota Press.

Lee RKK, Eaton RC, Zottoli SJ (1993). Segmental arrangement of reticulospinal neurons in the goldfish hindbrain. J Comp Neurol 329:539–556.

Lisberger SG, Miles FA, Optican LM, Eighmy BB (1981). Optokinetic response in the monkey: Underlying mechanisms and their sensitivity to long-term adaptive changes in vestibuloocular reflex. J Neurophysiol 45:869–890.

Lisberger SG, Pavelko TA, Bronte-Stewart HM, Stone LS (1994a). Neural basis for motor learning in the vestibuloocular reflex of primates: II. Changes in the responses of horizontal gaze velocity purkinje cells in the cerebellar flocculus and ventral paraflocculus. J Neurophysiol 72:954–973.

Lisberger SG, Pavelko TA, Broussard DM (1994b). Neural basis for motor learning in the vestibuloocular reflex of primates: I. Changes in the responses of brain stem neurons. J Neurophysiol 72:928–953.

Llinas R, Pare D (1994). Role of intrinsic neuronal oscillations and network ensembles in the genesis of normal and pathological tremors. In LJ Findley, WC Koller (eds), Handbook of Tremor Disorders. New York: Marcel Dekker. pp 7–36.

Llinas R, Yarom Y (1986). Oscillatory properties of guinea-pig inferior olivary neurones and their pharmalogical modulation: An in vitro study. J Physiol (Lond) 376:163–182.

Lumsden A, Clarke JDW, Keynes R, Fraser S (1994). Early phenotypic choices by neuronal precursors, revealed by clonal analysis of the chick embryo hindbrain. Development 120: 1581–1589.

Lumsden A, Keynes R (1989). Segmental patterns of neuronal development in the chick hindbrain. Nature 337:424–428.

Malicki J, Cianetti LC, Peschle C, McGinnis W (1992). A human HOX4B regulatory element provides head-specific expression in *Drosophila* embryos. Nature 358:345–347.

Manak JR, Scott MP (1994). A class act: Conservation of homeodomain protein functions. Development (Suppl):61–77.

Marín F, Puelles L (1995). Morphological fate of rhombomeres in quail/chick chimeras: A segmental analysis of hindbrain nuclei. Eur J Neurosci 7:1714–1738.

Marsh E, Pastor A, Baker R (1994). Cerebellar contribution to goldfish visuomotor adaptation. Soc Neurosci Abstr 20:858.

McCrea RA, Strassman A, May E, Highstein SM (1987). Anatomical and physiological characteristics of vestibular neurons mediating the horizontal vestibulo-ocular reflex of the squirrel monkey. J Comp Neurol 264:547–570.

McGinnis W, Krumlauf R (1992). Homeobox genes and axial patterning. Cell 68:283–302.

Metcalfe WK, Mendelson B, Kimmel CB (1986). Segmental homologies among reticulospinal neurons in the hindbrain of the zebrafish larva. J Comp Neurol 251:147–159.

Miles FA, Busettini C (1992). Ocular compensation for self-motion. In B Cohen, DL Tomko, F Guedry (eds), Sensing and Controlling Motion: Vestibular and Sensorimotor Function. New York: New York Academy of Sciences pp 220–232.

Neal HV (1898). The segmentation of the nervous system in *Squalus acanthias*. Bull Mus Comp Zool Harvard 31:147–294.

Neal HV (1918). The history of the eye muscles. J Morph 30:433–453.

Northcutt RG (1985). The brain and sense organs of the earliest vertebrates: Reconstruction of a morphotype. In RE Foreman, A Gorbman, JM Dodd, R Olsson (eds), Evolutionary Biology of Primitive Fishes. New York: Plenum, pp 81–112.

Northcutt RG, Gans C (1983). The genesis of neural crest and epidermal placodes: A reinterpretation of vertebrate origins. Q Rev Biol 58:1–28.

Orlovsky GN, Deliagina TG, Wallen P (1992). Vestibular control of swimming in lamprey: I. Responses of reticulospinal neurons to roll and pitch. Exp Brain Res 90:479–488.

Pastor AM, de La Cruz RR, Baker R (1992). Characterization and adaptive modifications of the goldfish vestibulo-ocular reflex by sinusoidal and velocity step vestibular stimulation. J Neurophysiol 68:2003–2015.

Pastor AM, de la Cruz RR, Baker R (1994a). Cerebellar role in adaptation of the goldfish vestibuloocular reflex. J Neurophysiol 72:1383–1394.

Pastor AM, de La Cruz RR, Baker R (1994b). Eye position and velocity integrators reside in separate brainstem nuclei in the goldfish hindbrain. Proc Natl Acad Sci USA 91:807–811.

Pastor AM, Marsh E, Baker R (1994). Role of the cerebellum in visuo-motor and vestibulo-ocular adaptation is independent of oculomotor performance in three orders of teleosts. Soc Neurosci Abstr 20:857.

Pombal MA, Rodicio MC, Anadón R (1994). The anatomy of the vestibulo-ocular system in lampreys. In JM Delgado-García, E Godaux, P-P Vidal (eds), Information Processing Underlying Gaze Control. Tokyo: Elsevier Science, pp 1–11.

Puelles L, Rubenstein JLR (1993). Expression patterns of homeobox and other putative regulatory genes in the embryonic mouse forebrain suggest a neuromeric organization. Trends Neurosci 16:472–479.

Raphan T, Cohen B (1985). Velocity storage and the ocular response to multidimensional vestibular stimuli. In A Berthoz, GM Jones (eds), Adaptive Mechanisms in Gaze Control. Reviews in Oculomotor Research. Amsterdam: Elsevier, pp 123–143.

Robinson DA (1989). Integrating with neurons. Annu Rev Neurosci 12:33–45.

Robinson DA (1992). Implications of neural networks for how we think about brain function. Behav Brain Sci 15:644–655.

Rovainen CM (1976). Vestibulo-ocular reflexes in the adult sea lamprey. J Comp Physiol [A] 112:159–164.

Rovainen CM (1982). Neurophysiology. In MW Hardisty, IC Potter (eds), Biology of Lampreys. London: Academic Press, pp 1–136.

Rubinson K, Cain H (1989). Neural differentiation in the retina of the larval sea lamprey (Petromyzon marinus). Vis Neurosci 3:241–248.

Ruddle FH, Bentley KL, Murtha MT, Risch N (1994). Gene loss and gain in the evolution of the vertebrates. Development (Suppl) 155–161.

Rudeberg S-I (1961). Morphogenetic studies on the cerebellar nuclei and their homologization in different vertebrates including man. Unpublished thesis, University of Lund.

Sasaki S, Shimazu H (1981). Reticulovestibular organization participating in generation of fast eye movement. Annu N Y Acad Sci 374:130–143.

Scott MP (1994). Intimations of a creature. Cell 79:1121–1124.

Scudder CA, Fuchs AF (1992). Physiological and behavioral identification of vestibular nucleus neurons mediating horizontal vestibulo-ocular reflex in trained rhesus monkey. J Neurophysiol 68:244–264.

Simpson JI (1984). The acessory optic system. Annu Rev Neurosci 7:13–41.

Simpson JI, Graf W (1985). The selection of reference frames by nature and its investigators. In A Berthoz, G Melvill Jones (eds), Adaptive Mechanisms in Gaze Control. Amsterdam: Elsevier, pp 3–16.

Slack JM, Holland PW, Graham CF (1993). The zootype and the phylotypic stage. Nature 361:490–492.

Solnica-Krezel L, Schier AF, Driever W (1994). Efficient recovery of ENU-induced mutations from the zebrafish germline. Genetics 136:1401–1420.

Sotelo C, Wassef M (1991). Cerebellar development: Afferent organization and Purkinje cell heterogeneity. Philos Trans R Soc Lond [B] Biol Sci 331:307–313.

Spencer RF, Wenthold RJ, Baker R (1990). Evidence for glycine as the putative inhibitory neurotransmitter of vestibular, reticular and prepositus hypoglossi neurons that project to the cat abducens nucleus. J Neurosci 9:2718–2736.

Stone LS, Lisberger SG (1990). Visual responses of Purkinje cells in the cerebellar flocculus during smooth-pursuit eye movements in monkeys: I. Simple spikes. J Neurophysiol 63:1241–1261.

Stoykova A, Gruss P (1994). Roles of Pax-genes in developing and adult brain as suggested by expression patterns. J Neurosci 14:1395—1412.

Tan K, LeDourarin M (1991). Development of the nuclei and cell migration in the medulla oblongata. Application of the quail-chick chimera system. Anat Embryol 183:321—343.

Tretjakoff D (1909). Das Nervensystem von Ammocoetes: II. Gehirn. Arch mikrosk Anat Entwicklungsgesch 74:636—779.

Ullen F, Orlovsky GN, Deliagina TG, Grillner S (1993). Role of dermal photoreceptors and lateral eyes in initiation and orientation of locomotion in lamprey. Behav Brain Res 54: 107—110.

Vaage S (1969). The segmentation of the primitive neural tube in chick embryos (*Gallus domesticus*). A morphological, histochemical and autoradiographical investigation. Ergeb Anat Entwicklungsgesch 41:1—88.

Walls GL (1962). The evolutionary history of eye movements. Vision Res 2:69—80.

Weiser M, Bass A, McElligot JG, Baker R (1988). Eye movement repertoire of the *Cabezon sculpin*. Biol Bull 175:308—309.

Weiser M, Marsh E, Baker R (1995). Brainstem eye velocity signals are necessary for visual and vestibular motor learning. Soc Neurosci Abstr 21:519.

Wicht H, Northcutt RG (1990). Retinofugal and retinopetal projections in the Pacific hagfish, *Eptatretus stouti* (Myxinoidea). Brain Behav Evol 36:315—328.

Wilkinson DG, Bhatt S, Cook M, Boncinelli E, Krumlauf R (1989). Segmental expression of Hox-2 homeobox-containing genes in the developing mouse hindbrain. Nature 341:405—409.

Young JZ (1935). The photoreceptors of lampreys: II. The functions of the pineal complex. J Exp Biol 12:254—270.

Zhang Y, Partsalis AM, Highstein SM (1995). Properties of superior vestibular nucleus flocculus target neurons in the squirrel monkey: I. General properties in comparison with flocculus projecting neurons. J Nurophysiol 73:2261—2278.

4 Adaptation of Automatic Postural Responses

Fay B. Horak

Rapid, automatic postural responses are evoked whenever there is an external perturbation to a body segment that causes disequilibrium or alters postural orientation (Horak and Macpherson, in press). Although these responses are quite rapid and stereotyped, to be functional they must adapt or change when biomechanical and sensory conditions change. Immediate changes in postural responses after a sudden change in biomechanical or sensory conditions can be attributed to altered sensory drive, but changes that occur slowly over many trials (when the sensory conditions are the same) are due to changes within the central nervous system (CNS) referred to as changes in *central set*. These changes alter the way in which the nervous system responds to identical stimulation over the course of repeated trials. Changes in central set form the basis for adaptive modification of automatic postural responses, thereby improving balance with practice, allowing postural coordination to be optimized with repeated exposure, and modifying postural responses when the intended goal of the task is altered. This chapter will review experimental evidence for several potential neural mechanisms responsible for adaptive modification of automatic postural responses.

The study of adaptation of postural control is not easy. One of the difficulties in studying adaptation of postural responses is that the transition between states often occurs within a very few trials compared to the prolonged period of adaptation reported for other motor responses (Lisberger, 1988; Demer, Porter, Goldberg, Jenkins, and Schmidt, 1989). Another difficulty is that it is technically difficult suddenly to change biomechanical or sensory constraints without the subject practicing the task prior to testing. For example, subjects "practice" balancing whenever they do any standing, even before they can be perturbed on a narrow beam or after space flight. The complexity of the biomechanics and sensorimotor control of postural control also makes it difficult to rule out such subtle changes in biomechanical or sensory constraints as initial body segment position, background levels of muscle activation, and the specific sensory signals triggering the response, all of which will alter postural responses independent of set-dependent adaptive changes.

In fact, there are many possible neural mechanisms that can account for changes in postural responses when the conditions change and, likewise, for the continued modification of responses with repeated perturbations when the current conditions have not changed. Much of the functional flexibility of postural coordination occurs both by sculpting of *afferent inflow* based on current conditions and by the particular parameters of the stimuli (Horak and Macpherson, in press). However, even when the afferent inflow is the same, the first response to an external perturbation will look quite different from a postural response to the same perturbation when it is predictable based on prior experienced. General arousal mechanisms affecting attention, anxiety, and startle-responses may promote overzealous responses to novel, difficult, or unexpected perturbations (Eysenck, 1964). Repetitive, monotonous sensory input is also associated with decreased attention and a gradual waning of response attributed to a generalized habituation. In simpler systems, habituation with repeated exposure to an initially novel set of stimuli has been shown to be mediated by local synaptic mechanisms (Kandel and Schwartz, 1982; Rothwell, Day, Berardelli, and Marsden, 1986). Some of the changes in postural responses with practice most probably involve true functional adaptation, in which the responses are shaped, or tuned, for the particular circumstances to optimize performance with the least amount of energy expenditure (Nashner, 1976; Brooks, 1984).

Adaptation involves the trial-by-trial adjustment of the magnitude of muscle activation (gain) or the gradual modification of the pattern and timing of muscles (synergy) activated by the perturbation (see also chapter 13, this volume). To gradually change a postural response to an identical stimulus, changes must occur in the nervous system to prepare for the upcoming, predicted stimulus. These changes have been attributed to a subset of central set called *sensorimotor set*, defined as "a state in which transmission parameters in various sensorimotor pathways have been adjusted to suit a particular task or context" (Prochazka, 1989). Set-dependent adaptation of postural response gain or synergies most likely involves higher centers such as the cerebellum, brainstem, and cortex (Evarts and Tanji, 1974; Evarts, 1975; Brooks, 1984; Prochazka, 1989). For postural control, this central sensorimotor set appears to be much more influenced by prior experience than by cognitive information such as intention or instruction.

It has been suggested that the study of set-dependent changes in postural responses to repeated, predictable perturbations is irrelevant because the purpose of the motor control system is to respond to sudden, unexpected perturbations to avoid a fall in the very first trials and because subjects seldom experience many exposures to identical perturbations (McIlroy and Maki, 1993b). Nevertheless, the postural control system ultimately depends on central set to "get it in the right ballpark," even for unanticipated perturbations. To organize and execute a complex postural act quickly, the nervous system preprograms much of postural responses, meaning that it triggers only a "best guess" for a particular situation which then is tuned by experience. It relies on prior experience to adjust transmission parameters gradually for changing tasks or contexts such as balancing when body parts are loaded, on alternative surface, characteristics, or when the postural goals change. Experience prepares the nervous system for a particular expected range of external perturbations such that postural responses, which appear so stereotyped and reflexive, can be optimized for different tasks and contexts.

This chapter will review behavioral evidence and possible mechanisms for short-term adaptation of postural coordination in response to external perturbations. It will not discuss the vast literature regarding how posture also adapts to changing sensory contexts by reweighting reliance on different sensory cues. It also will not review studies illustrating adaptation of postural coordination which accompany anticipated focal movements or studies of long-term motor learning of balance skills. The chapter is divided into six sections which discuss (1) the flexibility of postural responses due to afferent specificity, (2) the effects of repeated exposure on responses to postural perturbations, (3) the comparison of adaptive gain control and habituation, (4) the role of the cerebellum in adaptive gain control, (5) adaptation of postural strategies and synergies with a new model for understanding optimization of motor coordination, and (6) the effects of instruction or intention on postural set.

FLEXIBILITY FROM AFFERENT SPECIFICITY

When the support surface under a standing human is rapidly moved, muscles are activated throughout the body that oppose the perturbation and prevent loss of balance. Similarly, when an external force attempts to displace an intended postural orientation of a limb, a synergy of muscles is activated across many segments at comparable latencies (Crago, Houk, and Hasan, 1976; Gielen, Ramaekers, and van Zuylen 1988). The onset time of activation of automatic postural responses is in the medium latency range which is longer than monosynaptic loop time but shorter than voluntary reaction times; in the legs and trunk, latencies range from 70 to 180 ms, in the arms and hands latencies range from 50 to 80 ms, and in the neck they range from 45 to 70 ms. Although responses to whole-body perturbations could be triggered by vestibular, visual, proprioceptive, or cutaneous sensory information, evidence suggests that, like responses to single limb perturbations, muscle proprioceptors and cutaneous mechanoreceptors usually provide the shortest latency triggers for automatic postural responses (Mauritz, Dietz, and Haller, 1980; Inglis, Horak, Shupert, and Jones-Rycewicz, 1994; Horak, Nashner, and Diener, 1990; Horak and Macpherson, in press). Although these postural responses are probably triggered by the somatosensory system, the use of the term *functional stretch reflexes* to describe automatic postural responses has been questioned, as it is not always the stretched muscles which are activated (Nashner, 1976; Gielen et al., 1988). Triggered responses (Crago et al., 1976; Horak and Macpherson, in press) or preprogrammed responses

(Dewhurst, 1967) have been suggested as more appropriate descriptors, given the dependence of these responses on prior experience and their functional flexibility and adaptability to particular tasks and contexts.

Much of the functional flexibility of automatic postural coordination is a function of the particular sensory information specific to the impending perturbation. The specific patterns and magnitudes of muscles activated in response to an external perturbation depend on the initial support conditions (Nashner and Cordo, 1981; Schieppati and Nardone, 1991; Horak, Nutt, and Nashner, 1992), initial body positions (Horak and Moore, 1993), and the location and parameters of sensory stimuli triggering the response (Horak, Shupert, Dietz, and Horstmann, 1994). Postural responses always produce net forces approximately equal and opposite in direction to the perturbing forces, with a uniquely appropriate set of muscles activated for every direction of perturbation (Macpherson, 1995). Each muscle's activation is broadly tuned across a range of directions of perturbation but not necessarily maximally activated in the directions in which it is most stretched, loaded, or voluntarily activated (Keshner and Peterson, 1988; Macpherson, 1995). The pattern of sensory information from the initial conditions and triggering stimulus may determine largely the directional tuning of postural responses because errors in response direction have not been observed when the perturbation direction is unpredictable (Macpherson, 1995).

Any groups of muscles or any body segment can be used in a postural role, depending on the task and the nature of the disturbance (Marsden, Merton, and Mortan, 1977). For example, subjects perturbed while standing on their hands or while receiving support with their hands show directionally specific responses in fingers, hand, arms, shoulder, and trunk (Clement and Rezette, 1985; Macpherson, Horak, and Dunbar, 1989). If standing subjects hold a handle that is perturbed, segments in contact with both support surfaces (feet and hands) are activated first, suggesting that postural responses usually originate at the interface of the body and support surface (Nashner and Cordo, 1981). When initial support conditions or body positions are changed, the same surface perturbation will result in activation of a different set of muscles on the very first trial; muscles whose action is not effective in restoring equilibrium are not activated. For example, subjects translated while sitting show muscle activation in the trunk but not in the legs, and subjects supporting themselves on all four limbs show activation at the hips and shoulders but not at the ankles on the first four-limb trial (Macpherson et al., 1989; Horak, et al., 1992).

Likewise, if subjects assume an initially leaned position prior to a perturbation, trunk rather than ankle muscles are activated first (Horak and Moore, 1993). Although the ankle muscles are preloaded, preactivated, and prestretched by the initial lean, the perturbation which further stretches these ankle muscles results in less (and later) ankle muscle activation. Rapid hip flexion or extension is functionally appropriate in leaning trials because they can more quickly return the body center of mass to equilibrium to prevent a fall (Kuo, 1995). Thus, this switch in postural strategy cannot be predicted on the basis of the muscles that are stretched but rather on biomechanical constraints that affect attainment of the functional goal of preserving equilibrium (Kuo, 1995).

EFFECTS OF REPEATED EXPOSURE

Though much of the functional flexibility of postural coordination occurs by changes in the pattern of afferent inflow, automatic postural responses are also modified by repeated exposure to a particular perturbation. When subjects are repeatedly exposed to a particular postural perturbation, their automatic postural responses are gradually reduced in magnitude, and sometimes fewer or different muscles are activated as subjects change from a more vigorous to a less vigorous response. Initial postural responses to unexpected disturbances are larger than necessary and inefficiently executed with excessive muscle activation for the task. Nevertheless, they are unlikely simply startle-responses because the very first response to a disturbance always includes the appropriate spatiotemporal pattern of muscle activation for the particular stimulus parameters (Brown et al., 1991).

Reduction in the magnitude of postural responses with repeated exposure is demonstrated in figure 4.1A, which compares the first 10 and last 10 of 100 sequential automatic postural responses to a large (12-cm), fast (35-cm/s), backward surface translation. Initial responses included significant, early activation in all six recorded muscles. Although there was no change in muscle onset latency with repeated exposure, the magnitude of muscle activation decreased significantly, particularly in antagonist muscles that were eliminated with practice in some subjects. Figure 4.1B shows that agonist electromyogram (EMG) magnitudes, especially the stretched gastrocnemius, decreased the least (65–87 percent of initial values) whereas antagonist EMGs decreased the most (20–50 percent of initial values) during practice.

Performance improves with less effort after practice; the time it takes to reach a stable equilibrium position (t in figure 4.1A) decreases with practice, although subjects use progressively less torque against the surface to return to equilibrium. The peak center-of-pressure change in response to an identical backward surface translation significantly reduces from the first to eighth trial (figure 4.1C), suggesting that less effort is used to respond to the same perturbation with practice.

The postural sway traces in figure 4.1A also show that both the peak sway and the stable equilibrium position that humans (and cats) assume after repeated exposure to a surface perturbation gradually drifts as they practice (Diener, Horak, and Nashner, 1988; Horak, Diener, and Nashner, 1989; Maki and Whitelaw, 1993; McIlroy and Maki, 1993a; Macpherson, 1994a). Whereas initial postural responses to novel stimuli bring the center of body mass back near to its initial position, trials later in a session (over months of training and by trained athletes) show changes in preperturbation postural

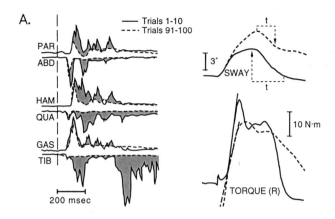

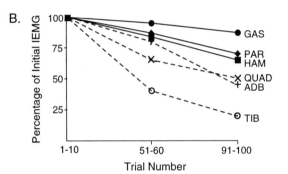

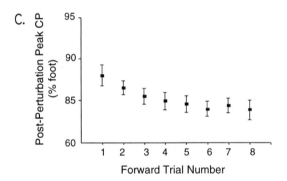

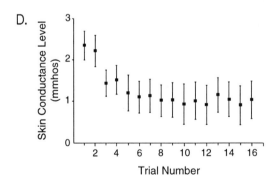

alignment. If the upcoming direction of perturbation is predictable, subjects lean in the direction of the induced sway; if the perturbation direction is unpredictable, subjects assume a forward-leaning equilibrium position (Horak et al., 1989; Maki and Whitelaw, 1993; McIlroy and Maki, 1993a). The final equilibrium position may drift with practice because response effort is reduced, thereby compromising initial alignment within boundaries of equilibrium. Alternatively, subjects may allow their postural alignment to drift to prepare for expected, upcoming perturbations. For example, subjects are known to spontaneously widen their base of support and lower their center of body mass by a crouch when a large postural perturbation is expected.

Subjects presumably adopt these postures because changing preperturbation equilibrium position may provide some performance benefit. If subjects move their center of foot pressure by only 2 percent of foot length (or about 6 mm), the change corresponds to an increase in plantar-flexor ankle torque of 4.2 N-m an average increase of 15 percent over baseline torques (Maki and Whitelaw, 1993; Horak and Moore, 1993; Shinha and Maki, 1993). Thus, even small leans increase the stiffness of the ankle joint and the effect might allow passive elastic properties and gravitational torques to assist with expected displacements (Shinha and Maki, 1993). Whether subjects can change the stiffness of their postural system based on central set, even without changes in initial position, has not been tested. However, it is clear that those examining the effects of set-dependent adaptation and neural habituation must take care in their studies to eliminate the effects of changes in initial position on automatic postural responses.

As the magnitude of the postural response reduces with repeated exposure, there occurs also a reduction in the tendency to use exaggerated strategies to maintain equilibrium (Maki, Whitelaw, and McIlroy, 1993; McIlroy and Maki, 1993a,b). For very fast perturbations, subjects often cannot resist stepping, shifting their feet, waving their arms, flexing their hips, or lifting their heels or toes to maintain balance. Repeated exposure to a perturbation may result in complete elimination of some muscle activations (e.g., early neck, hip, and arm muscles) and, thus, in a significant change in strategy (Debu and Woollacott, 1988; Keshner, Woolacott, and Debu, 1988; Horak et al., 1989). With repeated exposure to the same fast surface translation, subjects gradually

Figure 4.1 A. Reduction of EMG response, torque, and time to achieve equilibrium (t) with repetition of forward sway postural perturbation. Solid lines show average response of trials 1 to 10 and dashed lines show average response of trials 91 to 100. GAS, gastrocnemius; HAM, hamstrings; PAR, lumbar paraspinals; TIB, tibialis anterior; QUA, rectus femoris; ABD, rectus abdominis. B. Average reduction of integrated EMG (first 100 ms) in trials 51 to 60 and trials 91 to 100 as a percent of initial trials 1 to 10. C. Reduction of peak center of pressure (cp) response (expressed as a function of foot length) by prior testing experience. D. Change in galvanic skin response with repeated trials. Means and standard errors from six subjects. (A and B adapted from Horak et al., 1989; C and D reproduced from Maki and Whitelaw, 1993, with permission.)

Adaptation of Automatic Postural Responses

change from stepping or using large hip and arm movements to more and more erect posture with motion primarily at the ankle joints. As subjects reduce the vigor and forcefulness of their responses, they often report that the task becomes easier, and they may interpret this ease as a reduction in the perturbing stimulus rather than as a reduction in their response to the same stimulus.

It is difficult to distinguish among the many neural mechanisms (including arousal, habituation, and adaptation) that could contribute to the gradual reduction in automatic postural response magnitude to repeated, predictable perturbations. Arousal mechanisms involving attention, anxiety, and startle may be important in the first few trials. Anxiety or fear of falling may increase generalized arousal and promote overzealous responses in the first responses to a postural perturbation. Exposure to difficult, novel motor behaviors has been shown to cause increased arousal and the overshooting of desired targets (Eysenck, 1964). There is measurable autonomic arousal as indicated by high heart rate and the galvanic skin response (see figure 4.1D) in the first two to three trials of response to repeated postural perturbations (Hansen, Woolacott, and Debu, 1988; Maki, Holliday, and Topper, 1991; Maki and Whitelaw, 1993). In some cases, generalized startle-reflex responses may also summate with automatic postural responses because auditory startle responses activate leg muscles at times similar to those of automatic postural responses and are larger in stance than when sitting (Brown et al., 1991). Startle responses alone, however, cannot account for initial responses to unexpected perturbations because the correct, directionally specific muscle activation pattern is elicited in the first trial along with excessive muscle activation which is eliminated with practice.

ADAPTIVE GAIN CONTROL OR HABITUATION?

The gain, or magnitude, of a postural response to the same stimulus can be reduced either by habituation or by adaptive, central set effects. It is not easy to determine whether trial-by-trial adaptive changes in automatic postural responses may be due to a generalized habituation affect or to set-dependent adaptation. For example, Nashner (1976) reported gradual reduction of a stretch-induced gastrocnemius response in three to five trials when subjects were exposed to a slow-velocity, toes-up rotation of their support surface in stance (figure 4.2A). Because toes-up rotations followed prior experience with backward surface translations that produced a very large gastrocnemius response, the appearance of the functionally inappropriate gastrocnemius response to rotation was thought to be due to central set based on prior experience. The gradual reduction of the gastrocnemius over several trials and activation of the functionally appropriate, shortened tibialis was considered evidence of adaptive optimization of automatic postural responses.

However, other studies have shown that the presence of the gastrocnemius response does not depend on prior experience with surface translations and,

A.

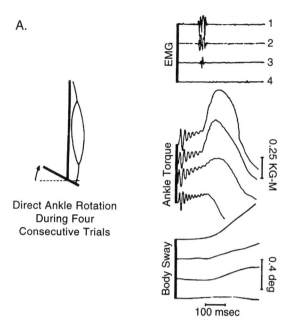

Direct Ankle Rotation
During Four
Consecutive Trials

B. Tibialis Response to Backward Sway

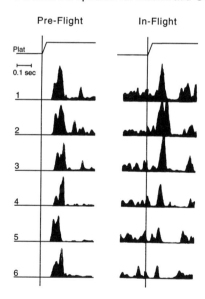

Figure 4.2 A. Reduction in gastrocnemius postural response and associated torque and body sway in response to four trials of upward surface rotation. (Reproduced from Nashner, 1976, with permission.) B. Reduction of tibialis postural response during six successive forward surface translations performed pre- and in-flight (day 2) with one astronaut. (Reproduced from Clement et al., 1985, with permission.)

thus, is probably not a set-dependent response (Hansen et al., 1988). The gradual reduction in gastrocnemius response to rotation may be a generalized habituation effect and not a specific, set-dependent adaptation, because the reduction in magnitude of other muscles (e.g., the functionally important tibialis response) habituates just as much as, or more than, the functionally inappropriate gastrocnemius response (Hansen et al. 1988; F.B. Horak, unpublished observation). In fact, early EMG responses to surface translations, or any novel postural stimulus, habituate just as much as early responses to surface rotations (Keshner, Allum, and Pfaltz, 1987; Hansen et al., 1988). A set-dependent gradual increase in gastrocnemius response to repeated platform translations following rotations would be good evidence for set-dependent adaptation, but this increase has not been repeated experimentally.

The amount and type of adaptive changes that are observed depend critically on the magnitude of the disturbance, because responses are more plastic when they are not driven by a very powerful peripheral sensory stimulus. The gastrocnemius response to faster rotations of the support surface do not change with practice (Keshner et al., 1987), and there is no gastrocnemius response at all to slower rotations. Furthermore, although the amount of ankle rotation may be similar for surface translations and rotations, it is difficult to rule out changes in other sensory stimuli that could account for changes in the postural response pattern. The relative activation of the gastrocnemius and tibialis in response to ankle dorsiflexion for surface translations and rotations, respectively, has been shown to depend on the amount of loading of the limbs in these two tasks, suggesting a role of load-dependent receptors in the context-specific switching of the postural patterns (Nardone, Corra, and Schiepati, 1990; Dietz, Gollhofer, Kleiber, and Trippel, 1992). The amount of knee and hip flexion also differs in response to surface translations and rotations and could contribute to modification of the response at the ankle (Allum and Honegger, 1992). Thus, the extent of set-dependent adaptive optimization in this postural task is still unclear.

The fine line between habituation and adaptive optimization can be seen in the study of postural response suppression in astronauts during repeated surface translations before and during space flight (figure 4.2B) (Clement, Gurfinkel, Lestienne, Lipshits, and Popov, 1985). Though there is some reduction in the response of tibialis to a forward surface translation with repeated preflight trials, the amount of suppression is much greater in flight, when the automatic postural response is no longer functional for the gravity-free environment. The tibialis burst in response to the translation was reduced or absent in space despite the fact that tibialis possessed a larger background tonic activity as the astronauts attempted to assume an "upright" standing posture with the feet fixed to the floor. The small reduction of the preflight response may be due to low-level habituation effects, whereas the large reduction during spaceflight may represent a set-dependent, functional adaptation for the new context by gradual minimization of the difference between expected and actual afference. Both the sensory and motor biomechanical constraints have changed in space, and it is not possible to differentiate among possible mechanisms underlying the reduction in postural response gain in this protocol.

One way to differentiate a set-dependent, adaptive effect from a generalized habituation effect is to observe a context-specific *increase* as well as decrease in response gain, depending on the nature of the prior experience. Even relatively simple responses to single-limb perturbations have been shown to be influenced by expectation, based on prior experience (Evarts and Tanji, 1974; Marsden et al., 1977; Hore and Villis, 1984). Setting aspects of the response in advance decreases the time it takes for the CNS to transform an eliciting stimulus into an appropriate response but leads to errors in response when the stimulus or external conditions unexpectedly change.

A good example of the use of central set for postural control is that subjects scale the magnitude of their initial postural responses to the amplitude of displacement that is expected, based on prior experience (Diener et al., 1988; Horak et al., 1989). Figure 4.3 shows that central control over response magnitude is important because postural responses are initiated before the availability of peripheral information characterizing the full nature of the stimulus. The magnitude of gastrocnemius response at 100-ms latency and the associated torque response against the surface are proportionately scaled to the amplitudes of translation, long before the amplitude of the current translation is known to the nervous system. Regressions through responses of 10 subjects to five different amplitudes of translation show scaling of the magnitude of postural responses when exposure to the translation amplitudes were blocked into groups of five like trials, and, therefore, were predictable but not when amplitudes were randomized and, therefore, unpredictable (figure 4.3B, from Horak and Diener, 1994).

Another way to demonstrate the effects of set-dependent adaptation of response gain is to observe the errors made in responses when subjects receive a different amplitude perturbation than they expect. For example, when subjects expect (based on prior experience with 7 to 12 previous exposures) a larger amplitude displacement than they actually receive, they underrespond, and when they expect a smaller amplitude than they actually receive, they overrespond to the same stimulus (figure 4.4A). The integrated EMG areas and the initial rate of change of torque responses in this figure show that responses to the same stimulus can be either increased or decreased, depending on what is expected based on immediate prior experience.

These amplitude-specific changes in response magnitude appear to rely on increasing or decreasing responsiveness (or loop gain) around a default response value which depends on the stimulus parameters responsible for triggering the response (Horak et al., 1989; Beckley, Bloem, Remler, Roos, and van Dijk, 1991). The histograms in Figure 4.4B show the same magnitude of the responses whether to a small- or large-amplitude perturbation when the actual and expected stimulus amplitude disagreed (were unexpected). This default value response was equivalent to a middle-range-amplitude response

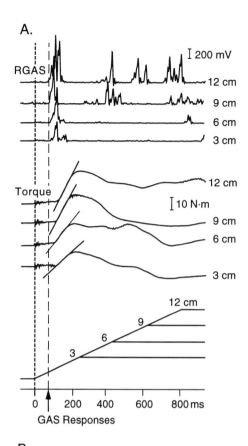

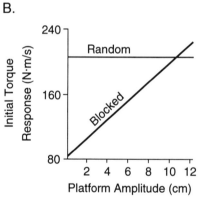

Figure 4.3 A. Initial right gastrocnemius (RGAS) burst with resulting torque occurs prior to completion of platform translations but is scaled to platform amplitude when they are predictable (each amplitude is presented as a block of 5 to 10 like trials). B. Set-dependent scaling of postural responses to amplitude of platform translation. Significant linear regression of initial torque responses from 10 normal subjects to platform amplitude disappears when amplitudes are presented randomly. (Adapted from Horak and Diener, 1994.)

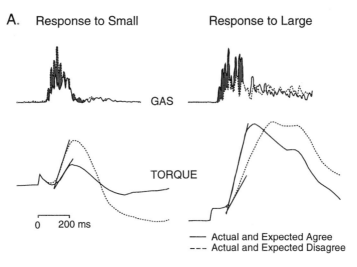

A. Response to Small   Response to Large

GAS

TORQUE

0   200 ms

—— Actual and Expected Agree
--- Actual and Expected Disagree

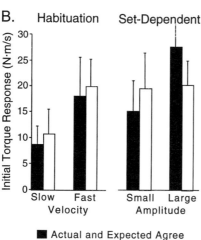

B.   Habituation   Set-Dependent

Slow   Fast   Small   Large
    Velocity   Amplitude

■ Actual and Expected Agree
□ Actual and Expected Disagree

Figure 4.4 A. Set-dependent effects on postural responses depending on expectation from prior experience. GAS-gastrocnemius. Differences in averaged gastrocnemius EMG and surface torque responses when a small and a large platform translation was presented in expected (solid line) and unexpected (dashed line) conditions. When subjects expected a 12-cm amplitude displacement but got a 1.2-cm displacement, they produced larger initial responses to a small-amplitude translation. When subjects expected a 1.2-cm displacement but got a 12-cm displacement, they produced smaller initial responses to a large-amplitude displacement. (Adapted from Horak et al., 1989.) B. Group means and standard deviations of initial rate of change of torque responses for expected (shaded bars) and unexpected (open bars) conditions from 10 subjects. Habituation effect is illustrated by overresponses to unexpected velocities whether they are unexpectedly large or small, indicating habituation when stimulus is repeated. Set-dependent adaptation is illustrated by directionally specific effects for unexpected amplitudes: Subjects overrespond when they expect a larger translation than that actually received but underrespond when they expect a smaller translation than that actually received.

(6 cm; 1.2 to 12-cm range presented); noteworthy is the fact that the size of the open histograms in figure 4.4B is similar for the fast velocity at 6 cm and for both unexpected amplitudes at 1.2 and 12 cm. When the perturbation amplitude was expected, the gain of the response to that constant velocity stimulus was increased or decreased approximately 20 percent, depending on whether a larger or smaller amplitude of translation was expected, based on prior experience.

Along with the early set-dependent changes in initial agonist EMG and force responses, later antagonist activity is also increased whenever the actual and expected perturbation disagree. This set-dependent antagonist activity is often reciprocally activated with agonists and appears to compensate for earlier agonist scaling errors due to set, and may involve both peripheral and central mechanisms (Hore and Villis, 1984; Horak and Diener, 1994).

Like set-dependent adaptation, habituation also can contribute to changes in postural response magnitude (Kandel and Schwartz, 1982). In contrast to central set effects, however, habituation effects are unidirectional. That is, initial responses to novel stimuli are always too large, regardless of the type of prior experience. An example of a habituation effect is repeated exposure to a particular perturbation velocity. As shown in figure 4.4B, whether subjects expect a slower or a faster perturbation than they actually receive, they always overrespond to the unexpected, or novel, velocity ($p < .01$; Horak et al., 1989). A gradual decrease in response magnitude then occurs whenever an initially novel stimulus is presented repeatedly. Although the stimulus stays the same, the magnitude of the automatic postural response gradually decreases over many trials. The magnitude of the postural response decreases with repeated exposure whether or not the perturbation direction is predictable, suggesting separate control of response direction and magnitude (Maki and Whitelaw, 1993). Habituation effects do not appear to influence the relative latencies or patterns of postural muscle activation and can affect some muscles more than others (Maki and Whitelaw, 1993; Macpherson, 1994b).

CEREBELLAR ROLE IN SET-DEPENDENT GAIN CONTROL

Though the cerebellum is likely involved in the coordination and temporal organization of multijoint movements (Thach, Goodkin, and Keating, 1992), it may play a more restricted role in postural responses. Even very severe cerebellar deficits do not appear to affect the latency or relative spatio-temporal pattern of postural responses to surface displacements (Horak and Diener, 1994). The ability to use on-line velocity feedback to scale the magnitude of postural responses also is not affected by cerebellar lesions. The midline cerebellum appears to be important for regulating the gain of automatic postural responses based on adaptive central set, though gain control involving habituation or arousal affects appears intact (Hore and Villis, 1984; Horak and Diener, 1994; Timmann and Horak, 1995).

The most obvious deficit of postural control in patients with cerebellar dysfunction is greater than normal magnitude of responses, or hypermetria. This hypermetria results in overshoots in initial position and a compensatory activation of antagonist muscles. Hypermetria has been observed in many types of movements and reflexes in cerebellar patients (Flament and Hore, 1986; Robinson, Straube, and Fuchs, 1993). Figure 4.5 shows that the initial rate of torque responses to platform translation velocities and amplitudes, as shown in figure 4.3, were consistently larger in cerebellar patients than in control subjects. Despite their large hypermetria, patients with cerebellar dysfunction are able to scale the magnitude of their postural responses with normal gain or slope of the stimulus-response curve based on on-line perturbation velocity information (figure 4.5A).

Although postural scaling based on peripheral sensory information is intact in cerebellar subjects, they cannot scale the magnitude of their postural responses to expected displacement amplitudes like normal subjects (figure 4.5B). In fact, cerebellar patients always use the same response magnitude, whether or not the displacement amplitude is predictable or randomized, suggesting that they have difficulty adjusting their response gain, based on prior experience.

The difficulty in scaling postural response gain to predicted displacement amplitudes was not due to a generalized inability to modify a fixed, large response gain. Amplitude scaling was still absent at lower displacement velocities when response magnitude was much reduced.

These results suggested that cerebellar dysfunction results in an inability to use central set to adjust postural response gain. As shown in the schematic in figure 4.5C, set-dependent changes in postural loop gain appear to involve shifting the threshold, rather than the slope, of somatosensory-triggered postural responses (Horak and Diener, 1994). When subjects expect, based on prior experience, either a larger (A_l) or smaller (A_s) displacement amplitude, they increase or decrease respectively the magnitude of their response, preserving the relative scaling (slopes) to displacement velocities.

To differentiate whether cerebellar disorders resulted in an inability to predict an upcoming postural stimulus or to adjust precisely the gain based on that prediction, responses to the same stimulus were compared when they were expected or unexpected. Average torque responses to the same perturbation amplitude were compared when they followed three to seven like-amplitudes and when they followed three to seven trials with a very different amplitude. Figure 4.6 shows that cerebellar subjects, like normal control subjects, made errors in the size of their responses because they were able to predict (based on prior experience) the impending amplitude of a perturbation. Like normal subjects, cerebellar patients overresponded to small-amplitude perturbations when they expected larger and underresponded to large-amplitude perturbations when they expected smaller perturbations.

If cerebellar subjects can use set to predict an upcoming stimulus amplitude, why do they have difficulty scaling response magnitude to predicted

A.

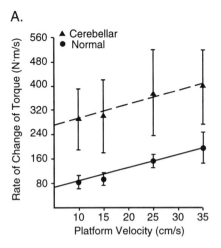

B.

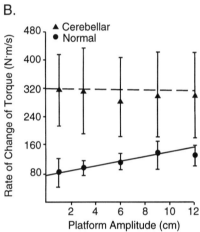

C.

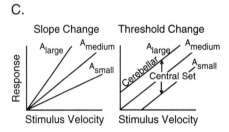

Figure 4.5 Scaling of initial torque responses to platform displacement characteristics in normal subjects (circles) and cerebellar patients (triangles). A. Reactive scaling to displacement velocity. B. Predictive scaling to displacement amplitudes. Cerebellar patients scale responses to platform velocity but not to platform amplitude, which must be predicted based on prior experience. The mean ±SD of torque responses and the average linear regression for all 10 subjects in each group are indicated. C. Schematic representation of the effect of central set on the threshold rather than the gain (slope) of the stimulus-response relation, depending on expected amplitudes of displacement. (Adapted from Horak and Diener, 1994.)

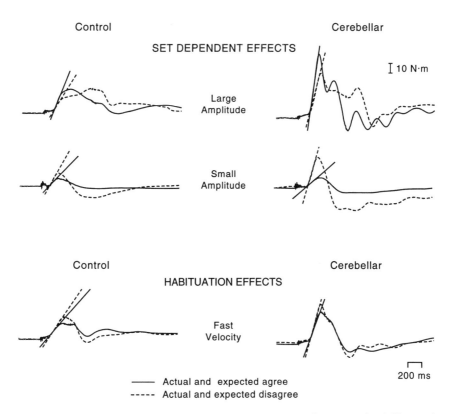

Control   Cerebellar

SET DEPENDENT EFFECTS

⊥ 10 N·m

Large
Amplitude

Small
Amplitude

Control   Cerebellar

HABITUATION EFFECTS

Fast
Velocity

200 ms

—— Actual and expected agree
----- Actual and expected disagree

Figure 4.6 Differences in averaged torque responses represented in expected (solid line) and unexpected (dashed line) conditions are similar for cerebellar and normal subjects, although cerebellar subjects show hypermetric responses. (Top) Set-dependent effects of small and large expected displacement amplitudes on torque response. (Bottom) Habituation effects in which subjects overrespond to unexpectedly fast displacement velocities and then habituate responses with repetition. (Adapted from Timmann and Horak, in press.)

stimulus amplitudes? We suggest that cerebellar patients' difficulty with scaling postural responses to predicted displacement amplitudes is due to their difficulty in modifying precisely response gain based on set. We repeated the predicted amplitude–scaling experiment as shown in figure 4.5 with another group of cerebellar patients who were not as severely hypermetric. Figure 4.7 shows the extremely large trial-to-trial response magnitude variability in cerebellar patients compared to control subjects when the patients are attempting to scale responses to displacement amplitudes that are presented sequentially. Though the cerebellar patients exhibit a tendency to scale responses to anticipated perturbation amplitudes, their large response variability does not allow for significant scaling when only five to seven sequential trials are provided. In fact, the patients with the greatest hypermetria showed the greatest difficulty in predictive scaling, although they also showed larger than normal differences to expected and unexpected amplitudes. Thus, the cerebellum appears essential for precisely adapting (based on

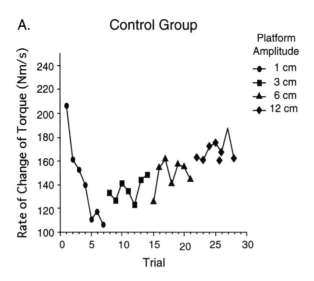

A. **Control Group**

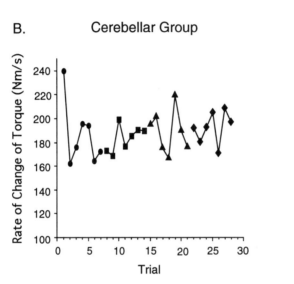

B. **Cerebellar Group**

Figure 4.7 Larger trial-to-trial variability of set-dependent magnitude of torque response for serial presentation of four different displacement amplitudes for 15 cerebellar patients compared to 15 control subjects. Habituation of response in first few trials is seen for both the control (A) and cerebellar (B) group. (Adapted from Timmann and Horak, submitted for publication.)

central set) the gain of postural responses, although it may not be essential for generating the predictive central set.

The cerebellum does not appear to be essential for simple reduction in postural responses with repetition that depends on habituation and arousal mechanisms. Habituation mechanisms are intact because cerebellar patients, like normal subjects, reduce the magnitude of their responses when stimulus velocity is expected, based on prior experience (see figure 4.6, bottom).

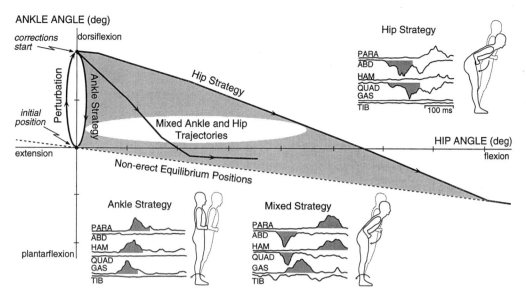

Figure 4.8 Ankle-to-hip strategy continuum for automatic postural response strategies to anterior-posterior surface translations in standing humans. The shaded area in the ankle angle versus hip angle plot shows the range of trajectories in the sagittal plane angle-angle space for the ankle, the hip, and mixed ankle and hip strategies. The perturbation, a backward translation, induces forward sway primarily about the ankle joints toward dorsiflexion on the upward-going ankle angle axis. Subjects can respond with a pure ankle strategy, a pure hip strategy, or any combination to the same perturbation depending on central set. The insets show the patterns of EMG activity typical for the various strategies. PARA = paraspinals; ABD = abdominals; HAM = hamstrings; QUAS = quadriceps; GAS = gastrocnemius; TIB = tibialis. (Adapted from Horak and Macpherson, in press.)

Like normal subjects, they overrespond to unexpected perturbation velocities (even when the prior experience predicts that the stimulus will be slower than the actual stimulus) and then gradually habituate the magnitude of their responses with repetition (Timmann and Horak, 1995). Large reduction of postural responses over the very first few trials (perhaps due to arousal affects) is also intact in cerebellar patients as seen in figure 4.7b. Thus, cerebellar disorders result in deficits in the precision of modifying the gain of automatic postural responses based on predictive sensorimotor set, although postural response magnitude can still be modulated by on-line velocity information and by habituation and arousal.

ADAPTATION OF POSTURAL STRATEGIES AND SYNERGIES

Not only the gain but also the movement strategy (or muscle synergy) of postural responses may adapt with prior experience. Subjects can use a continuum of postural movement strategies between a "pure ankle" and a "pure hip" strategy when responding to sagittal plane—surface translations with the feet in place (Horak and Nashner, 1986; figure 4.8). The ankle strategy

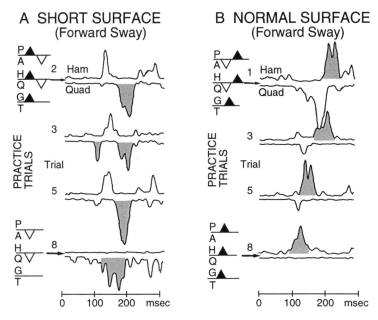

Figure 4.9 Adaptation of muscle patterns during practice trials after change of support surface from normal to beam (A) and from beam to normal (B). Hamstrings and quadriceps EMG activity from individual responses (trials 2, 3, 5, and 8) to forward sway displacements with schematic pattern of all recorded muscles at left. G, gastrocnemius; T, tibialis; H, hamstrings; Q, quadriceps; A, abdominis; P, paraspinals. Early trials of practice show complex patterns including dorsal ankle strategy muscles (dark triangles) and ventral hip strategy muscles (open triangles). A. Transition from ankle strategy pattern with early hamstrings to hip strategy with early quadriceps by trial 8. B. Transition from hip strategy with early quadriceps to ankle strategy with early hamstrings by trial 8. (Adapted from Horak and Nashner, 1986.)

involves active torque about the ankles with relatively little hip motion and is associated with a distal-to-proximal muscle activation pattern (e.g., gastrocnemius, hamstrings, and paraspinals) in response to forward sway (figure 4.9). In contrast, the hip strategy involves active torque about the hips and is associated with early proximal muscle activation (e.g., rectus abdominis and rectus femoris) in response to forward sway. The ankle strategy is normally used in response to slow, small surface translations on a firm support surface, whereas the hip strategy is normally used in response to fast translations in which stepping correction is not allowed or when ankle torque is limited.

In response to external displacements, postural movement strategies to recover equilibrium adapt or change gradually over several trials following a sudden change in biomechanical conditions. For example, sudden changes in the width of the support surface result in gradual changes in both the kinematics and EMG patterns and amplitudes in response to surface translations as subjects switch from an ankle to a hip movement strategy or vice versa. In the first trials following a change in surface width, subjects make errors by persisting in the movement pattern optimal for the previous condition. Specifically, in the first trials on a normal, flat surface following trials standing on a narrow beam, subjects use excessive hip motions, surface shear forces, and early hip EMG bursts which were appropriate for the narrow surface (Horak and Nashner, 1986). Over the next 5 to 20 trials with the same conditions, the strategy gradually changes until the temporal pattern of muscle activation stabilizes for the particular task conditons.

Figure 4.9 illustrates two examples of typical progressive shifts between the ankle and hip strategy following changing in surface length. During the second trial following a shift to the short surface in figure 4.9A, early hamstrings activation (consistent with an ankle strategy) preceded quadriceps activation (consistent with a hip strategy). Over the next six trials, the hamstring's burst of EMG gradually reduced and then disappeared, and quadriceps activation occurred 55 ms earlier than it did in the first trial. Likewise, following shifts to the normal surface (figure 4.9B), the transition from the hip to the ankle strategy involved a gradual decrease in the inappropriate quadriceps activity until it was absent by the eighth trial; at that point, hamstrings, consistent with the ankle strategy, were activated 60 ms earlier than during the first trial. During early adaptation trials, the relative amplitudes of the muscle bursts appeared to change gradually, whereas the relative timing of muscle bursts changed abruptly between sequential and interdigitated activation of antagonists, suggesting a neural constraint limiting the possible combinations of complex muscle activation patterns (McCollum, Horak, and Nashner, 1984).

Horak and Nashner (1986) suggested that the continuum of ankle-hip strategy trajectories could be synthesized from the combination of "hybrid" blends between the ankle and hip central patterns. The synthesis of complex motor actions from interactions among simpler behavioral units has been suggested for gait transitions from walk, trot, and gallop (Collins and Stewart, 1993; Collins and Richmond, 1995) and for hybrid blends of the dorsal and ventral scratch reflex at boundary areas in turtles (Stein, Camp, Robertson and Mortin, 1986). An advantage to combining two existing strategies, instead of creating a new strategy for each novel condition, is that balance can be attained within seconds because new, complex strategies can be created quickly by manipulating relatively few temporal and spatial parameters (Bernstein, 1967; Greene, 1972).

Though the processes underlying adaptation of complex balancing behaviors can be inferred only, it is clear that these processes do occur automatically and do not require intervention of higher cortical levels or conscious activity. In the past, it was argued that more complex postural behaviors, such as standing or walking on a narrow beam, involved higher-level, learned mechanisms and that the automatic reflex mechanisms were inactivated (Roberts, 1978). All studies examining such complex postural behaviors as learning to balance across narrow beams (Horak and Nashner, 1986), responding to perturbations during gait (Nashner and Forssberg, 1986), and even balancing upside down on hands (Clement and Rezette, 1985) show no changes in postural response latency, suggesting that postural adaptation takes place within the automatic postural control system itself. Thus, the short-term trial-to-trial adaptation appears to depend on automatic processes using both prior experience and current conditions to get postural responses in the right ballpark and then to "tune" the behavior by reducing the difference between actual and desired (optimal) performance (Greene, 1972).

A recently developed optimal control model of human postural coordination predicts the gradual transition between the ankle and hip strategies for control of sagittal sway (Kuo, 1992). By combining vectors representing acceleration of the ankle, knee, and hip resulting from activation of each of 14 leg muscles, the model shows that the set of biomechanically possible leg-trunk actions is surprisingly limited, a finding that suggests that the choices available to the nervous system are equally limited (Kuo, 1995). However, the choice of a strategy depends not only on biomechanical constraints but also on the postural variables (or objectives) that are optimized (e.g., energy expenditure, center of body mass position, head stability, and vertical alignment of the trunk). These objectives are satisfied by a linear quadratic Gaussian optimal controller that resolves redundancies through minimization of "error" functions. Thus, when the center of mass objective is highly weighted, the model predicts that a hip strategy will be observed in response to a perturbation, whereas when a high priority is placed on vertical alignment of the trunk, the model predicts an ankle strategy.

A change from one strategy to another can occur in the model because it includes a control selection center (figure 4.10). This center uses both the

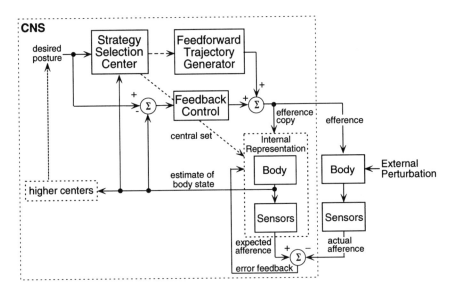

Figure 4.10 Optimal control model predicting transitions from ankle to hip strategy for sagittal plane postural control. The model includes a strategy selection center with both feed-forward and feedback control which can be modified by differences between expected and actual sensory afference resulting from external perturbations to posture. (Adapted from Kuo, 1992.)

initial mechanical state and the desired state specified by higher centers to preselect the type of response necessary; it also chooses the appropriate feedback gain and feed-forward trajectory in advance of a perturbation. This center further specifies an internal representation of body biomechanics and sensory dynamics based on central set, thereby providing a prediction of expected afferent input. The difference between the expected and actual sensory information is used to adjust the internal representation of body state, which is then used to adjust feedback gain and feed-forward trajectories. Thus, the model predicts separate mechanisms for adapting feedback gain and muscle activation patterns, both of which depend on feed-forward control. In this view, postural adaptation involves the gradual optimization of motor performance—given task-specific objectives or goals, by trial-to-trial matching of expected and actual afference. Of course, this idea is not new (Borah, Young, and Curry, 1988). Bernstein (1967) argued, "Coordination lies basically not in the character and accuracy of a tetanic effector impulse but in the accuracy of some sort of preparatory effector impulses which organize and prepare the periphery for the reception of the right impulse at the right moment."

Selection of a postural movement strategy (e.g., a compensatory step, ankle, or hip strategy) and its magnitude appears partly to occur prior to triggering of automatic postural responses. Strategy selection can be influenced by central set based on prior experience (Horak and Nashner, 1986), order of testing related to arousal effects (Maki and Whitelaw, 1993), and by sensory information specific to the characteristics of the perturbing stimulus and environment. Compared to central set effects, the influence of precued prior information or prior instruction (cognitive set) on modifying postural response synergies or gain is more subtle.

EFFECTS OF INSTRUCTION OR INTENTION

Voluntary attempts to alter an automatically triggered postural response using cognitive set are often unsuccessful because voluntary reaction times have a significantly longer latency than postural responses. There is no significant effect on postural response gain or muscle selection when subjects are given prior visual information regarding the relative size or direction of an upcoming surface rotation or translation (Diener, Horak, Stelmach, Guschlbauer, and Dichgans, 1991; Maki and Whitelaw, 1993). When subjects are instructed to respond voluntarily and quickly to a surface displacement with an other-than-automatic movement strategy, the automatic postural response occurs first at 100 ms, followed by their voluntary reactions at 180 ms (Nashner and Cordo, 1981). Fast, voluntary reactions to a postural trigger are faster than a normal visual or auditory reaction time but never as fast as an automatic postural response (McIlroy and Maki, 1993a; Shupert, Horak, and Black, 1994; Burleigh, Horak, and Malouin, 1995).

However, recent studies have shown that automatic postural responses can be suppressed by a subject's intention (M. Do, personal communication; Burleigh, Horak, and Malouin, 1995). When subjects are instructed to step rather than remain in place in response to a backward surface translation, their initial response can be an asymmetrical weight shift for stepping instead of the normal symmetrical weight shift for an in-place, automatic postural response. The EMG latencies for intentional step initiation, however, are longer than for an automatic postural response, suggesting that voluntary (or cortical) mechanisms have been substituted for automatic postural mechanisms, which are suppressed (Do, Breniere, and Bouisset, 1988; McIlroy and Maki, 1993b; Burleigh et al., 1995).

When a conflict arises between a voluntary response to a surface perturbation and an automatic postural response, the automatic postural response can be suppressed in a selective, task-specific manner even though the voluntary muscle activity occurs 50 to 100 ms later than the automatic postural response (McIlroy and Maki, 1993a; Burleigh et al., 1995; Burleigh and Horak 1995). For example, when subjects are instructed to respond to a backward surface translation with a forward step, the automatic postural response of the gastrocnemius, which is in conflict with the intent to move the center of mass forward for the step, can be suppressed up to 95 percent in the stance leg. The specificity of the effects of this cognitive set can be seen by the suppression of soleus in both legs but lack of suppression of gastrocnemius in the intended swing leg in which plantarflexion activation is required later for push-off (Burleigh et al., 1995).

To determine whether suppression of the automatic postural response was due primarily to the subject's intention to step or to changes in central set, based on anticipation of the displacement characteristics, the amount of suppression was compared when subjects were presented with unpredictable (random) versus predictable (blocked) displacement velocities. Figure 4.11 shows that although there was a trend to suppress early gastrocnemius activity when the displacement velocities were unpredictable, most of the suppression occurred when the displacement velocities could be predicted, based on prior experience. Prediction of perturbation velocity resulted in a lower response magnitude (bias) without affecting the gain (slope) of the response with increasing velocities. Prediction of perturbation velocity was not required for suppression of the later period of gastrocnemius activity corresponding to the onset of step-related tibialis muscle activity, suggesting a collision between the descending step commands and the triggered automatic response rather than a set-dependent suppression.

Thus, although a subject's intention, or cognitive set, can interfere partially with the expression of an automatic postural response or suppress its gain, voluntary intervention cannot preselect new postural responses at the shortest latencies. Cognitive set does not appear to be as powerful as central sensorimotor set in modifying automatic postural responses.

Intended Stance Limb Gastroc

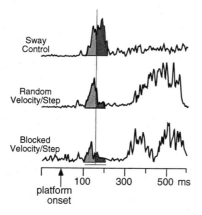

Early Gastroc (0-50ms)

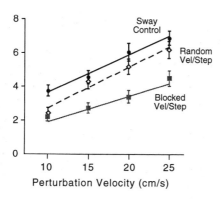

Late Gastroc (51-100ms)

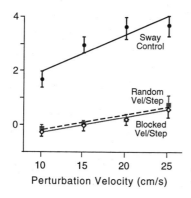

Figure 4.11 Suppression of gastrocnemius (Gastroc) response to backward platform translation when subjects intend to step. Early gastrocnemius activity (0–50 ms) shows larger suppression when platform velocity is predictable (blocked) than when it is randomized. Suppression of late gastrocnemius activity (51–100 ms) is not dependent on prediction.

Adaptation of Automatic Postural Responses

CONCLUSIONS

Automatic postural responses are modified immediately with changes in context and then continue to change or adapt with repeated exposure to perturbations, even when the conditions remain the same. It is often difficult to differentiate the many neural mechanisms contributing to functional modification of postural responses (including changing sensory drive, arousal, habituation, and set-dependent adaptation). Adaptation, or functional optimization of postural responses, that depends on the nature of prior experience can affect both the gain and the temporal synergy of the responses. The cerebellum appears to be a critical contributor to adaptive gain modification of postural responses based on sensorimotor set. Central somatosensory set based on prior experience appears to be much more powerful for modifying postural responses than arousal mechanisms, habituation, or cognitive set. Set-dependent adaptation is critical for optimization and functional modification of fast, automatic postural responses to disequilibrium in varying contexts and environments. Future studies will need to determine what variables are optimized by postural adaptation and whether the optimized variables can vary depending on the specific task, context, subject's intentions, and central set.

ACKNOWLEDGMENTS

These studies have been supported by grants from the National Institute on Aging (AG06457), the National Institute on Deafness and Other Communication Disorders (DC01849), and the National Institute on Deafness and Other Communication Disorders-National Aeronautics and Spare Administration (960-DC02072).

REFERENCES

Allum JHJ, Honegger F (1992). A postural model of balance-correcting movement strategies. J Vestib Res 2:323–347.

Beckley DJ, Bloem BR, Remler MP, Roos RAC, van Dijk JG (1991). Long latency postural responses are functionally modified by cognitive set. Electroencephalogr Clin Neurophysiol 81:353–358.

Bernstein N (1967). The Coordination and Regulation of Movement. London: Pergamon Press.

Borah J, Young LR, Curry RE (1988). Optimal estimator model for human spatial orientation. Annu N Y Acad Sci 545:51–73.

Brooks VB (1984). The cerebellum and adaptive tuning of movements. Exp Brain Res Suppl. 9:170–183.

Brown P, Day BL, Rothwell JC, Thompson PD, Marsden CD (1991). The effect of posture on the normal and pathological auditory startle reflex. J Neurol Neurosurg Psychiatry 54:892–897.

Burleigh AL, Horak FB (in press). Influence of predicted and actual velocity information on perturbed step initiation. J Neurophysiol.

Burleigh AL, Horak FB, Malouin F (1995). Modification of postural responses and step initiation: Evidence for goal directed postural interactions. J Neurophysiol 72:2892–2902.

Clement G, Gurfinkel VX, Lestienne F, Lipshits MI, Popov KE (1985). Changes of posture during transient perturbations in microgravity. Aviat Space Environ Med 56:666–671.

Clement G, Rezette D (1985). Motor behavior underlying the control of an upside-down vertical posture. Exp Brain Res 59:428–484.

Collins JJ, Richmond SA (1994). Hard-wired central pattern generators for quadrupedal locomotion. Biol Cybern 71:375–385.

Collins JJ, Stewart I (1993). Hexapodal gaits and coupled nonlinear oscillator models. Biol Cybern 68:287–298.

Crago PE, Houk JC, Hasan Z (1976). Regulatory actions of human stretch reflex. J Neurophysiol 39:925–935.

Debu B, Woollacott M (1988). Effects of gymnastics training on postural responses to stance perturbations. J Motor Behav 20:273–300.

Demer JL, Porter FI, Goldberg J, Jenkins HA, Schmidt K (1989). Adaptation to telescopic spectacles: Vesibulo-ocular reflex plasticity. Invest Ophthalmol Vis Sci 30:159–170.

Dewhurst DJ (1967). Neuromuscular control system. IEEE Trans Biomed Eng 3:167–171.

Diener HC, Horak FB, Nashner LM (1988). Influence of stimulus parameters on human postural responses. J Neurophysiol 59:1888–1895.

Diener HC, Horak FB, Stelmach G, Guschlbauer B, Dichgans J (1991). Direction and amplitude precuing has no effect on automatic posture responses. Exp Brain Res 84:219–223.

Dietz V, Gollhofer A, Kleiber M, Trippel M (1992). Regulation of bipedal stance: Dependency on "load" receptors. Exp Brain Res 89:229–231.

Do MC, Breniere Y, Bouisset S (1988). Compensatory reactions in forward fall: Are they initiated by stretch receptors? Electroencephalogr Clin Neurophysiol 69:448–452.

Evarts EV (1975). Changing concepts of central control of movement. Can J Physiol Pharmacol 53:191–201.

Evarts EV, Tanji J (1974). Gating of motor cortex reflexes by prior instruction. Brain Res 71:479–494.

Eysenck HJ (1964). Experiments in Motivation. Oxford: Pergamon.

Flament D, Hore J (1986). Movement and electromyographic disorders associated with cerebellar dysmetria. J Neurophysiol 55:1221–1232.

Gielen CCAM, Ramaekers L, van Zuylen EJ (1988). Long-latency stretch reflexes as coordinated functional responses in man. J Physiol (Lond) 407:275–292.

Greene P (1972). Problems of organization of motor systems. Prog Theor Biol 2:304–338.

Hansen PD, Woollacott MH, Debu B (1988). Postural responses to changing task conditions. Exp Brain Res 73:627–636.

Horak FB, Diener HC, Nashner LM (1989). Influence of central set on human postural responses. J Neurophysiol 62:841–853.

Horak FB, Diener HC (1994). Cerebellar control of postural scaling and central set in stance. J Neurophysiol 72:479–493.

Adaptation of Automatic Postural Responses

Horak FB, Macpherson JM (in press). Postural orientation and equilibrium. In JL Rowell, J Shepard (eds), Handbook of Physiology: Section 12, Integration of Motor, Circulatory, Respiratory and Metabolic Control During Exercise. New York: Oxford University Press.

Horak FB, Moore SP (1993). The effect of prior leaning on human postural responses. Gait Posture 1:203–210.

Horak FB, Nashner LM (1986). Central programming of postural movements: Adaptation to altered support surface configurations. J Neurophysiol 55:1369–1381.

Horak FB, Nashner LM, Diener HC (1990). Postural strategies associated with somatosensory and vestibular loss. Exp Brain Res 82:167–177.

Horak FB, Nutt J, Nashner LM (1992). Postural inflexibility in parkinsonian subjects. J Neurol Sci 111:46–58.

Horak FB, Shupert CL, Dietz V, Horstmann G (1994). Vestibular and somatosensory contributions to responses to head and body displacements in stance. Exp Brain Res 100:93–106.

Hore J, Villis J (1984). Loss of set in muscle response to limb perturbations during cerebellar dysfunction. J Neurophysiol 51:1137–1148.

Inglis JT, Horak FB, Shupert CL, Jones-Rycewicz C (1994). The importance of somatosensory information in triggering and scaling automatic postural responses in humans. Exp Brain Res 101:159–164.

Kandel ER, Schwartz JH (1982). Molecular biology of learning: Modulation of transmitter releases. Science 218:433–443.

Keshner EA, Allum JHJ, Pfaltz CR (1987). Postural coactivation and adaptation in the sway stabilizing responses of normals and patients with bilateral vestibular deficit. Exp Brain Res 69:77–92.

Keshner EA, Peterson BW (1988). Motor control strategies underlying head stabilization and voluntary head movements in humans and cats. In O Pompeiano, JHJ Allum (eds), Progress in Brain Research, Elsevier, Amsterdam: pp 329–339.

Keshner EA, Woollacott MH, Debu B (1988). Neck, trunk and limb muscle responses during postural perturbations in humans. Exp Brain Res 71:455–466.

Kuo, AD (1992). Visualization techniques for analyzing control of human movement: Affine mappings between multi-dimensional spaces. Unpublished doctoral dissertation, Stanford University.

Kuo A (1995). An optimal control model for analyzing human postural balance. IEEE Trans Biomed Eng 42:87–101.

Lisberger SG (1988). The neural basis for learning of simple motor skills. Science 242:728–735.

Macpherson JM (1994a). The force constraint strategy for stance is independent of prior experience. Exp Brain Res 101:397–405.

Macpherson JM (1994b). Changes in a postural strategy with inter-paw distance. J Neurophysiol 71:931–940.

Macpherson JM (1995). Strategies that simplify the control of quardrupedal stance: II. Electromyographic activity. J Neurophysiol 60:218–231.

Macpherson JM, Horak FB, Dunbar DC (1989). Stance dependence of automatic postural adjustments in humans. Exp Brain Res 78:557–566.

Maki BE, Holliday PJ, Topper AK (1991). Fear of falling and postural performance in the elderly. J Gerontol 46:M123–M131.

Maki BE, Whitelaw RS (1993). Influence of expectation and arousal on center-of-pressure responses to transient postural perturbations. J Vestib Res 3:25–39.

Maki BE, Whitelaw RS, McIlroy WE (1993). Does frontal-plane assymetry in compensatory postural responses represent preparation for stepping? Neurosci Lett 149:87–90.

Marsden CD, Merton PA, Morṭan HB (1977). Anticipatory postural responses in the human subject. J Physiol 275:47P–48P.

Mauritz K-H, Deitz V, Haller M (1980). Balancing as a clinical test in the differential diagnosis of sensory-motor disorders. J Neurol Neurosurg Psychiatry 43:407–412.

McCollum G, Horak F, Nashner LM (1984). Parsimony in neural calculations for postural movement. In J Bloedel, J Dichgans, W Precht (eds), Cerebellar Functions. Berlin: Springer-Verlag, pp 52–66.

McIlroy WE, Maki BE (1993a). Changes in early automatic postural responses associated with the prior-planning and execution of a compensatory step. Brain Res 631:203–211.

McIlroy WE, Maki BE (1993b). Task constraints on foot movement and the incidence of compensatory stepping following perturbation of upright stance. Brain Res 616:30–38.

Nardone A, Corra T, Schieppati M (1990). Different activations of the soleus and gatrocnemii muscles in response to various types of stance perturbation in man. Exp Brain Res 80:323–32.

Nashner LM (1976). Adapting reflexes controlling the human posture. Exp Brain Res 26:59–72.

Nashner LM, Cordo PJ (1981). Relation of automatic postural responses and reaction-time voluntary movements of human leg muscles. Exp Brain Res 43:395–405.

Nashner LM, Forssberg H (1986). Phase-dependent organization of postural adjustments associated with arm movements while walking. J Neurophysiol 55–6:1382–1394.

Prochazka A (1989). Sensorimotor gain control: A basic strategy of motor systems? Prog Neurobiol 33:281–307.

Roberts TDM (1978). Neurophysiology of Postural Mechanisms. London: Butterworth.

Robinson FR, Straube A, Fuchs AF (1993). Role of the caudal fastigial nucleus in saccade generation: II. Effects of muscimol inactivation. J Neurophysiol 70:1741–1758.

Rothwell JC, Day BL, Berardelli A, Marsden CD (1986). Habituation and conditioning of the human long-latency stretch reflex. Exp Brain Res 63:197–204.

Schieppati M, Nardone A (1991). Free and supported stance in Parkinson's disease: The effect of posture and 'postural set' on leg muscle responses to perturbation, its relation to the severity of the disease. Brain 114 (3):1227–1244.

Shinha T, Maki B (1993). Effect of lean on postural dynamics: Identification of a posture control model. IEEE Trans Biomed Eng 15:1179–1180.

Shupert CL, Horak FB, Black FO (1994). Hip sway associated with vestibulopathy. J Vestib Res 4:231–244.

Stein PGS, Camp AW, Robertson GA, Mortin LI (1986). Blends of rostral and caudal scratch reflex motor patterns elicited by simultaneous stimulation of two sites in the spinal turtle. J Neurosci 6:2259–2266.

Thach WT, Goodkin HG, Keating JG (1992). The cerebellum and the adaptive coordination of movement. Annu Rev Neurosci 15:403–442.

Timmann D, Horak FB (1996). Prediction and set-dependent scaling of early postural responses in cerebellar patients. Manuscript submitted for publication.

II Conditioned Reflexes

5 The Brain Substrates of Classical Eyeblink Conditioning in Rabbits

Joseph E. Steinmetz

Classical conditioning of the rabbit nictitating membrane-eyeblink response has been adopted by a number of researchers as a standard behavioral paradigm for studying the neural substrates of a simple form of motor learning and memory. Classical conditioning involves presenting a conditioned stimulus (CS) just before an unconditioned stimulus (US). Initially, presentation of the CS fails to elicit overt behavioral responses, whereas the US reliably produces a reflexive response called the *unconditioned response* (UR). After several CS-US pairings, the CS begins to elicit the eyeblink response (or *conditioned response*, CR) even on trials when no US is presented. A tone or light normally is used as the CS for rabbit classical eyeblink conditioning, whereas corneal air puffs or mild periorbital shocks (both of which cause discrete eyeblinks) are used as the US. With continued CS-US pairings, the rabbit learns to execute an anticipatory eyeblink response to the tone or light CS before presentation of the air puff or shock US. Moreover, the rabbit learns to time the anticipatory eyeblink response optimally so that its eyelids are maximally closed at the time when the air puff is presented. Due largely to the efforts of Gormezano and associates (e.g., Gormezano, Schneiderman, Deaux, and Fuentes, 1962, Gormezano, Kehoe, and Marshall-Goodell, 1983), a great deal of behavioral data are available concerning this basic paradigm.

EVIDENCE FOR THE INVOLVEMENT OF THE CEREBELLUM IN CLASSICAL EYEBLINK CONDITIONING

Over the last 15 years, a number of researchers have investigated the involvement of the cerebellum in this very simple motor learning task. McCormick, Lavond, Clark, Kettner, Rising, and Thompson, (1981); McCormick, Clark, Lavond, and Thompson (1982a); and McCormick, Guyer, and Thompson (1982b) first reported that aspiration or electrolytic lesions of the cerebellum (including portions of the deep nuclei) abolished CRs that were learned prior to the lesion. Cerebellar lesions placed before training prevented acquisition of the classically conditioned eyeblink response (Lincoln, McCormick, and Thompson, 1982). This basic effect has been replicated by a number of laboratories using electrolytic lesions (e.g., Yeo, Hardiman, and Glickstein, 1985a; Weisz and LoTurco, 1988; Lavond, Logan, Sohn, Garner, and Kanzawa, 1990; Steinmetz, Lavond, Ivkovich, Logan, and Thompson, 1992a; Steinmetz, Logue, and Steinmetz, 1992b), chemical lesions (e.g., Lavond, Hembree, and Thompson, 1985), and reversible lesions (e.g., Chapman, Steinmetz, Sears, and Thompson, 1990; Clark, Zhang, and Lavond, 1992; Krupa, Thompson, and Thompson, 1993). However, some investigators have reported post-lesion sparing of CRs under some training conditions (Welsh and Harvey, 1989; Kelly, Zuo, and Bloedel, 1990). It appears that a rather discrete lesion of the dorsolateral anterior interpositus nucleus disrupts eyeblink conditioning (Lavond et al., 1985; Steinmetz et al., 1992b). Lesions of the cerebellar cortex have produced a wider range of effects including reports of complete response abolition (Yeo, Hardiman, and Glickstein, 1985b; Yeo and Hardiman, 1992) and reports of varying degrees of response impairments (Lavond, Steinmetz, Yokaitis, and Thompson, 1987; Lavond and Steinmetz, 1989; Hardiman and Yeo, 1992; Harvey, Welsh, Yeo, and Romano, 1993). These deep nuclear and cerebellar cortical lesion data provide strong evidence in support of a critical role for the cerebellum in eyeblink conditioning.

Cerebellar recording data lend support to the lesion data. Multiple unit recordings from the cerebellar cortex and the interpositus nucleus revealed neuronal discharge patterns that formed amplitude/time-course models that were highly correlated with execution of the learned behavioral responses (e.g., McCormick and Thompson, 1984). Moreover, the onsets of these neuronal models preceded the behavioral eyeblink response by 30 to 60 ms, a time period consistent with synaptic delays present from the cerebellar nuclei to the red nucleus to the cranial nerve nuclei that control facial musculature responsible for the eyeblink response. Single-unit analyses of interpositus nucleus activity revealed a number of patterns of neuronal discharge, including units that responded to presentation of either the CS or the US and units that discharged in relation to the behavioral response (Berthier and Moore, 1990). Cerebellar cortical activity also has been studied (McCormick and Thompson, 1984; Berthier and Moore, 1986), and such studies found Purkinje cells that responded to the CS and US and Purkinje cells that displayed spiking patterns that appeared to be related to generation of the behavioral responses. Two basic patterns of behavior-related Purkinje cell activity were observed: Neurons that increased their discharge rate after CS presentation and neurons that decreased their discharge rate after CS presentation.

We have extensively studied ways in which the CS and US might be projected to the cerebellum from the periphery. Based on a variety of lesion, stimulation, and recording data, we have hypothesized that a tone CS is projected from the periphery by way of a number of primary auditory areas in the brainstem to several sites in the lateral regions of the basilar pontine nuclei (Steinmetz, Rosen, Chapman, Lavond, and Thompson, 1986; Steinmetz,

Logan, Rosen, Thompson, Lavond, and Thompson, 1987; Steinmetz, 1990b). Tone information is then thought to be projected to the cerebellar cortex and the deep nuclei via mossy fibers that originate in the pontine nuclei (Steinmetz and Sengelaub, 1992; Gould, Sears, and Steinmetz, 1993). In another series of lesion, stimulation, and recording experiments, we have traced potential US pathways and have hypothesized that an air puff US is projected from the cornea of the eye through the trigeminal nucleus to well-defined regions of the dorsal accessory inferior olive (McCormick, Steinmetz, and Thompson, 1985; Sears and Steinmetz, 1991). The US information is then projected to the cerebellar cortex and the deep nuclei via climbing fibers that originate in the dorsal accessory olive (Yeo, Hardiman, and Glickstein, 1985c; Mauk, Steinmetz, and Thompson, 1986; Yeo, Hardiman and Glickstein, 1986). This may not be the only route to the cerebellum for US information. We have some data that show that air puff USs also activate mossy fiber input to the cerebellum (see following). Axons originating in the trigeminal nucleus are known to project directly to the cerebellar cortex and nuclei and also to project indirectly to the cerebellar cortex and nuclei via the pontine nuclei (Van Ham and Yeo, 1992). Although not widely studied, this source of input to the cerebellum may also be important for eyeblink conditioning. Figure 5.1 provides a summary of the neuronal circuitry hypothesized to be involved in eyeblink conditioning.

In addition to studies conducted to delineate neural pathways and networks that carry conditioning-related activity to and from the cerebellum, a number of experiments have varied basic parameters of the standard rabbit eyeblink conditioning paradigm in an attempt to establish the generality of the involvement of the cerebellum in similar motor learning procedures. The involvement of the cerebellum is not restricted to classical conditioning procedures involving a tone CS and air puff US. Cerebellar lesions and middle cerebellar peduncle sections disrupted eyeblink conditioning when tactile or visual stimuli were used as CSs and also when periorbital shock was used as US (Yeo et al., 1985a,b; Lewis, LoTurco, and Solomon, 1987). Lesions of the cerebellum were effective in abolishing conditioned responding when a variety of interstimulus intervals (ISIs) were used in conjunction with standard delay conditioning and when trace conditioning was given (Steinmetz, 1990a; Stotler, Miller, and Steinmetz, 1990). In standard delay conditioning, the CS and the US overlap, whereas in trace conditioning a time period elapses between CS offset and US onset. Lesions of the cerebellum effectively abolished CRs formed with an avoidance-conditioning procedure (Polenchar, Patterson, Lavond, and Thompson, 1985). In this study, paired CS and US presentations were given as in standard eyeblink conditioning. However, in the avoidance procedure, the US was withheld if the rabbit performed a CR during the CS-US period (i.e., the rabbit could avoid presentation of the air puff if a CR was executed). Cerebellar involvement has been extended to the classical conditioning of other skeletal muscle response systems. For example,

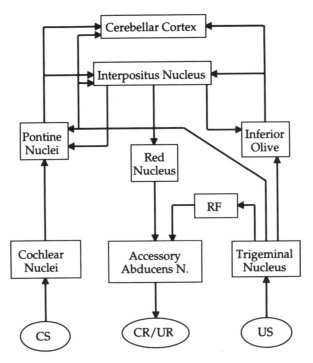

Figure 5.1 Schematic diagram showing brain and cerebellar areas hypothesized to be involved in classic eyeblink conditioning (see text for details). RF, reticular formation; CS, conditioned stimulus; CR-UR, conditioned response/unconditioned response; US, unconditioned stimulus.

lesions that encompass medial portions of the interpositus nucleus abolished leg flexion conditioning established with a tone CS and shock delivered to the hindlimb as a US (Donegan, Lowry, and Thompson, 1983). Further, involvement of the cerebellum in aversive classical conditioning has been demonstrated in a number of species besides rabbits, including rats (Skelton, 1988), cats (Voneida, Christie, Bogdanski, and Chopko, 1990), and humans (Daum, Schugens, Ackermann, Lutzenberger, Dichgans, and Birbaumer, 1993).

It seems clear from the data presented above that the cerebellum is importantly involved in the acquisition and performance of the classically conditioned eyeblink response. However, the precise role of the cerebellum in this simple motor learning task is far from understood. In the remaining portion of this chapter, we will raise and attempt to address three current issues that we are currently investigating, all of which concern the involvement of the cerebellum in classical eyeblink conditioning. These issues include (1) the relative roles of the cerebellar cortex and the deep nuclei in acquisition and performance of the conditioned eyeblink response, (2) the limitations of the involvement of the cerebellum in classical conditioning, and (3) the localized versus distributed nature of the neural network involved in eyeblink conditioning.

THE ROLES OF CEREBELLAR CORTEX AND DEEP NUCLEI IN CLASSICAL EYEBLINK CONDITIONING

Early lesion experiments used rather large, unilateral aspiration and electrolytic lesions to demonstrate that the cerebellum was critically involved in classical eyeblink conditioning (McCormick et al., 1981; Lincoln et al., 1982). These lesions often incorporated extensive regions of the interpositus and dentate nuclei and also relatively large areas of the white matter and cerebellar cortex dorsal to the deep nuclei. Over the years, a variety of experiments have attempted to define more precisely the regions of the cerebellum involved in eyeblink conditioning.

Electrolytic lesions confined to the interpositus nucleus have abolished retention of the eyeblink CR (e.g., Steinmetz et al., 1992a). The abolition seems permanent. Rabbits given more than 20,000 postlesion paired trials over a 10-month period failed to show reacquisition of the eyeblink CR on the side of the lesion even though they could readily learn the eyeblink CR when training was given to the nonlesioned side (Steinmetz et al., 1992b). These electrolytic lesions, however, undoubtedly caused damage to fibers of passage enroute to the cerebellar cortex along with damage to the nuclear cells, thus making it difficult to assess the relative involvement of cerebellar cortex and the deep nuclei in conditioning. Using kainic acid, which destroys cell bodies while leaving fibers of passage intact, Lavond et al. (1985) defined a relatively small area (about 1 mm^3) in the lateral dorsal anterior interpositus nucleus that was critical for retention of the eyeblink CR. This rather restricted area was destroyed in all previous electrolytic lesion experiments and is a likely candidate for a region of CS-US convergence during conditioning. Recording studies from our laboratory support this idea: We found cells in this region of the interpositus nucleus that could be activated by electrical stimulation of the lateral region of the pontine nuclei and the inferior olive, the origins of our hypothesized CS and US pathways to the cerebellum, respectively (Gould et al., 1993).

Reversible lesions of this area of the interpositus nucleus produced temporary abolition of conditioned responding. Loss of the CR during the inactivation period resulted from the infusion into the interpositus nuclei of well-trained rabbits of such substances as lidocaine, a local anesthetic (Chapman et al., 1990), bicuculline, a gamma amino butyric acid (GABA) antagonist (Mamounas, Thompson, and Madden, 1987), and muscimol, a GABA agonist (Krupa et al., 1993). These reversible lesion agents have also been infused into the interpositus nucleus during the acquisition phase of conditioning as a means of evaluating the contributions of the nucleus to the conditioning process. The major assumption underlying these experiments is that critical plasticity processes that occur during the acquisition of the conditioned eyeblink response are blocked during infusion of the reversible lesioning compound. No "savings" in acquisition should be seen once the infusion is discontinued (i.e., the rabbits should learn at the same rate as rabbits that have received no training trials). The results of the use of lidocaine have been mixed. Welsh and Harvey (1991) reported some saving in their rabbits after lidocaine infusion was stopped. Conversely, Nordholm, Thompson, Dersarkissian, and Thompson, (1993) reported no savings in rabbits trained for several days while lidocaine was infused into the nuclei. The difference in these results could be due to a difference in placement of the infusion cannula within the nucleus or possibly due to differences in training procedures (e.g., Welsh and Harvey used a light CS in addition to a tone CS in their experiment). Infusion of muscimol during initial acquisition training prevented CR formation, and rabbits showed no signs of savings when compared to appropriate controls (Krupa et al., 1993). Infusion of muscimol into the red nucleus (a target for interpositus nucleus projections) during acquisition training prevented expression of CRs during training but failed to prevent savings from occurring. These muscimol results have been supported strongly by a series of experiments involving another type of reversible lesion—temporary lesions induced by a cold probe device used to inactivate specific brain regions by cooling. Abolition of eyeblink CRs was seen when the interpositus was cooled after rabbits were trained, and rabbits showed no savings of training when the interpositus was cooled during acquisition training (Clark et al., 1992). Cooling of the red nucleus (Clark and Lavond, 1993) or cranial nerve nuclei and reticular formation areas involved in response production (Zhang and Lavond, 1991) during training prevented the expression of CRs but failed to prevent a savings effect. These reversible lesion data argue strongly for a critical role of the interpositus nucleus in the acquisition and performance of the classically conditioned eyeblink response.

The effects of lesions of cerebellar cortex on eyeblink conditioning have been somewhat inconsistent. Yeo et al. (1985b) conditioned rabbits with light and white noise CSs paired with periorbital shock USs and then induced unilateral aspiration lesions of the cortex that spared the underlying white matter and deep nuclei. They reported that rather restricted lesions that incorporated Larsell's sixth hemispheric lobule (HVI) abolished CRs to both CSs, whereas larger lesions that failed to incorporate lobule HVI had no effect. Lavond et al. (1987) used rather extensive unilateral aspiration lesions to assess the involvement of cerebellar cortex in retention of the eyeblink CR. Although the rabbits initially showed no postlesion CRs, they eventually relearned the task with additional training. Lavond and Steinmetz (1989) also lesioned the cerebellar cortex of naive rabbits, then trained them on the eyeblink conditioning task. Rabbits with lesions confined to the cerebellar cortex were able to learn with the eye ipsilateral to the lesion, but many more sessions were required to learn relative to naive controls. In addition, the CR amplitudes were greatly reduced as compared to controls. Yeo and Hardiman (1992) reexamined the effects of cortical lesions using extended postoperative conditioning and tone and light CSs paired with periorbital shock USs. Combined lesions of lobule HVI and the ansiform lobe abolished CRs, but extended retraining enabled a slight recovery of CR frequency. Smaller lesions also initially abolished CRs but allowed more complete recovery of CRs during retraining. Although these data do not reveal as consistent a lesion effect as seen in the interpositus nucleus lesion data, the data suggest that the cerebellar cortex is importantly involved in the classical eyeblink conditioning in process.

In an attempt to define better the respective roles of cerebellar cortex and the interpositus nucleus during eyeblink conditioning, we have adopted the strategy of varying the basic conditioning procedure while recording multiple- and single-unit activity from the two cerebellar areas. In this manner, we hope to define specific features of the conditioning process encoded by the two areas. Specifically, we have studied cerebellar activity during extinction

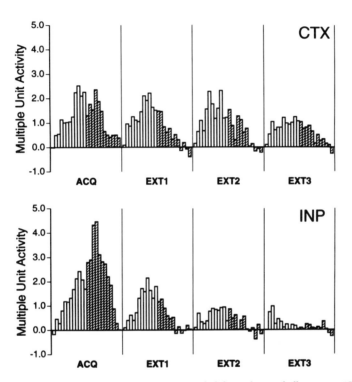

Figure 5.2 Multiple-unit activity recorded from the cerebellar cortex (CTX) and the interpositus nucleus (INP) on the last day of paired acquisition training (ACQ) and on three days of CS-alone extinction training (EXT1–EXT3). EXT1 and EXT2 show data recorded on the first and second half of the first extinction session, whereas EXT3 shows data recorded on the final day of extinction training. Standardized scores of unit activity are depicted (see Sears and Steinmetz, 1990, 1991, for computational procedures). The 24 bars of each histogram represent standard scores calculated for 20-msec periods of time from CS onset to the end of the trial (total trial length = 480 m). For session ACQ, the clear bars represent unit activity recorded between CS and US onset (i.e., the CS period), whereas the stippled bars represent activity recorded after US onset (i.e., the US period). For sessions EXT1–EXT2, no US was presented, but the CS and US periods are shown. This figure shows that even though behavioral CRs have been extinguished, learning-related cerebellar cortical activity is still present. Conversely, learning-related activity in the interpositus nucleus rapidly disappears as CRs are extinguished.

Brain Substrates of Classical Eyeblink Conditioning

training, during backward and unpaired presentations of the CS and US, and during discrimination and reversal conditioning. In our extinction experiments, rabbits were trained to a conditioning criterion with CS-US paired trials and then given CS-alone presentations across many days until the CRs fell below 5 percent (Gould and Steinmetz, 1996). Cerebellar cortical and deep nuclear recordings were made during the extinction phase (figures 5.2 and 5.3). Our recordings revealed a different pattern of activation across extinction at the cortical and interpositus sites. The characteristic CR-related activity in the interpositus nucleus was observed only when CRs were present (i.e., as extinction occurred, CR-related activity disappeared). This was not observed at all recording sites within the cortex. At a number of cortical sites, training-related activity persisted for several days after CRs had disappeared, thus demonstrating that the cerebellar cortical neuronal response could be dissociated from the behavioral response.

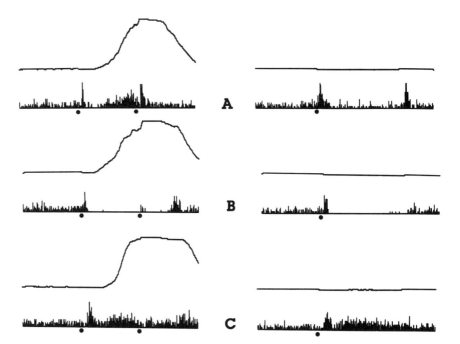

Figure 5.3 Examples of eyeblink responses (top traces) and corresponding single unit activity (bottom histograms) recorded from the cerebellar cortex during 10 paired CS-US trials (left column) and 10 CS-alone extinction trials (right column). A total of 750 msec from trial onset to trial offset are shown. Onsets of the CS and US are indicated by filled circles under the histograms. A. During paired trials when CRs were present, this unit discharged to both the CS and the US and also showed activity that was related to the behavioral response. After extinction, the behavior-related activity disappeared, but the CS-related activity was still present. B. During paired training, this unit decreased its discharge rate during the CS and US periods. This spiking pattern continued after behavioral extinction occurred. C. During paired training, activity related to presentation of the tone CS was observed, as was activity related to the behavioral response. This pattern was still present after behavioral extinction occurred during CS-alone training.

We also have recorded cerebellar activity during backward and explicitly unpaired presentations of the tone CS and air puff US normally used during eyeblink conditioning (Gould and Steinmetz, 1996). During five sessions of backward paired training, the US was presented before the CS, thereby giving the rabbits experience with paired presentations of the stimuli used during conditioning in a situation where overt behavioral CRs were not seen. During five sessions of explicitly unpaired presentations of the CS and US, the stimuli were never paired, thus giving the rabbits experience with the conditioning stimuli in a situation where the stimuli do not overlap. Forward paired training was given after the unpaired training. Because pilot work demonstrated that interpositus nucleus activity was not altered during the backward and unpaired training procedures, we concentrated our recording efforts on the cerebellar cortex. Recordings from the cerebellar cortex during backward training showed a number of interesting patterns of activation even though CRs were not learned (figure 5.4). As expected, a number of Purkinje cells responded to presentations of the tone or air puff. Some increased their

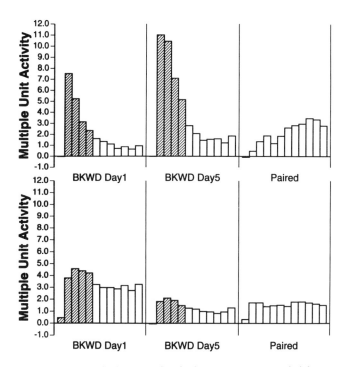

Figure 5.4 Standard scores of multiple-unit activity recorded from cerebellar cortex during the first (BKWD Day 1) and fifth (BKWD Day 5) sessions of backward pairing (i.e., US-CS pairings) and during the last day of forward pairing (Paired). Activity recorded between US and CS presentation is depicted by stippled bars, whereas activity after CS presentation is depicted by open bars. Two basic patterns of activity were seen: Some sites showed increases in unit activity across the backward training days (top histograms). These sites eventually showed CR-related activity during forward pairing. Other sites showed decreases in unit activity over backward training (bottom histograms) and these sites failed to show CR-related activity during forward training.

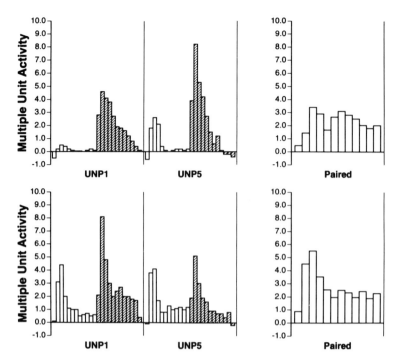

Figure 5.5 Standard scores of multiple-unit activity recorded from the cerebellar cortex during the first (UNP1) and fifth (UNP5) sessions of unpaired CS and US presentations and during the last day of forward paired presentations (Paired). Activity recorded on CS-alone trials is depicted by open bars whereas activity recorded on US-alone trials is depicted by stippled bars. The two types of trials have been combined here for presentation purposes. Two basic patterns of activity were seen: Some sites showed CS- and US-related increases in unit activity across the unpaired training days (top histograms). These sites eventually showed CR-related activity during forward pairing. Other sites showed no change in unit activity across unpaired training (bottom histograms), and these sites did not show CR-related activity during forward training.

firing rate, whereas others decreased their firing rate. Over the course of backward training, however, the spiking patterns changed. Again, both increases and decreases in firing rates over baseline levels were seen. We even observed changes in cerebellar cortical activity during unpaired CS and US presentations (figure 5.5). Many recording sites showed CS- or US-evoked patterns of activation or both. Some of these sites showed an increase in CS or US activation over the unpaired training sessions, whereas other sites showed no changes or, slight decreases in activity at most. Interestingly, the recording sites that showed significant increases in CS- or US-evoked activity during unpaired training showed CR-related patterns of activity when training was switched to forward pairing (i.e., the same cortical neurons seemed to alter their firing patterns predictably during both unpaired and forward paired training situations). These data also revealed an interesting feature of the US-evoked activity: Although the Purkinje cells showed complex spike discharges when the air puff US was presented during both the backward and unpaired training sessions, many of the Purkinje cells responsive to the air puff also showed trains of US-evoked simple spikes. Moreover, the alterations in activity over the course of backward training noted in most Purkinje cells involved the US-evoked simple spike patterns. These data suggest that US projections from the trigeminal nucleus to the cerebellar cortex arriving by way of the mossy fiber system may be importantly involved in eyeblink conditioning. The involvement of these projections most certainly deserves a closer analysis.

We have also monitored multiple-unit activity in the cerebellar cortex and the interpositus nucleus during the many sessions required to produce classical discrimination followed by reversal eyeblink conditioning (Gould and Steinmetz, 1994). During discrimination training, we presented two tones of different frequencies. One tone (the CS$^+$) was always followed by an air puff US whereas the other tone (the CS$^-$) was never followed by the US. During reversal training, the CS$^+$ and the CS$^-$ were switched. In the course of these procedures, the rabbits first learned to blink to the CS$^+$ and withhold responding to the CS$^-$ (the discrimination phase). They then learned to blink to the former CS$^-$ while witholding responding to the former CS$^+$ (the reversal phase). During both phases of conditioning, similar patterns of activity were observed in the cerebellar cortex: CR-related activity was present on CS$^+$ trials but not on CS$^-$ trials. Activity in the interpositus nucleus differed during the two conditioning phases. After the discrimination criterion was reached, CR-related activity was present on CS$^+$ but not CS$^-$ trials. After reversal training, however, only a very weak activation of the interpositus nucleus was seen on CS$^+$ trials, with no activation present on CS$^-$ trials.

Observed differences in cerebellar cortical and nuclear activities when variations of the basic conditioning procedures are introduced suggest that the cerebellar cortex and interpositus nucleus may play different roles in classical eyeblink conditioning. With the exception of reversal conditioning after discrimination training, the interpositus nucleus seems consistently to demonstrate activity related to acquisition and performance of the behavioral CR. When a CR is present, CR-related activity in the interpositus nucleus is seen. When CRs are absent, no such activity is seen. Cerebellar cortex, on the other hand, shows a variety of neuronal spiking patterns that are, at times, unrelated CR production. In situations where no behavioral CRs are present (e.g., during extinction training, backward training, and unpaired CS and US training), CS- and US-related activity can be seen and, more importantly, the patterns of this activity change systematically over the course of these training situations. From these data, we have hypothesized that synaptic arrangements in these two cerebellar areas support different types and degrees of plasticity induced by CS and US activation (Gould and Steinmetz, 1994). Plasticity involving the interpositus nucleus seems to be limited to situations were the CS is presented before the US, whereas plasticity involving cerebellar cortical cells seems to occur in a variety of stimulus arrangements. In other words, the interpositus nucleus requires a rather specific ordering and timing of CS and US inputs, whereas the cerebellar cortex is responsive to a wider variety of patterns of CS and US inputs. From this observation, we have hypothesized that basic excitability changes that are necessary for activating brainstem nuclei (responsible for generating the eyeblink CR to CS input) occur in the interpositus nucleus in a very pairing-specific manner. More general, nonpairing-specific excitability changes occur in the cerebellar cortex, and these changes are responsible for modulating the pairing-specific alteration in activity in the interpositus nucleus. The cortical activity may be responsible for the specific refinements of CR or UR topographies (or both), including contributing input to shape the optimal gain and the optimal timing of the eyeblink CR.

Lesion and recording data support these roles for the cerebellar cortex and interpositus nucleus. Several experiments have demonstrated the recovery of CRs after cerebellar cortical lesions (Lavond et al., 1987; Lavond and Steinmetz, 1989; Harvey et al., 1993). However, the postlesion appearance of the CRs typically required some period of reacquisition training, and any CRs that were seen were generally of reduced amplitude. Lesions of the interpositus nucleus have generally produced complete CR abolition even for long periods of postlesion observation (Steinmetz et al., 1992a,b) although, under some training circumstances, postlesion CRs have been reported (Welsh and Harvey, 1989; Kelly et al., 1990). These data are consistent with the idea that the interpositus nucleus undergoes critical pairing-specific plasticity to promote CR formation and performance, whereas the cortex provides a modulatory input possibly involved in CR gain. There are also recent data suggesting a role for the cerebellar cortex in CR timing. Perrett, Ruiz, and Mauk (1993) used an ISI discrimination task coupled with cerebellar cortical lesions to demonstrate an involvement of the cerebellar cortex in CR timing. In this procedure, two tones of different frequencies were used to signal two different ISIs, a long ISI (e.g., 750 ms) and a short ISI (e.g., 250 ms). Under these training conditions, rabbits learned to time their CRs to the appropriate ISI signaled by each tone to the extent that their eyeblink responses were maximal at the time when the air puff was presented. Perrett et al. (1993) showed that lesions that incorporated anterior portions of the cerebellar hemisphere abolished the rabbit's ability to generate optimally timed CRs; the rabbits tended to perform all CRs quite early in the ISI period. We recently have used this same behavioral procedure to analyze the activity of Purkinje cells under shifting ISI conditions (Allen and Steinmetz, 1994). We found many cells that showed CR-related activity during this discrimination task, and all these cells effectively encoded both ISIs. When the tone frequency signaled a short ISI, optimally timed CRs for the short ISI were executed, and the Purkinje cell showed spiking patterns with onsets and distributions that were highly correlated with the timing of the CRs. When the tone frequency signaled a long ISI, optimally timed CRs for the long ISI were executed, and the same Purkinje cell showed spiking patterns with onsets and distributions that were highly correlated with the timing of the longer latency CRs. These cerebellar cortical lesion and recording data support a role for cerebellar cortex in modulating the timing of the CR. Furthermore, these data, together with the results of a variety of other experiments, support the idea that the interpositus nucleus and the cerebellar cortex, acting in concert yet likely encoding different aspects of the conditioning process, comprise a critical portion of the neural circuitry involved in classic eyeblink conditioning.

LIMITATIONS OF THE INVOLVEMENT OF THE CEREBELLUM IN CLASSICAL CONDITIONING

One potentially useful approach for delineating further the role of the cerebellum in motor learning is to attempt to identify limitations concerning the involvement of the cerebellum in classical eyeblink conditioning and similar learning paradigms. In other words, a careful description of those associative learning conditions that do not appear to critically engage the cerebellum should advance our understanding of the nature of the learning tasks that are mediated through the cerebellum.

Experiments to date have shown that interpositus lesions abolish eyeblink conditioning and other forms of classical conditioning that involve skeletal muscle responses. These same lesions, however, have been shown not to affect autonomic conditioning, such as the decelerations of heart rate that are observed with paired presentations of a tone CS and air puff US (Lavond, Lincoln, McCormick, and Thompson, 1984). Although some experiments have shown an important involvement of the vermis in autonomic conditioning in the rat (e.g., Supple and Leaton, 1990), the exact nature of this involvement is still under investigation. These data suggest that the involvement of the cerebellum in classical conditioning may be limited to conditioning of skeletal muscle responses.

The complexity of the skeletal motor response required for a given learning task might to some extent determine the degree of cerebellar involvement in the conditioning. The conditioned eyeblink and conditioned leg flexion responses that have been demonstrated to be dependent on cerebellar processing are highly discrete responses. To date, no data have shown the critical involvement of the cerebellum in conditioning tasks that require more complex movements. In collaboration with M. Gabriel et al., we recently evaluated the effects of interpositus nucleus lesions on two conditioning tasks using a within-subject design (Steinmetz, Sears, Gabriel, Kubota, Poremba, and Kang, 1991). Rabbits were given bilateral interpositus nucleus lesions, then trained on two tasks that differed in the movement required for learning, classical eyeblink conditioning, and discriminative avoidance conditioning. In the discriminative avoidance conditioning, rabbits were placed in a wheel and presented with a tone CS that was followed after a period of time by a mild foot shock. The rabbits could avoid the foot shock by rotating the wheel via a stepping motion. One of the major differences between these behavioral paradigms is the complexity of the motor response required; the eyeblink is unilateral and very discrete, whereas the response required for wheel rotation involves coordinated, bilateral limb movements. Results of the bilateral interpositus nucleus lesions were unequivocal. The lesions completely prevented acquisition of the classically conditioned eyeblink response on both the left and right sides. However, these same rabbits showed normal acquisition rates of the conditioned avoidance response. These data show a differential involvement of the interpositus nucleus in these associative learning paradigms: The learning of a simple, discrete conditioned response was blocked by the cerebellar lesion, whereas the learning of a more complicated conditioned movement was unaffected.

Other data suggest that the cerebellum may be involved only in aversive conditioning. In general, classical and instrumental conditioning paradigms are divided into two categories: aversive conditioning (which involves learning with presentation of noxious stimuli) and appetitive conditioning (which involves learning with reinforcement or reward). Research by Gibbs (1992) suggests that the cerebellum may be involved only in aversive conditioning. Gibbs assessed the effects of cerebellar lesions on eyeblink conditioning (an aversive task) and jaw-movement conditioning (an appetitive task) in rabbits. Jaw-movement conditioning involves presentation of a tone or light CS just prior to a squirt of a sweet liquid into the oral cavity (the US). The presentation of liquid causes a rhythmic jaw movement associated with a rewarding consummatory response. Though the cerebellar lesions blocked performance of the aversively motivated conditioned eyeblink response, the lesions had no effect on conditioning of the appetitively motivated conditioned response. Recently we have demonstrated a similar selective involvement of the cerebellum in aversive conditioning using a signaled bar-press task in rats, a task that has some similarities to classical conditioning (Steinmetz, Logue, and Miller, 1993). In these signaled bar-press tasks, rats were presented with a tone for a period of time. If the rats pressed a response bar during the tone period, they received a food pellet reward (the appetitive consequence), or they successfully avoided a mild foot shock (the aversive consequence). Bilateral cerebellar lesions completely prevented learning of the aversive task but had no affect on the acquisition and performance of the appetitive task even though the same rats (with the same lesions) were run in both tasks.

Whereas CSs activate common brain areas during appetitive and aversive conditioning, the USs used during appetitive and aversive tasks undoubtedly activate different brain systems. During appetitive procedures, CR acquisition and performance are most likely dependent on the activation of reward systems in the brain caused by presentation of the appetitive US. Many studies have identified forebrain areas as involved chiefly in reward processes (e.g., Gallistal, Gomita, Yadin, and Campbell, 1985). It seems likely that the cerebellum is not involved critically in the US-mediated activation of the reward system but rather that regions of the forebrain receive the necessary convergent information from the neutral CS and appetitive US for CR production. The noxious stimuli that are commonly used during aversive classical conditioning seem to share one feature in common: They activate somatosensory inputs to the brain (e.g., corneal afferents, the skin overlying the forepaws, the skin overlying the hindlimbs). The cerebellum receives multiple sources of input from the somatosensory system and is a likely point of convergence for information that arises from the neutral CS and the aversive US. The cerebellum may therefore be involved in aversive conditioning but not in appetitive conditioning because it receives convergent information about the CS and US during aversive conditioning but not during appetitive conditioning.

Many researchers have demonstrated an inverted U-shaped function that describes the relationship between the length of the ISI and the rate or magnitude of eyeblink conditioning (see Gormezano et al., 1983, for review). In general, conditioning does not occur with ISIs of less than 50 to 80 msec or with ISIs greater than 4 to 5 s, and training is fastest and most robust when the ISI is between 200 and 400 ms. The ISI function demonstrates a fundamental behavioral restriction of classical eyeblink conditioning: CR acquisition occurs only when the time between CS onset and US onset falls within a relatively narrow range (i.e., 100 ms–5 s). Because the cerebellum is known to be important for this type of learning, it seems possible that cerebellar anatomy and physiology impose this temporal restriction (i.e., the neural circuitry of the cerebellum is equipped to process converging input from the two sources of peripheral input only when the two inputs arrive at the cerebellum within the window of time defined by the ISI function). Furthermore, the optimal ISI (i.e., the range of ISIs that produces the most rapid and robust conditioning) may be determined by cerebellar processing. Assuming that the cerebellum plays a major role in aversive classical conditioning of discrete responses, it is possible that optimal conditioning may occur when the timings of the CS and US inputs are optimized for cerebellar function and that this may correspond to an ISI between 200 and 400 ms. A testable prediction that directly follows from this hypothesis is that at nonoptimal ISIs, noncerebellar brain areas (e.g., hippocampus, neostriatum) become importantly, if not essentially, involved in the acquisition and retention of well-timed CRs.

There are variations of classical and instrumental conditioning procedures and related associative learning paradigms employing ISIs that extend well beyond the 5-s upper limit for the ISI established in studies of classical eyeblink conditioning (see Hearst, 1988, for review). The lack of conditioning of discrete responses when the ISI is greater than 5 s may make sense from an ethological point of view. When a long interval elapses between a signaling stimulus and an aversive stimulus, discrete responses may not be the best way to avoid or alleviate the aversive stimulus. Rather, more complex behaviors such as locomotion may be a more effective way of dealing with the aversive event. Therefore, it is reasonable to conclude that these types of associative learning would not critically involve the cerebellum but rather brain areas involved in generating the more complex behaviors.

Given the limitations just described, it is possible to speculate about the precise conditions under which the cerebellum becomes engaged during associative learning and how the cerebellum might encode the learning. The cerebellum seems to become critically involved in simple motor learning when (1) discrete, aversively motivated responses are involved; (2) the learning involves the pairing of two stimuli; a neutral stimulus preceding a second stimulus that activates somatosensory inputs into the brain; and (3) the temporal lag between the stimuli is no greater than 4 to 5 s and no less than 50 to 80 ms.

As depicted in figure 5.1, we can hypothesize that the aversive, somatosensory input used as an US is projected into the cerebellum along at least two sources of input: climbing fibers that arise from neurons in the dorsal accessory inferior olive and mossy fibers that arise from brainstem nuclei that relay information about US presentation. The US input produces a rather discrete reflex (called the *UR*) by activating brainstem nuclei or spinal cord areas responsible for generating a response that corresponds to the somatosensory input used to elicit the response (e.g., an eyeblink to a corneal air puff, a forepaw flexion to electrical stimulation of the forepaw skin, a hindlimb flexion to electrical stimulation of the foot pad). The neutral, signaling stimulus designated as the *CS* is projected into the cerebellum by way of axons that originate in the pontine nuclei. For conditioning to occur, the CS and US inputs must arrive in the cerebellum and associated brain stem circuitry within the time window defined by the ISI function. In this model of conditioning, the CS input of a given modality would remain invariant across conditioning paradigms. For example, a tone CS would be expected to activate the same cerebellar and brainstem areas during eyeblink conditioning as during forepaw conditioning. Cerebellar representation of the US input, however, would depend on the location on the body where the US was applied, a topography that is defined by the patterns of somatosensory input from climbing fibers or mossy fibers activated by the US. In this manner, a rather fixed region of the cerebellum would be activated by the CS, whereas the region of the cerebellum activated by the US would depend on where on the body the US was applied. Neuronal plasticity associated with the various types of classical conditioning could then occur in any area of the cerebellum (cerebellar cortex or deep nuclei) that received overlapping CS and US input. As discussed earlier, although the precise roles of cerebellar cortical and deep nuclear plasticities in eyeblink conditioning have not been defined, it seems clear that together these brain areas are critically involved in the acquisition and performance of a major category of aversive, classically conditioned skeletal muscle responses.

THE LOCALIZED VERSUS DISTRIBUTED NATURE OF THE BRAIN SUBSTRATES OF CLASSICAL EYEBLINK CONDITIONING

With the possible exception of data from studies that involved inactivation of the cerebellum during initial acquisition of the eyeblink CR (Clark et al., 1992; Krupa et al., 1993), no data exist that directly prove that critical plasticity necessary for eyeblink conditioning occurs within regions of the cerebellum. Indeed, a controversy has existed in this research area over the last several years about the role of the cerebellum in eyeblink conditioning. Speculation has ranged from a role for the cerebellum in only performance aspects of conditioning with critical sites of learning-related plasticity assumed to be located elsewhere in the brain (e.g., Welsh and Harvey, 1989) to a role for the cerebellum as a critical structure in which plasticity necessary for acquisition and storage of the eyeblink CR occurs (e.g., Thompson, 1986). Even if one assumes that converging CS and US inputs produce plasticity in the cerebellum, there remains the question as to whether this plasticity alone is sufficient to support eyeblink conditioning or if there are other important (if not necessary) brain regions activated during eyeblink conditioning. In other words, one might ask if the site or sites of plasticity critical for eyeblink conditioning are localized to the cerebellum or if critical sites of plasticity are distributed to other regions of the brain. Several brainstem areas are potential sites of conditioning-related plasticity (including the red nucleus, the cranial nerve nuclei responsible for eyeblink reflexes, the trigeminal nucleus, the cochlear nuclei, the basilar pontine nuclei, and the inferior olive). Data concerning plasticity processes in these structures are presented here, with emphasis on those data that relate to classical eyeblink conditioning.

Tsukahara, Oda, and Notsu (1981) have explored the involvement of the red nucleus in classical forelimb flexion conditioning in cats. They showed that the red nucleus, which receives projections directly from the interpositus nucleus, was critically involved in classical leg flexion conditioning. Cats were trained with a microstimulation CS applied to the cerebral peduncle and a shock US applied to the skin of the forelimb. The involvement of the red nucleus in classical eyeblink conditioning in rabbits has been well established. Conditioned response-related activity has been recorded from this structure during rabbit eyeblink conditioning (e.g., Haley, Thompson, and Madden, 1988; Chapman et al., 1990), and red nucleus lesions have produced complete CR abolition (e.g., Rosenfield and Moore, 1983). Data from reversible lesion experiments suggest, however, that the CR-related activity is likely projected to the red nucleus from other brain areas, such as the interpositus nucleus. Lidocaine injections (Chapman et al., 1990) and brain cooling (Clark et al., 1992) of the red nucleus have been done concomitantly with recordings from the interpositus nucleus. In both cases, inactivation of the red nucleus caused abolition of CRs. Relatively normal levels of CR-related activity were still recorded in the interpositus nucleus even though behavioral CRs were blocked by the red nucleus inactivation. These data indicate that the CR-related activity in the red nucleus likely originates in the interpositus nucleus. The role of the red nucleus may be to route this activity to brainstem motor nuclei as well as to other regions of the brain.

A number of studies have delineated the cranial nerve nuclei involved in generating eyeblink responses (i.e., eyelid and nictitating membrane movement) (e.g., Cegavske, Thompson, Patterson, and Gormezano, 1976). Similar to red nucleus recordings, CR-related activity is generated in these nuclei, Young, Cegavske, and Thompson (1976) demonstrated tone-induced changes in excitability in motoneurons that make up part of the path responsible for nictitating membrane (NM) extension in rabbits. They tested the excitability of the NM response to air puff and the excitability of abducens motoneurons (neurons partially responsible for NM extension) to electrical stimulation delivered at various times after presentation of a 350-ms tone. The excitability to air puff increased at tone onset and gradually decreased following tone offset. This same function was observed when the excitability of abducens motoneurons was tested. During paired training involving a tone CS and air puff US, no increases in excitability of abducens motoneurons were noted as CR developed. However, rabbits given tone-abducens stimulation testing showed large savings during subsequent tone–air puff training. These data showed that although tonic increases in excitability of this cranial nerve nucleus did not occur when CRs formed, the nucleus was nevertheless plastic, showing rapid changes in excitability during CS-US pairings. More recent evidence supports the idea that the eyeblink motor nuclei receive CR-related input from other brain regions and that CRs are not simply the result of plasticity within these nuclei (Disterhoft, Quinn, Weiss, and Shipley, 1985; Steinmetz et al., 1992a). In these experiments, rabbits received standard classical eyeblink conditioning followed by lesions of the accessory abducens nucleus. Immediately after the lesions, very large reductions in CR and UR amplitude and frequency were noted. With additional training, CR amplitude recovered (presumably through the activation of other eyeblink-related motoneurons) whereas UR amplitudes remained suppressed for the duration of training. These data are consistent with the hypothesis that CR-related activity is generated in the cerebellum and projected down onto a variety of motor nuclei responsible for eyeblink conditioning. However, the Young et al. (1976) study suggests that the motor nuclei are more than passive receivers of the cerebellar input during paired training. These nuclei appear to show phasic excitability changes related to paired CS-US training, changes that could shape performance of the conditioned and reflex responses.

The cochlear nuclei and trigeminal nucleus contain the first synapses in the brain for both auditory information arising from the tone CS and somatosensory information arising from the air puff US, respectively. Both of these brain regions are therefore candidate sites for plasticity associated with eyeblink conditioning. Woody et al. recorded single-unit activity from the dorsal cochlear nuclei (Woody, Wang, Gruen, Landeira-Fernandez, 1992) before and after classical conditioning in the cat. Conditioning was established with an acoustic CS and glabellar-tap US. After conditioning, they observed an increase in the percentage of units that responded to the auditory CS. Similar results were found when ventral cochlear recordings were performed (Woody, Wang, and Gruen, 1994). These data demonstrate conditioning-related plasticity at early, precerebellar synapses involved in transmitting auditory CSs into the brain. Though similar recording studies have not been done in the trigeminal nucleus, it is possible that conditioning-related changes in the trigeminal could affect US inputs to cerebellar and other brain stem areas. For example, Bracha, Wu, Cartwright, and Bloedel (1990) showed that alterations of activity in the trigeminal nucleus affected CR and UR production. Lidocaine infused into the region of the trigeminal nucleus of previously trained rabbits altered CR or UR frequency and amplitude (or both) depending on the site of the infusions. Though these studies show that conditioning-related activity occurs in brainstem nuclei located very early in the pathways thought to be involved in projecting the CS and US to the cerebellum, there are data that suggest that these regions are not necessary for eyeblink conditioning. First, lesions of the pontine nuclei (Steinmetz et al., 1987) and inferior olive (McCormick et al., 1985; Yeo et al., 1986) abolished conditioning, thus demonstrating that plasticity in the cochlear and trigeminal nucleus could not support eyeblink conditioning independently. Second, we produced eyeblink conditioning in rabbits by using microstimulation of the pontine nuclei as a CS and microstimulation of the inferior olive as a US (Steinmetz, Lavond, and Thompson, 1988). In this preparation, the cochlear and trigeminal nuclei were bypassed, and stimulation was delivered directly to the cerebellar afferents hypothesized to project CS and US information into the cerebellum. Even though eyeblink conditioning can be established without activating the cochlear and trigeminal nuclei, plasticity in the auditory and air puff relay systems normally may occur during eyeblink conditioning with peripheral stimuli, perhaps supporting increased attentiveness to the conditioning stimuli, as has been suggested by Woody et al., (1994) for the cochlear nuclei.

The pontine nuclei and the inferior olive are other potential sites of plasticity during classical eyeblink conditioning. As shown in figure 5.1, we have hypothesized that these sites are involved in relaying the CS and US into the cerebellum during conditioning. Recording studies have shown that both of these brain regions change their patterns of firing over the course of conditioning. We have shown that cells in the lateral region of the basilar pontine nuclei are responsive to auditory input; auditory-related discharges can be seen in this region when tone CSs are presented (Steinmetz et al., 1987). We also have preliminary (unpublished) data that indicate that this auditory-evoked activity increases significantly over the course of training, possibly reflecting changes occuring in the pontine nuclei or changes occuring afferent to the pons (e.g., in the cochlear nuclei). Furthermore, Gohl, Clark, and Lavond (1993) have shown that in addition to the auditory-related discharge, some pontine sites develop CR-related activity over the course of paired training. The CR-related activity may be projected to the pontine nucleus via axons that originate in the interpositus nucleus. Lesions of the interpositus nucleus abolish the CR-related component of the pontine recordings but do not affect the auditory-evoked responses. We also have recorded from the dorsal accessory olive over the course of eyeblink conditioning (Sears and Steinmetz, 1991). No auditory-related activity was observed but, as predicted, evoked responses to the air puff US were recorded early in training. Surprisingly, the evoked responses decreased as the rabbits acquired the conditioned eyeblink response until little if any air puff–evoked activity was present in the inferior olive when CRs were near 100 percent. The air puff–evoked responses were present, however, on US-alone trials that were given at the end of each session. We have speculated that as CR-related activity builds in the interpositus nucleus, an increase in inhibition of olivary cells occurs either through direct (Anderson et al., 1988) or indirect (Weiss et al., 1990) sources of inhibitory input to the olive. The pontine and olivary recording data show that activity in the nuclei hypothesized to send input to the cerebellum during eyeblink conditioning is not static throughout training. Rather, the activities in these structures change as a result of conditioning. Because these two sites are afferent to the cerebellum, changes in there sites could provide a powerful modulatory effect on the input into the cerebellum, an effect that likely contributes to plasticity processes associated with classical eyeblink conditioning.

Neural plasticity generated by classical conditioning is certainly not confined to the cerebellum and brainstem but also can be seen in areas such as the hippocampus, thalamus, and neostriatum. Over the years. a variety of experiments have shown that amplitude/time-course models of behavioral CR are formed in the hippocampus (Berger and Thompson, 1978) though this activity seems to be dependent in some fashion on activity in the interpositus nucleus (Clark, McCormick, Lavond, and Thompson, 1984; Sears and Steinmetz, 1990). Under some conditions, the hippocampus is necessary for classical trace conditioning; lesions of the hippocampus have been shown to impair or abolish trace conditioning (Moyer, Deyo, and Disterhof, 1990). We have recorded CR-related activity in the thalamic region that receives projections from the cerebellar nuclei, and we have shown that lesions of the interpositus nucleus —but not red nucleus lesions—abolish the behavior-related activity (Sears, Logue, and Steinmetz, in press). We have hypothesized that the thalamus relays information from the interpositus nucleus to a number of higher brain areas, perhaps to integrate the learned eyeblink response into the ongoing behavior of the animal. Other researchers have shown that conditioning-related plasticity occurs within the thalamus independent of lower brain areas (Rispal-Padel and Meftah, 1992). Finally, we have done extensive recordings from the rabbit neostriatum during eyeblink conditioning and observed a variety of neuronal responses including evoked activity to the CS and US and neurons that modeled the behavioral CR (White, Miller, White, Dike, Rebec, and Steinmetz, 1994). These data suggest a role for the neostriatum in eyeblink conditioning and suggest that this paradigm may be useful for advancing our understanding of interactions between the basal ganglia and cerebellum.

CONCLUSIONS

A rather impressive array of data argue for the critical involvement of the cerebellum in acquisition and performance of discrete, aversive, classically conditioned, skeletal muscle responses. We are currently operating under the assumption that plasticity occurs in the cerebellar cortex and the deep nuclei owing to convergent CS and US input. The plasticity is assumed to play a major role in producing the well-timed learned responses that are characteristic of this type of conditioning. The data reviewed herein, however, also argue strongly that the cerebellum is not the only brain structure to show alterations in activity related to classical eyeblink conditioning. A variety of other structures seem to be involved in coding this very simple type of motor learning. However, still to be examined is the relative independence of each structure in establishing plasticity during eyeblink conditioning. Such examination may be accomplished in future studies by inactivating areas know to be critical for normal conditioning, such as the interpositus nucleus, while recording activity in target structures before, during, and after conditioning. Areas of the brain that show independent changes in excitability could then be studied more closely for their independent contributions to the conditioning process.

The preceding data speak to the localized versus distributed nature of the neural substrates of classic eyeblink conditioning. There is no doubt that the total neural network involved in eyeblink conditioning is distributed widely across the brain, encompassing cerebellar, brainstem, and forebrain areas. It is likely that the involvement of all these areas allows the learning and memory of this class of relatively simple behaviors under a variety of stimulus parameters, timing conditions, contexts, and response demands. However, the data also argue that a rather localized core brain network, comprised of the cerebellum (cortex and nuclei) and associated brainstem areas, is necessary for the acquisition and performance of this type of conditioning. Future experiments designed to study the particulars of the cerebellar-based network—and how this smaller neural network operates within the confines of the larger brain network known to be involved in encoding this and other forms of learning —should advance our understanding of the brain substrates of motor learning and adaptation.

ACKNOWLEDGMENTS

I acknowledge a number of graduate students who have worked with me at Indiana University and whose data are, in part, presented here. These students include Lonnie Sears, Thomas Gould, Daniel Miller, M. Todd Allen, Wesley White, and Ilsun White. I also thank Donald Katz for helpful comments on an earlier version of this text. Our research was supported by National Institute of Mental Health grant MH44052, funds from the Indiana University Research Fund and the Indiana University Graduate School, and funds from the Indiana University Center for the Integrative Study of Animal Behavior.

REFERENCES

Allen MT, Steinmetz JE (1994). Cerebellar single-unit activity during discrimination learning to different CS-US intervals in the classically conditioned rabbit eyeblink paradigm. Soc Neurosci Abstr 20:795.

Anderson G, Garwicz M, Hesslow G (1988). Evidence for a GABA-mediated cerebellar inhibition of the inferior olive in the cat. Brain Res 472:450−456.

Berger TW, Thompson RF (1978). Neuronal plasticity in the limbic system during classical conditioning of the rabbit nictitating membrane response: I. The hippocampus. Brain Res 145:323−346.

Berthier NE, Moore JW (1986). Cerebellar Purkinje cell activity related to the classically conditioned nictitating membrane response. Exp Brain Res 63:341−350.

Berthier NE, Moore JW (1990). Activity of deep cerebellar nuclear cells during classical conditioning of nictitating membrane extension in rabbits. Exp Brain Res 83:44−54.

Bracha V, Wu JZ, Cartwright M, Bloedel JR (1990). Selective effects of lidocaine microinjections into the region of the spinal trigeminal nucleus on the conditioned and unconditioned responses of the rabbit nictitating membrane reflex. Soc Neurosci Abstr 16:474.

Cegavske CF, Thompson RF, Patterson MM, Gormezano I (1976). Mechanisms of efferent neuronal control of the reflex nictiating membrane response in rabbit (*Oryctolagus cuniculus*). J Comp Physiol Psychol 90:411−423.

Chapman PF, Steinmetz JE, Sears LL, Thompson RF (1990). Effects of lidocaine injection in the interpositus nucleus and red nucleus on conditioned behavioral and neural responses. Brain Res 537:149−156.

Clark RE, Lavond DG (1993). Reversible lesions of the red nucleus durig acquisition and retention of a classically conditioned behavior in rabbits. Behav Neurosci 107:264−270.

Clark GA, McCormick DA, Lavond DG, Thompson RF (1984). Effects of lesions of cerebellar nuclei on conditioned behavioral and hippocampal neuronal responses. Brain Res 291:125−136.

Clark RE, Zhang AA, Lavond DG (1992). Reversible lesions of the cerebellar interpositus nucleus during acquisition and retention of a classically conditioned behavior. Behav Neurosci 106:879−888.

Daum I, Schugens MM, Ackermann H, Lutzenberger W, Dichgans J, Birbaumer N (1993). Classical conditioning after cerebellar lesions in humans. Behav Neurosci 107:748−756.

Disterhoft JF, Quinn KJ, Weiss C, Shipley MT (1985). Accessory abducens nucleus and conditioned eye retraction/nictitating membrane extension in rabbit. J Neurosci 5:941−950.

Donegan NH, Lowry RW, Thompson RF (1983). Effects of lesioning cerebellar nuclei on conditioned leg-flexion responses. Soc Neurosci Abstr 9:331.

Gallistal CR, Gomita Y, Yadin E, Campbell KA (1985). Forebrain origins and termination of the medial forebrain bundle metabolically activated by rewarding stimulation or by reward blocking doses of pimozide. J Neurosci 5:1246−1261.

Gibbs CM (1992). Divergent effects of deep cerebellar lesions on two different conditioned somatomotor responses in rabbits. Brain Res 585:395−399.

Gohl EB, Clark RE, Lavond DG (1993). Learning related unit activity in the lateral pontine nuclei is abolished with reversible inactivation of the interpositus nucleus. Soc Neurosci Abstr 19:1000.

Gormezano I, Kehoe EJ, Marshall-Goodell BS (1983). Twenty years of classical conditioning research with the rabbit. In JM Sprague, AN Epstein (eds), Progress in Physiological Psychology. New York: Academic, vol 10, pp 197–275.

Gormezano I, Schneiderman N, Deaux EG, Fuentes I (1962). Nictitating membrane classical conditioning and extinction in the albino rabbit. Science 138:33–34.

Gould TJ, Sears LL, Steinmetz JE (1993). Possible CS and US pathways for rabbit classical eyelid conditioning: Electrophysiological evidence for projections from the pontine nuclei and inferior olive to cerebellar cortex and nuclei. Behav Neurol Biol 60:172–185.

Gould TJ, Steinmetz JE (1994). Multiple-unit activity from rabbit cerebellar cortex and interpositus nucleus during classical discrimination/reversal eyelid conditioning. Brain Res 652: 98–106.

Gould TJ, Steinmetz JE (1996). Changes in rabbit cerebellar cortical and interpositus nucleus activity during acquisition, extinction and backward classical eyelid conditioning. Neurobiol Learn Mem. 65:17–34.

Haley DA, Thompson RF, Madden J IV (1988). Pharmacological analysis of the magnocellular red nucleus during classical conditioning of the rabbit nictictating membrane response. Brain Res 454:131–139.

Hardiman MJ, Yeo CH (1992). The effect of kainic acid lesions of the cerebellar cortex on the conditioned nictitating membrane response in the rabbit. Eur J Neurosci 4:966–980.

Harvey JA, Welsh JP, Yeo CH, Romano AG (1993). Recoverable and nonrecoverable deficits in conditioned responses after cerebellar cortical lesions. J Neurosci 13:1624–1635.

Hearst E (1988). Fundamentals of learning and conditioning. In RC Atkinson, J Herrnstein, G Lindzey, RD Luce (eds), Stevens' Handbook of Experimental Psychology, 2nd ed New York: Wiley, vol 2, pp 3–109.

Kelly TM, Zuo C-C, Bloedel JR. (1990). Classical conditioning of the eyeblink reflex in the decerebrate-decerebellate rabbit. Behav Brain Res 38:7–18.

Krupa DJ, Thompson JK, Thompson RF (1993). Localization of a memory trace in the mammalian brain. Science 260:989–991.

Lavond DG, Hembree TL, Thompson RF (1985). Effects of kainic acid lesions of the cerebellar interpositus nucleus on eyelid conditioning in the rabbit. Brain Res 326:179–182.

Lavond DG, Lincoln JS, McCormick DA, Thompson RF (1984). Effects of bilateral lesions of the dentate and interpositus cerebellar nuclei on conditioning of heart-rate and nictitating membrane/eyelid responses in the rabbit. Brain Res 305:323–330.

Lavond DG, Logan CG, Sohn JH, Garner WDA, Kanzawa SA (1990). Lesions of the cerebellar interpositus nucleus abolish both nictitating membrane and eyelid EMG conditioned responses. Brain Res 514:238–248.

Lavond DG, Steinmetz JE (1989). Acquisition of classical conditioning without cerebellar cortex. Behav Brain Res 33:113–164.

Lavond DG, Steinmetz JE, Yokaitis MH, Thompson RF (1987). Reacquisition of classical conditioning after removal of cerebellar cortex. Exp Brain Res 67:569–593.

Lewis JL, LoTurco JJ, Solomon PR (1987). Lesions of the middle cerebellar peduncle disrupt acquisition and retention of the rabbit's classically conditioned nictitating membrane response. Behav Neurosci 101:151–157.

Lincoln JS, McCormick DA, Thompson RF (1982). Ipsilateral cerebellar lesions prevent learning of the classically conditioned nictitating membrane/eyelid response of the rabbit. Brain Res 242:190–193.

Mamounal LA, Thompson RF, Madden J (1987). Cerebellar GABAergic processes: Evidence for critical involvement in a form of simple associative learning in the rabbit. Proc Natl Acad Sci USA 84:2101–2105.

Mauk MD, Steinmetz JE, Thompson RF (1986). Classical conditioning using stimulation of the inferior olive as the unconditioned stimulus. Proc Natl Acad Sci USA 83:5349–5353.

McCormick DA, Clark GA, Lavond DG, Thompson RF (1982a). Initial localization of the memory trace for a basic form of learning. Proc Natl Acad Sci USA 79:2731–2742.

McCormick DA, Guyer PE, Thompson RF (1982b). Superior cerebellar peduncle lesions selectively abolish the ipsilateral classically conditioned nictitating membrane/eyelid response of the rabbit. Brain Res 244:347–350.

McCormick DA, Lavond DG, Clark GA, Kettner RE, Rising CE, Thompson RF (1981). The engram found? Role of the cerebellum in classical conditioning of nictitating membrane and eyelid responses. Bull Psychon Soc 18:103–105.

McCormick DA, Steinmetz JE, Thompson RF (1985). Lesions of the inferior olivary complex cause extinction of the classically conditioned eyeblink response. Brain Res 359:120–130.

McCormick DA, Thompson RF (1984). Neuronal responses of the rabbit cerebellum during acquisition and performance of a classically conditioned nictitating membrane-eyelid response. J Neurosci 4:2811–2822.

Moyer JR, Deyo RA, Disterhoft JF (1990). Hippocampectomy disrupts trace eyeblink conditioning in rabbits. Behav Neurosci 104:243–252.

Nordholm AF, Thompson JK, Dersarkissian C, Thompson RF (1993). Lidocaine infusion in a critical region of cerebellum completely prevents learning of the conditioned eyeblink response. Behav Neurosci 107:882–886.

Perrett SP, Ruiz BP, Mauk MD (1993). Cerebellar cortex lesions disrupt learning-dependent timing of conditioned eyelid responses. J Neurosci 13:1708–1718.

Polenchar BE, Patterson MM, Lavond DG, Thompson RF (1985). Cerebellar lesions abolish an avoidance response in rabbit. Behav Neur Biol 44:221–227.

Rispal-Padel L, Meftah E-M (1992). Changes in motor responses induced by cerebellar stimulation during classical forelimb flexion conditioning in cat. J Neurophysiol 68:908.

Rosenfield ME, Moore JW (1983). Red nucleus lesions disrupt the classically conditioned nictitating membrane response in rabbits. Behav Brain Res 10:393–398.

Sears LL, Logue SF, Steinmetz JE (in press). Involvement of the ventrolateral thalamic nucleus in rabbit classical eyeblink conditioning. Behav Brain Res.

Sears LL, Steinmetz JE (1990). Acquisition of classically conditioned-related activity in the hippocampus is affected by lesions of the cerebellar interpositus nucleus. Behav Neurosci 104:681–692.

Sears LL, Steinmetz JE (1991). Dorsal accessory inferior olive activity diminished during acquisition of the rabbit classically conditioned eyelid response. Brain Res 545:114–122.

Skelton RW (1988). Bilateral cerebellar lesions disrupt conditioned eyelid responses in unrestrained rats. Behav Neurosci 102:586–590.

Steinmetz JE (1990a). Classical nictitating membrane conditioning in rabbits with varying interstimulus intervals and direct activation of cerebellar mossy fibers as the CS. Behav Brain Res 38:97–108.

Stenmetz JE (1990b). Neuronal activity in the rabbit interpositus nucleus during classical NM-conditioning with a pontine-nucleus-stimulation CS. Pyschol Sci 1:378–382.

Steinmetz JE, Lavond DG, Ivkovich D, Logan CG, Thompson RF (1992a). Disruption of classical eyelid conditioning after cerebellar lesions: Damage to a memory trace system or a simple performance deficit? J Neurosci 12:4403–4426.

Steinmetz JE, Lavond DG, Thompson RF (1988). Classical conditioning in rabbit using pontine nucleus stimulation as a conditioned stimulus and inferior olive stimulation as an unconditioned stimulus. Synapse 3:225–233.

Steinmetz JE, Logan CG, Rosen DJ, Thompson JK, Lavond DG, Thompson RF (1987). Initial localization of the acoustic conditioned stimulus projection system to the cerebellum essential for classical eyelid conditioning. Proc Natl Acad Sci USA 84:3531–3535.

Steinmetz JE, Logue SF, Miller DM (1993). Using signaled barpressing tasks to study the neural substrates of appetitive and aversive learning in rats: Behavioral manipulations and cerebellar lesions. Behav Neurosci 107:941–954.

Steinmetz JE, Logue SF, Steinmetz SS (1992b). Rabbit classically conditioned eyelid responses do not reappear after interpositus nucleus lesion and extensive post-lesion training. Behav Brain Res 51:103–114.

Stenmetz JE, Rosen DJ, Chapman PF, Lavond DG, Thompson RF (1986). Classical conditioning of the rabbit eyelid response with a mossy fiber stimulation CS: I. Pontine nuclei and middle cerebellar peduncle stimulation. Behav Neurosci 100:871–880.

Steinmetz JE, Sears LL, Gabriel M, Kubota Y, Poremba A, Kang E (1991). Cerebellar interpositus nucleus lesions disrupt classical nictitating membrane conditioning but not discriminative avoidance learning in rabbits. Behav Brain Res 45:71–80.

Steinmetz JE, Sengelaub DR (1992). Possible conditioned stimulus pathway for classical eyelid conditioning in rabbits: I. Anatomical evidence for direct projections from the pontine nuclei to the cerebellar interpositus nucleus. Behav Neurol Biol 57:103–115.

Stotler J, Miller DP, Steinmetz JE (1990). Cerebellar interpositus nucleus lesions and limbic system activity during classical eyelid conditioning in rabbits. Soc Neurosci Abstr 16:762.

Supple WF, Leaton RN (1990). Cerebellar vermis: Essential for classically conditioned bradycardia in the rat. Brain Res 509:17–23.

Thompson RF (1986). The neurobiology of learning and memory. Science 223:941–947.

Tsukahara N, Oda Y, Notsu T (1981) Classical conditioning mediated by the red nucleus in the cat. J Neurosci 1:72–79.

Van Ham JJ, Yeo CH (1992). Somatosensory trigeminal projections to the inferior olive, cerebellum and other precerebellar nuclei in rabbits. Eur J Neurosci 4:302–317.

Voneida T, Christie D, Bogdanski R, Chopko B (1990). Changes in instrumentally and classically conditioned limb-flexion responses following inferior olivary lesions and olivocerebellar tractotomy in the cat. J Neurosci 10:3583–3593.

Weiss C, Houk JC, Gibson AR (1990). Inhibition of sensory responses of cat inferior olive neurons produced by stimulation of red nucleus. J Neurophysiol 64:1170–1185.

Weisz DJ, LoTurco JJ (1988). Reflex facilitation of the nictitating membrane response remains after cerebellar lesions. Behav Neurosci 102:203–209.

Welsh JP, Harvey JA (1989). Cerebellar lesions and the nictitatig membrane reflex: Performance deficits of the conditioned and unconditioned response. J Neurosci 9:299–311.

Welsh JP, Harvey JA (1991). Pavlovian conditioning in the rabbit during inactivation of the interpositus nucleus. J Physiol (Lond) 444:459–480.

White IM, Miller DP, White W, Dike GL, Rebec GV, Steinmetz JE (1994). Neuronal activity in rabbit neostriatum during classical eyelid conditioning. Exp Brain Res 99:179–190.

Woody CD, Wang X-F, Gruen E (1994). Response to acoustic stimuli increases in the ventral cochlear nucleus after stimulus pairing. Neuroreport 5:513–515.

Woody CD, Wang X-F, Gruen E, Landeira-Fernandez J (1992). Unit activity to click CS changes in dorsal cochlear nucleus after conditioning. Neuroreport 3:385–388.

Yeo CH, Hardiman MJ (1992). Cerebellar cortex and eyeblink conditioning: A reexamination. Exp Brain Res 88:623–638.

Yeo CH, Hardiman MJ, Glickstein M (1985a). Classical conditioning of the nictitating membrane response of the rabbit: I. Lesions of the cerebellar nuclei. Exp Brain Res 60:87–98.

Yeo CH, Hardiman MJ, Glickstein M (1985b). Classical conditioning of the nictitating membrane response of the rabbit: II. Lesions of the cerebellar cortex. Exp Brain Res 60:99–113.

Yeo CH, Hardiman MJ, Glickstein M (1985c). Classical conditioning of the nictitating membrane response of the rabbit: III. Connections of cerebellar lobule HVI. Exp Brain Res 60: 114–126.

Yeo CH, Hardiman MJ, Glickstein M (1986). Classical conditioning of the nictitating membrane response of the rabbit: IV. Lesions of the inferior olive. Exp Brain Res 63:81–92.

Young RA, Cegavske CF, Thompson RF (1976). Tone-induced changes in excitability of abducens motoneurons and of the reflex path of nictitating membrane response in rabbit (*Oryctalagus cuniculus*). J Comp Physiol Psychol 90:424–434.

Zhang AA, Lavond DG (1991). Effects of reversible lesions of reticular or facial neurons during eyeblink conditioning. Soc Neurosci Abstr 17:869

6

Learning and Performance: A Critical Review of the Role of the Cerebellum in Instrumental and Classical Conditioning

John A. Harvey and John P. Welsh

Since the publication of theoretical articles by Marr (1969) and Albus (1971), there have been recurring discussions concerning the possible role of the cerebellum in the acquisition of skilled movements—that is, motor learning (for recent reviews see Thach, Goodkin, and Keating, 1992; Welsh and Harvey, 1992; Bloedel and Bracha, 1995; see also chapters 11 and 13). More recently, it has been suggested that the anterior interpositus nucleus is the site of the neuronal changes underlying acquisition of the nictitating membrane (NM) response and the site of memory storage for learned responses (e.g., see Thompson, 1986; Thompson and Krupa, 1994). However, the recent suggestions that plasticity of cerebellar activity forms the basis for either motor learning or for acquisition of the NM response remain highly controversial.

To evaluate the literature in this area, one must take into account three important facts. First, learning is not a uniform construct; there are many forms of learning. Second, no consistent terminology has been applied to the different forms of learning that have been employed to gain insight into cerebellar regulation of learned behaviors. Indeed, the frequent use of improper definitions has tended to blur important issues. For example, as will be described further, the majority of studies that have examined the role of the cerebellum in learning have not employed procedures that would provide an explicit measure of motor learning. Moreover, the classically conditioned NM response is not an example of motor learning but rather of associative learning. Third (and perhaps most important) no consistent attempt has been made to carry out control studies that would indicate the degree to which changes in acquisition or retention of conditioned responses (CRs) can be attributed to a role of the cerebellum in learning or in the performance of a learned movement. This chapter will emphasize the current literature dealing with the role of the cerebellum in learning and performance, and attempt to address these issues. Because of their historical importance, some of the earlier papers in this area also have been reviewed (for a more detailed historical review, see Welsh and Harvey, 1992). Research dealing with the role of the cerebellum in regulating the vestibuloocular reflex will not be reviewed because its modification via learning is neither instrumental nor classical, and this unique form of adaptational learning has been reviewed recently (du Lac, Raymond, Sejnowski, and Lisberger, 1995; see also chapter 2).

INSTRUMENTAL AND CLASSICAL CONDITIONING

For animal experimentation, the convention of dividing learning into instrumental and classical (Pavlovian) forms remains appropriate for understanding the role of the cerebellum in learning. Instrumental conditioning is accomplished by defining a desired response and bringing it under stimulus control. For example, pressing a lever or turning left in a T-maze might be rewarded with the presentation of a positive stimulus (food for a hungry animal) or with the escape from or avoidance of an aversive stimulus (cold water or electric shock). The important aspect of this form of conditioning is that the reward cannot occur until the identified response has been produced by the animal; this is the basic feature that distinguishes instrumental from classical conditioning (see table 6.1). In classical conditioning, the experimenter defines a target response and then chooses an unconditioned stimulus (US) that will elicit that response as an unconditioned response (UR) and a conditioned stimulus (CS) that does not initially elicit that target response. Acquisition of CRs to the CS depends solely on the appropriate temporal pairing of the CS and US in a situation in which the animal has no control over the delivery of either the CS or US or over their temporal relationship. For example, during instrumental conditioning of leg flexion, an animal can flex its leg to the CS and thus avoid receiving the shock US or flex its leg to the US and thus escape from further shocks. By contrast, in classical conditioning, the shock is delivered at the same time after CS onset regardless of whether a leg flexion has or has not occurred. Indeed, classical conditioning can occur in the absence of any responses made by the animal (see Welsh and Harvey, 1991, 1992). Thus, procedures that block the occurrence of the CR and UR will not prevent the acquisition of a classically conditioned response but would, of course, totally prevent the acquisition of instrumental responses. Because classical conditioning requires only that there is a temporal pairing of two stimuli (the CS and US), it provides a measure of associative learning but not of motor learning as defined here (see table 6.1).

Table 6.1 Types of Learning and Their Characteristics

Response Characteristics	Instrumental Learning		Classical Pavlovian
	Motor Learning	Not Motor Learning	
Response is followed by reward.	Yes	Yes	No
Response is required for learning.	Yes	Yes	No
Changes in response topography are rewarded and measured.	Yes	No	No

INSTRUMENTAL CONDITIONING AND MOTOR LEARNING

Instrumental conditioning can be subdivided based on the degree to which exteroceptive and interoceptive stimuli come to control the targeted response. For exteroceptive stimuli, animals may be required to depend on spatial cues within the environment (spatial learning) or on auditory and visual stimuli explicitly provided by the experimenter (simple or conditional discriminations). The actual motor acts involved in these forms of instrumental learning are often in the repertoire of the animal (e.g., pecking a key for a pigeon, licking for a rat, ambulating). In this context, the experimenter may define learning to be the increasingly efficient use of these exteroceptive stimuli by the animal so as to produce the response targeted by the investigator. However, such an instrumental paradigm is not necessarily a paradigm of motor learning, because it is not the type of behavior per se that is of interest to the experimenter, but rather the increased use of the exteroceptive stimulus.

For an instrumental conditioning procedure to be a measure of motor learning, a specific response topography must be defined by the experimenter. Further, the achievement of this criterion response must result from the differential reinforcement that allows the animal gradually to shape its motor acts to produce the correct response topography and thus to maximize an extrinsic or intrinsic reward. In such a paradigm, the animal usually will need to rely on interoceptive stimuli to produce responses that are temporally and spatially coordinated. For example, animals will need to depend on internal temporal cues (and also on kinesthetic, vestibular, and cutaneous cues) because to learn to traverse a maze skillfully, press a lever efficiently, flex a limb rapidly, or escape quickly from shock usually requires that the animal adjust its posture and coordinate its movements. It is the heightened use of temporal, kinesthetic, vestibular, and cutaneous cues to refine a movement that forms the hallmark of motor learning. These interoceptive cues normally are not under the control of the experimenter but are used by animals to increase the efficiency of their responses and thus to optimize the receipt of a reward. Acquiring an effective tennis or golf stroke for humans or a specific arm movement in a monkey defines motor learning, as does learning to balance on a high wire for a human or on a rotorod for a rodent.

Surprisingly, in spite of the continued interest in the role of the cerebellum in motor learning, only a few studies have employed an instrumental paradigm that provides an explicit measure of motor learning. For example, maze learning does not depend necessarily on the production of a highly specified response topography to obtain a reward, and therefore may not provide a reliable measure of motor learning. Animals with a variety of motor impairments can perform correctly because it does not matter whether the animal crawls, walks, or rolls through the maze as long as its movements take it into the correct arm of a maze. This aspect of instrumental conditioning procedures is best illustrated by a description of the behavior of a female rat following cerebellectomy.

Thirty days after operation the motor symptoms were still pronounced. She walked as if drawing a heavy weight, with fore and hind legs extended forward and dragging her along in a series of lunges. At this time she was tested in the maze and made a perfect retention record (Lashley and McCarthy, 1926, p. 428).

It should be recognized that the considerable degrees of freedom allowed the animal to shape its instrumental response (i.e., travel through the maze) precluded any accurate assessment of motor learning. It also should be clear that the female rat in the previously described study might not have been able to demonstrate its retention of the learned maze habit if the retention score depended on the animal's ability to execute a fixed response topography. Thus, a measure of the acquisition or retention of CRs depends completely on what the experimenter has chosen to define as the criterion performance. This raises the broader issue of how one can distinguish between performance and learning. Clearly in the maze situation described, one would conclude that the animal showed significant motor impairments but had retained a memory of the maze habit. However, if the experimenter had demanded a specific posture for traversing the maze, or required that the rat not touch any of the walls of the maze, one would conclude that the animal had failed to demonstrate retention, perhaps due to its significant motor impairments. Without an independent assessment of motor function, and especially when a stringent response criterion is employed, a conclusion that the memory of the maze had been degraded by the cerebellar lesion would be premature. Thus, the difficulty in demonstrating an impairment in learning is proportional to the difficulty of the motor task; this is especially true when considering the effects of lesions to the cerebellum, in which case the experimenter must differentiate between the deficits in performance due to an impaired ability to learn versus an impaired ability to move.

The example taken from Lashley and McCarthy (1926) also illuminates the fact that the effects of damage to the motor system can be masked by various strategies employed by the animal to produce a response that will be rewarded. It is noteworthy that such strategies may vary from animal to animal. Thus, in some cases, motor impairments (as in humans) may be observed only when response requirements are made more stringent, so that compensation is no longer possible. For example, one can degrade stimulus control or increase response complexity.

THE LEARNING-PERFORMANCE DICHOTOMY

It is important to maintain a distinction between the terms *acquisition* and *learning*, and this is especially critical for lesion studies. Acquisition is what we observe, and it refers to a change in performance across training trials as measured by the frequency of responses, latency to respond, correct versus incorrect response, or any other measures that may be employed. Learning is something we infer when we have ruled out other possibilities. Thus, changes in acquisition do not always mean that learning has been affected; rather, the changes may be due to any number of parameters that can alter performance (e.g., motivation, sensory capacity, motor ability, and temporal organization of behavior). Similarly, an altered retention of a previously learned response may not necessarily imply a loss of memory. A good example is that a well-fed animal will not usually demonstrate retention of an instrumental response that had been rewarded by food, although simply depriving the animal of food will reinstate the response. These distinctions between performance and learning factors are important because, as shown below, changes in motivation, motoric abilities and the ability to time responses are a common effect of cerebellar damage and can influence the performance of both instrumental and classically conditioned responses.

THE EFFECT OF CEREBELLAR LESIONS ON ACQUISITION AND RETENTION OF INSTRUMENTALLY CONDITIONED RESPONSES

Table 6.2 summarizes the studies that have examined the effects of lesions of the cerebellar cortex, of its deep nuclei, and of the inferior olive on the acquisition or retention (and reacquisition) of instrumental aversive (avoidance) conditioning and appetitive conditioning, and on the acquisition of motor learning in which the animal had to acquire the ability to maintain balance or to acquire specific response topographies. We were able to locate 30 publications dating from 1917 to 1995 that report a total of 37 experiments. All but one (Steinmetz, Logue, and Miller, 1993) of the 37 experiments reported that animals with damage to cerebellar circuitry demonstrated a significant acquisition or significant retention and reacquisition of instrumental CRs (marked *Yes* in table 6.2). As summarized in table 6.2, these studies employed pigeons, mice, rats, rabbits, cats, dogs, monkeys, and humans, and involved a variety of reversible and irreversible lesions to cerebellar circuitry (including cerebellectomies, partial or near total destruction of the cerebellar cortex, lesions of the fastigial, interposed, or dentate nuclei, and lesions of the inferior olivary nucleus). In addition, two mutant mouse strains were employed: The lurcher mouse, which demonstrates a genetically determined degeneration of Purkinje cells and a secondary loss of granule and inferior olive cells, and the metabotropic glutamate receptor (mGluR1) mutant, which lacks a subtype of the mGluR1 that is abundant in Purkinje cells. In addition, the experiments employed a variety of stimuli, motor responses, and conditioning paradigms.

Taken together, the majority of these studies (n = 27) found that though animals did demonstrate significant acquisition or retention of CRs (see table 6.2), they were impaired relative to controls. Eight experiments reported no effect of cerebellar damage on acquisition or retention, one experiment reported an accelerated rate of acquisition, and one experiment reported no acquisition.

Figure 6.1 illustrates some of the findings obtained in the experiments (see table 6.2) that examined acquisition of the avoidance response. Dahhaoui,

Table 6.2 Acquisition or Retention of Instrumental Conditioning

Measure	Method	Lesion	Species	Acquired or Retained CRs	Reference
Avoidance conditioning					
SPD	Morris water maze		Lurcher mouse	Yes-A*	Lalonde et al., 1988
VID	Morris water maze		Lurcher mouse	Yes-A*	Lalonde et al., 1993
VID	T-maze	Cerebellar cortex	Rat	Yes-A*	Buchtel, 1970
VID	Shuttle box	Cerebellar cortex	Rat	Yes-A*	Bleek and Peters, 1974
VID	One-way box	Cerebellar coetex	Rat	Yes-A**	Bleek and Peters, 1974
VICS	Shuttle box	Inferior olive	Rat	Yes-A*	Denk et al., 1968
AUCS	Pole climbing	Cerebellar cortex	Rat	Yes-A*	Langer and Klingberg, 1969
AUCS	Shuttle box	Cerebellectomy	Rat	Yes-A*	Dahhaoui et al., 1990
AUCS	Leg flexion	Inferior olive	Cat	Yes-A*	Voneida et al., 1990
AUD	Running wheel	Interpositus	Rabbit	Yes-A**	Steinmetz et al., 1991
AUCS	Shuttle box	Dentate and lateral interpositus	Rat	Yes-A**	Fish et al., 1979
AUCS	Shuttle box	Fastigial and medial interpositus	Rat	Yes-A***	Fish et al., 1979
AUCS	Leg flexion	Cerebellectomy	Dog	Yes-R*	Popov, 1929
AUCS	Shuttle box	Cerebellectomy	Rat	Yes-R*	Dahhaoui et al., 1990
AUD	Leg flexion	Cerebellectomy	Dog	Yes-R*	Gambaryan, 1960
VICS	Lever pressing	Dentate and interpositus	Rat	No-A	Steinmetz et al., 1993
Appetitive learning					
Timing behavior	Lever pressing	Paleocerebellum	Rat	Yes-A*	Kirk et al., 1982
VID	Lever pressing	Cerebellar cortex	Rat	Yes-A*	Buchtel, 1970
VICS	Lever pressing	Dentate and interpositus	Rat	Yes-A**	Steinmetz et al., 1993

VID	Lever pressing	Cerebellar cortex	Cat	Yes-A*	Rubia et al., 1969
VID	Lever pressing	Cerebellar cortex	Cat	Yes-A*	Davis et al., 1970
AUCO	Grasping	Cerebellar damage	Human	Yes-A*	Holmes, 1917
VID	Lever pressing	Cerebellar cortex	Cat	Yes-R**	Rubia et al., 1969
VID	Key pecking	Vermis	Pigeon	Yes-R**	Monjan and Peters, 1970
Match to sample	Key pecking	Vermis	Pigeon	Yes-R**	Monjan and Peters, 1970
AUD	Lever pressing	Vermis	Cat	Yes-R**	Munson and Monjan, 1967
VICS, AUCS, or somesthetic CS	Arm flexion or extension	Dentate nucleus	Monkey	Yes-R*	Spidalieri et al., 1983
SPD	Maze	Cerebellectomy	Rat	Yes-R*	Lashley and McCarthy, 1926
Motor learning					
Equilibrium	Tilt platform		Lurcher mouse	Yes-A*	Lalonde, 1994
Equilibrium	Stationary rotorod		mGluR1 mutant mouse	Yes-A*	Aiba et al., 1994
Equilibrium	Rotating rod	Cerebellectomy	Rat	Yes-A*	Auvray et al., 1989
CFM		Deep nuclei	Cat	Yes-A*	Shimansky et al., 1994
VM		Cerebellar damage	Humans	Yes-A*	Timman et al., 1994
Tongue extension		Inferior olive	Rat	Yes-A*	Welsh, 1994
BIAF		Cerebellar cortex, deep nuclei, or inferior olive	Monkey	Yes-R*	Soechting et al., 1976
Step-tracking, hold-and-resist arm movements		Inferior olive	Monkey	Yes-R*	Kennedy et al., 1982
RM		Interpositus	Cat	Yes-R*	Bloedel and Bracha, 1995

SPD, spatial discrimination; VID, visual discrimination; VICS, visual conditioned stimulus; AUD, auditory discrimination; AUCS, auditory conditioned stimulus; AUCO, auditory command; CFM, complex forelimb movement; VM, visuomotor movement; BIAF, ballistically initiated arm flexion; RM, reaching movement; Yes-A, animals demonstrated acquisition; Yes-R, animals demonstrated retention and reacquisition; No-A, animals demonstrated no acquisition; *, acquisition or retention inferior to controls; **, acquisition or retention equal to controls; ***, acquisition or retention superior to controls.

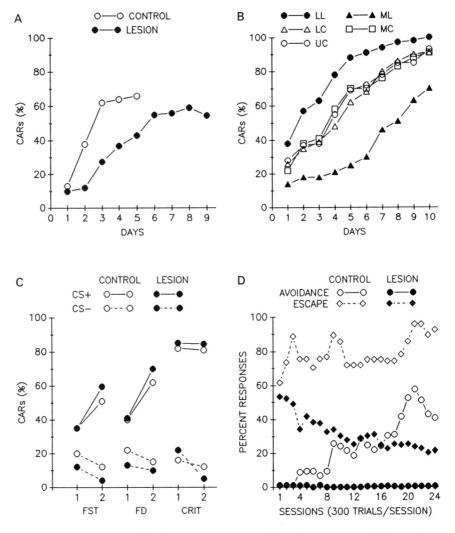

Figure 6.1 Effect of cerebellar lesions on acquisition of avoidance responses. A. Percentage of conditioned avoidance responses (CARs) as a function of days of training for control and cerebellectomized rats. (Adapted from Dahhaoui et al., 1990, with permission from Elsevier Science.) B. Percentage of CARs as a function of days of training for lesions of the dentate plus lateral portion of the interpositus nucleus (LL), lesions of the fastigial plus medial portion of the interpositus nucleus (ML), sham-operated control for LL (LC), sham-operated control for ML (MC), and unoperated control rats (UC). (Based on data presented in Fish et al., 1979 with permission.) C. Percentage of CARs as a function of stages of acquisition of an auditory discrimination in the rabbit. FST, the first conditioning session; FD, the first session during which discriminative avoidance conditioning was observed; CRIT, first session during which the criterion for achievement of a discrimination occurred. The numbers 1 and 2 refer to the first and second block of 60 trials during that session. The CS+ and CS− were 1- or 8-kHz tones. Lesions were placed in the anterior interpositus nucleus. (Adapted from Steinmetz et al., 1991, with permission from Elsevier Science.) D. Percent avoidance (circles) and percent escape (diamonds) responses as a function of 24 conditioning sessions in control rats (open symbols) and rats receiving lesions of the dentate and interpositus nuclei (closed symbols). (Adapted from Steinmetz et al., 1993, Copyright © 1993 by the American Psychological Association.)

Caston, Auvray, and Reber, (1990) found that cerebellectomized rats demonstrated a significant acquisition of a conditioned avoidance response to a tone CS but at a rate that was significantly slower than the acquisition demonstrated by sham-operated controls (see figure 6.1A). Rats with bilateral lesions of the fastigial and medial portions of the interposed nucleus also demonstrated a significant but retarded acquisition of a conditioned avoidance response to a tone CS; however, lesions of the dentate and lateral portions of the interposed nucleus produced an accelerated acquisition (see figure 6.1B; Fish et al., 1979). Rabbits with bilateral damage to the anterior portions of the interpositus nucleus did not differ from controls in their acquisition of a discriminated avoidance response involving a CS^+ and CS^- that differed in frequency (see figure 6.1C; Steinmetz et al., 1991).

The data taken from the only study that failed to observe acquisition of an instrumental avoidance response after a cerebellar lesion (Steinmetz et al., 1993) are presented in figure 6.1D. However, there were a number of problems in this study that make an interpretation of this negative outcome difficult. In this study, rats had to press a lever within 5 s of tone onset to turn off a tone and thus avoid a shock. If they failed to respond to the tone by 5 s, they began to receive foot shocks. A lever press could terminate shock delivery and allow the animal to escape from the shock. If no escape response occurred, the animal would receive a total of four shocks. It should be noted that both the avoidance response and the escape response are learned instrumental behaviors involving the same movement, a lever press. Although rats whose dentate and interpositus nuclei were lesioned failed to demonstrate any evidence of conditioned avoidance responses, they did demonstrate more than 50 percent of escape responses during the first two sessions (comprising a total of 600 trials). Thus, these lesions did not block the ability of the animal to acquire the lever press response per se.

An additional problem with this study is that the acquisition of the avoidance response by control rats was quite slow in that they demonstrated only 40 percent of CRs by the last (twenty-fourth) session (i.e., after 7,200 trials). Because many of the studies cited in table 6.2 reported that animals with damage to cerebellar circuitry demonstrated acquisition but at an impaired rate relative to controls, it is quite possible that more trials might have been needed to observe acquisition by the lesioned animals. The presence of escape responses makes this a more likely conclusion. It should be noted that the decrease in escape responses demonstrated by the lesioned animals is consistent with the acquisition of learned helplessness characteristic of situations in which an animal receives as large number of shocks. Because each failure to escape resulted in the presentation of 4 shocks, we can estimate that lesioned animals have received between 540 and 960 shocks per day.

Figure 6.2 presents some other conditioning paradigms used to examine the effects of damage to the cerebellum. In appetitive tasks employing visual discriminations, lesions of the cerebellar cortex in the rat (see figure 6.2A; Buchtel, 1970) or cat (see figure 6.2B; Davis et al., 1970) retarded but did not

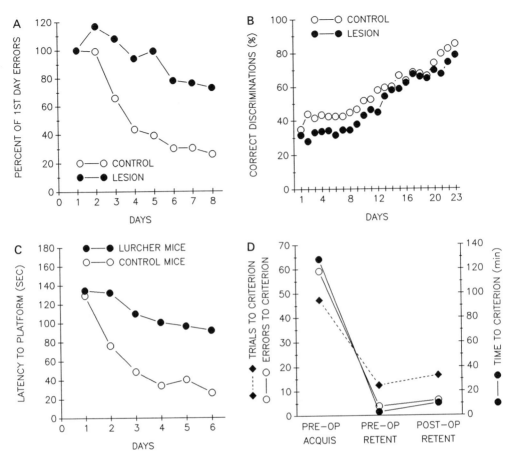

Figure 6.2 Effect of cerebellar lesions on visual discriminations and spatial learning. A. Errors during acquisition of a visual discrimination (plotted as percent of errors committed on the first day of acquisition) are plotted versus days of training for control rats and rats with lesions of the cerebellar cortex. (Adapted from Buchtel, 1970, with permission. Copyright © 1970 by the American Psychological Association.) B. The percent correct discriminations are plotted versus days of training for cats with cerebellar cortical lesions and their controls. (Adapted from Davis et al., 1970, with permission.) C. The acquisition of an avoidance response based on spatial cues. Mice were tested in the Morris water maze, which contains a submerged platform that cannot be seen because the water has been made opaque. The graph presents the latency to reach the platform by lurcher mice who lack Purkinje cells and control mice as a function of days of training. (Adapted from Lalonde et al., 1988.) D. Rats were trained in a maze containing eight culs de sac and then were cerebellectomized. Data are presented in terms of performance as measured by the number of trials to criterion performance (10 consecutive errorless trials), errors to criterion and time to criterion (i.e., time taken to run the maze). Data are presented after acquisition (PRE-OP ACQUIS), 10 days later during a preoperative retention test (PRE-OP RETENT), and 10 days after being cerebellectomized (POST-OP RETENT). (Based on data from mean values reported by Lashley and McCarthy, 1926.)

prevent acquisition of a correct discrimination. In the study by Buchtel (1970), deficits in appetitive conditioning produced by cerebellar damage were related to an altered sensitivity to high levels of motivation. Lesioned rats were retarded in their ability to acquire the visual discrimination when they were in a high motivational state (as shown in figure 6.2A), but acquired at the same rate as controls when they were in a low motivational state (see Buchtel, 1970). It is not clear to what extent motivational effects of cerebellar damage might have affected the outcome of the other studies employing appetitive conditioning.

Lurcher mice with degenerated Purkinje cells in the cerebellar cortex demonstrated acquisition of spatial learning in the Morris water maze but at a rate slower than that in controls (see figure 6.2C; Lalonde et al., 1988). The retention of spatial learning using food reinforcement was also only slightly impaired in cerebellectomized rats (see figure 6.2D; Lashley and McCarthy, 1926).

Figure 6.3 presents three of the eight experiments that measured the acquisition of a motor skill (see table 6.2). In each of these studies, animals had to acquire the ability to maintain their equilibrium on a moving base, a task in which cerebellar patients demonstrate significant impairments (see chapter 4). In one study (Auvray, Caston, Reber, and Stelz, 1989), rats were required to maintain their balance on a rotating rod (see figure 6.3). Normal control rats do not demonstrate acquisition of this motor skill until some time between 18 and 21 days of age. In agreement with this, young rat pups that were cerebellectomized at 10 days of age and immediately trained on a rotating rod showed no acquisition as measured by time spent on the rotorod until approximately age 18 days (see figure 6.3A). Beginning at 18 days, lesioned rats demonstrated significant acquisition but this was greatly retarded relative to their age-matched controls. Cerebellectomies performed at age 20 days, when the animal had developed the ability to acquire this task, had a less severe effect, with lesioned animals demonstrating criterion acquisition but still at a rate slower than that of controls (see figure 6.3B). Finally, cerebellectomies carried out at age 24 days had a small but nonsignificant effect on the rat's ability to maintain its equilibrium on the rotorod (see figure 6.3C). Thus, cerebellar damage produced before the development of a functional circuitry that allows an animal to adjust its posture on a moving surface has the greatest effect on acquisition of this form of motor learning.

The findings in rats were consistent with studies in the lurcher mouse and the mGluR1 mutant mouse, both of which are born with significant cerebellar deficits. Figure 6.3D presents data for lurcher mice that were required to maintain their balance on a tilting platform (Lalonde, 1994). It can be seen that the mice were able to improve their time on the platform over the 6 days of training but remained significantly inferior to control mice. The deficit in acquisition demonstrated by the lurcher mice (see figure 6.3D) was essentially equivalent in severity to the deficit observed in rats cerebellectomized at 10 days of age (see figure 6.3A). The mGluR1 mutant mouse demonstrated even

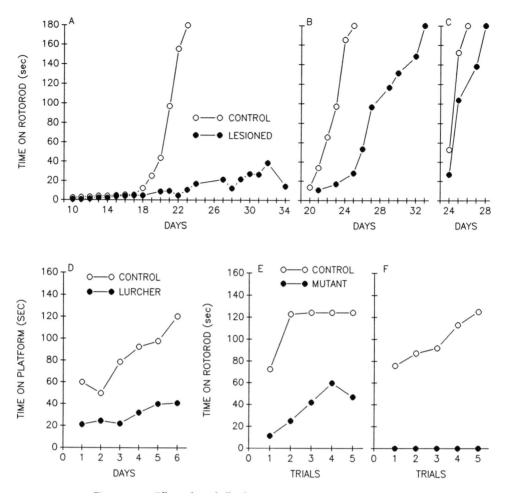

Figure 6.3 Effect of cerebellar lesions on motor learning. Rats were required to maintain their balance on a rotating rod, and the time taken to fall from the rod is plotted as a function of the age of the animals in days. Rats received sham surgery or cerebellectomies at age 10 days (A), 20 days (B), or 24 days (C). Acquisition training began immediately after surgery (at 10, 20, and 24 days) with criterion performance considered to be reached when the animal could maintain its balance on the rotating rod for 180 seconds. (Adapted from Auvray et al., 1989, with permission from Elsevier Science.) D. Lurcher mice and control mice were required to maintain their balance on a tilting platform, and the time taken to fall from the platform is plotted as a function of days of training. Lurcher mice are retarded in acquisition but do demonstrate significant acquisition. (Based on data presented in Lalonde, 1994.) (E, F) mGluR1 mutant mice were required to maintain their balance on a stationary (E) or rotating (F) rotorod. (Adapted from Aiba et al., 1994, with permission.)

more severe deficits in its ability to maintain its posture (Aiba, Kano, Chen, Stanton, Fox, Herrup, Zwingman, and Tonegawa, 1994). Thus, although these mutant mice were able to improve their time on a stationary rotorod, their performance was far below that of control mice (see figure 6.3E), and they were not able to acquire the ability to stay on a rotating rotorod (see figure 6.3F). This latter finding with the mGluR1 mutant mouse emphasizes again the importance of determining whether motor deficits have prevented acquisition during tests of motor learning. The fact that these mutant mice could demonstrate improvement on a stationary rod indicates that motor learning was not eliminated, whereas their lower initial performance on the stationary rod emphasizes that impaired motor ability prevented them from staying on the more challenging rotating rod and thereby demonstrating any significant learning. Similar conclusions were reached in the other studies of motor learning (see table 6.2) that examined acquisition or retention of motor learning involving tongue movements in the rat (Welsh, 1994) and limb movements in the cat (Shimansky, Wang, Bloedel, and Bracha, 1994; Bloedel and Bracha, 1995), monkey (Soechting, Ranish, Palminteri, and Terzuolo, 1976; Kennedy, Ross, and Brooks, 1982), or human (Timmann, Shimansky, Larson, Wunderlich, Stelmach, and Bloedel, 1994).

EFFECT OF CEREBELLAR LESIONS ON THE TEMPORAL ORGANIZATION OF BEHAVIOR

A number of studies cited in table 6.2 presented evidence that damage to the cerebellum may produce changes in acquisition of instrumental behavior due to an impairment in the temporal organization of behavior. In one study, rats could receive a food reward but only if they had waited 20 s before making a lever response (Kirk, Berntson, and Hothersall, 1982). Responses occurring less than 20 s after a previous response were not rewarded and delayed the possibility of a lever press being rewarded by another 20 s. The acquisition of this instrumental task was significantly retarded (but not prevented) in rats receiving lesions of the paleocerebellum (figure 6.4A). Acquisition in part A is measured by the number of reinforcements (food pellets) obtained by the rat per lever press. By the fourth week, this ratio was approximately 0.6 for control rats, indicating that they were pressing the lever approximately 1.7 times for one reward. By contrast, lesioned rats were making approximately 3.3 responses per reward. The basis for this slower acquisition by lesioned animals was reflected by the interresponse times for both control and lesioned rats (see figure 6.4B). It can be seen that the control animals show an orderly distribution of interresponse times, with approximately 60 percent of their responses being spaced the required 20 or more seconds apart. However, the distribution of interresponse times was shifted to the left for lesioned animals, so that only about 30 percent of their responses were spaced 20 or more seconds apart. This result strongly suggests that the cerebellar lesions had affected the timing ability of the animals.

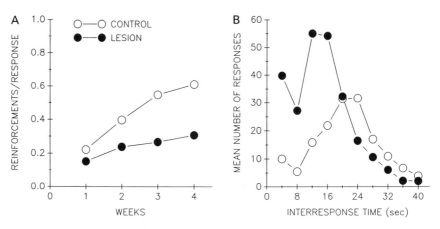

Figure 6.4 Effects of cerebellar lesions on timing behavior. Rats were trained on a differential reinforcement of low rates schedule which requires spacing responses at least 20 seconds apart in order to receive a food reward (see text for further details). A. Acquisition of timing behavior in rats with paleocerebellar lesions and their controls (expressed as the ratio of number of reinforcements received per response) as a function of weeks of training. B. The number of responses as a function of their interresponse times. Note that the modal time between responses was 20 to 24 seconds for controls but 12 to 16 seconds for lesioned animals. (Reprinted with permission from WT Kirk, GB Bernston, D Hothersau, Effects of paleocerebellar lesions on DRL performance in the albino rat. J Comp Physiol Psychol 96:348–360, 1982. Copyright © 1982 by the American Psychological Association.)

A recent study using a novel paradigm of motor learning showed that the olivocerebellar system was required for the temporal organization of behavior but not for associative or motor learning (Welsh, 1994). In an associative learning phase of this study (employing autoshaping), rats were trained to associate a tone CS with a US that was an injection of water into the mouth. The rats acquired a small tongue-protrusion CR to the tone CS over six sessions of associative training. In a motor learning phase of the study, the receipt of the water US was made contingent on the rat's extending its tongue a criterion distance out of its mouth so as to hit a target that could deliver the water onto the tongue. The criterion protrusion distance for receipt of the water was gradually increased over sessions until the rats would extend their tongue 6 mm in response to the tone CS. Neither the acquisition of the tone CS–water US association (figure 6.5A), nor the ability to learn to make lengthened tongue-protrusion CRs (see figure 6.5B) was affected by prior neurotoxic destruction of the inferior olive with 3-acetylpyridine. Both normal rats and rats without their inferior olive (and thus without climbing fiber inputs to Purkinje cells and deep cerebellar nuclei) required about 12 conditioning sessions to acquire the 6-mm tongue-protrusion CR. In contrast, the timing of the tongue-protrusion CR was significantly altered by inferior olive destruction, as evidenced by a significantly increased latency to hit the target after tone onset during the associative learning phase (seè figure 6.5C) and during motor learning (see figure 6.5D) as well as a significantly increased variability in the latency to initiate the response.

CR FREQUENCY

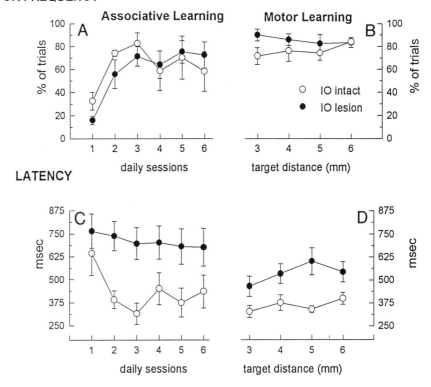

Figure 6.5 Role of the olivocerebellar system in the temporal organization of a learned behavior. A. Frequency of conditioned tongue-protrusion responses (CRs) over six daily sessions of associative (autoshaping) conditioning. Target distance was 2.5 mm. B. Asymptotic frequency of protrusion responses at target distances of 3–6 mm during motor learning. IO = inferior olive. C. Latency from tone onset of tongue-protrusion responses for normal and olivary-lesioned rats over six daily sessions of autoshaping. D. Latencies of tongue protrusion during motor learning when the target was progressively moved away from the mouth. Olivary-lesioned rats took significantly longer to reach the target during both stages of the paradigm (both $p \leq .01$). Control (white circle, $n = 5$) and 3-acetylpyridine-treated (black circles, $n = 8$) rats. Error bars represent 1 standard error of the mean (Welsh, 1994).

An alteration in the temporal organization of behavior was also obtained in a visual matching-to-sample task (Monjan and Peters, 1970). In that study, lesions of the cerebellar cortex in the pigeon had no effect on the number of errors committed during a matching-to-sample task; however, the latency distribution of their responses indicated a significant shift to longer latencies during performance of this task. Increases in reaction times for arm movements were also reported as a result of cerebellar damage in humans (Holmes, 1917; Timmann et al., 1994), cerebellar cortical lesions in squirrel monkeys (Soechting et al., 1976); deep nuclear lesions in the cat (Shimansky et al., 1994) and monkey (Soechting et al., 1976; Kennedy et al., 1982; Spidalieri, Busby, and Lamarre, 1983); and olivary lesions in the cat (Voneida, Christie, Bogdonski, and Chopko, 1990) and monkey (Soechting et al., 1976). Indeed, the past 200 years of research have clearly established that damage to the cerebellum alters the topography and timing of responses (for review see Welsh and Harvey, 1992, and Bloedel and Bracha, 1995).

In summary, the results of the studies presented in table 6.2 are quite consistent. They demonstrate that damage to various portions of cerebellar circuitry impairs but does not abolish an animal's ability to acquire instrumental responses (including motor learning), nor does it abolish an animal's ability to demonstrate retention of previously learned responses. We can conclude thereby that the cerebellum, its deep nuclei, and the inferior olive are not essential for learning and memory of instrumental responses. The question that remains is whether the impaired acquisition observed in the majority of studies simply reflects a motor deficit or whether there is a motor deficit combined with some deficits in learning. Future research should concentrate on this issue. However, at the moment, given the variety of performance deficits after cerebellar lesions due to alterations in motivational, temporal, and motor functions, the most consistent and parsimonious view is that the cerebellum is important for the occurrence of motor behavior coordinated in space and time, and that damage to such a system will produce varying degrees of impairment in instrumental conditioning not attributable to a change in the ability to learn or remember.

THE EFFECT OF CEREBELLAR LESIONS ON ACQUISITION AND RETENTION OF CLASSICALLY CONDITIONED RESPONSES

There is a long history of research examining the effects, on classical conditioning, of damage to the cerebellar cortex or its deep nuclei and these studies have provided a reasonably clear set of results (a review of this history is presented in Welsh and Harvey, 1992, and Bloedel and Bracha, 1995). In general, studies of classical conditioning have confirmed the results obtained with instrumental conditioning: The ability of animals to make an association is not dependent on cerebellar circuitry. Agreement with this view is not currently unanimous because (as in the case of instrumental conditioning) there is confusion as to the relevant measures required to indicate an involvement of the cerebellum in learning as opposed to performance.

The role of the cerebellum in the classical conditioning of eyeblink reflexes has been a focus of research in the last decade. Damage to the cerebellar cortex (especially the cortical zones were microstimulation produced eyeblinks [Hesslow, 1994a]), retarded but did not prevent the acquisition of the conditioned NM response (Lavond and Steinmetz, 1989). Animals with cerebellar cortical lesions also demonstrated an impairment in the retention of previously acquired CRs that was followed by a rapid reacquisition of CRs with further training (Lavond, Steinmetz, Yokaitis, and Thompson, 1987; Harvey, Welsh, Yeo, and Romano, 1993). These cortical lesions did alter the performance of the conditioned and unconditioned NM reflex. Removal of the eyeblink microzones, though not preventing learning, always produced an enduring 50-percent reduction in the amplitude of the CR (Harvey et al., 1993) and increased UR amplitude (hypermetria) above control values (Yeo and Hardiman, 1992). Similarly, the mGluR1 mutant mouse that lacks a metabotropic glutamate receptor located on Purkinje cells (Aiba et al., 1994) demonstrated a significant acquisition of CRs but approximately a 30-percent decrease in CR amplitude. Interruption of climbing fiber inputs to Purkinje cells also failed to block retention and reacquisition of limb flexion CRs in the cat but did reduce the amplitude of the CRs (Voneida et al., 1990; see also Bloedel and Bracha, 1995).

In contrast to cerebellar cortical lesions, lesions of the cerebellum that included the anterior interpositus nucleus prevented CR acquisition (Lincoln, McCormick, and Thompson, 1982), abolished retention, and prevented reacquisition (McCormick and Thompson, 1984; Yeo, Hardiman, and Glickstein, 1985). Considerable debate was generated when it was demonstrated that some rabbits with lesions of the anterior interpositus initiated CRs only at latencies outside the CS-US interval (Welsh and Harvey, 1989b)—reproducing one of the classical neurological symptoms of cerebellar damage: delayed initiation of movement (Holmes, 1917). As in the case of instrumental conditioning described earlier, cerebellar lesions have been repeatedly demonstrated to alter the temporal organization of classically conditioned responses. For example, using CS-alone test trials, cerebellar patients undergoing eyeblink conditioning were found to produce most of their CRs after the time at which the US would have been presented. Consequently, cerebellar patients demonstrated only approximately 7.5 percent of CRs within the CS-US interval but 26 percent outside this interval (Topka, Valls-Solé, Massaquoi, and Hallett, 1993). Similarly, cats that had received inferior olive lesions (Voneida et al., 1990) and cerebellectomized dogs (Fanardjian, 1961) also demonstrated dysmetric CRs.

These observations of a performance deficit in the CR as measured by a reduced amplitude and increased onset latency lead to the hypothesis that cerebellar lesions produce deficits in the performance of CRs but not in associative learning. In a heroic attempt to disprove this classic neurological interpretation, Steinmetz, Logue, and Steinmetz, (1992a) trained three rabbits for 200 days after an anterior interpositus lesion and never observed any CRs, much less any CRs performed at long latency. Nevertheless, their robustly negative result still did not provide any additional insight into the role of the anterior interpositus nucleus in learning, because a large degree of motor impairment after deep nuclear damage is lifelong (Holmes, 1939) and could have prevented those rabbits from responding.

Classical conditioning of the eyeblink response is characterized by the elicitation of CRs by a tone or light stimulus that is initially subliminal (i.e., incapable of eliciting the response overtly) whereas the US is often a suprathreshold stimulation of the cornea that has direct, disynaptic and multisynaptic pathways for UR elicitation. After learning, the tone CS nearly always elicits CRs, but these are produced with far less force than the UR elicited by the US employed during conditioning (Welsh, 1992). Only by decreasing the intensity of the US do the kinematics of the UR more closely resemble those of the CR. Despite initial reports (McCormick and Thompson, 1984; Rosenfield and Moore, 1985), it is now clear that inactivation of the anterior interpositus nucleus (Welsh and Harvey, 1989a,b; Welsh, 1992; Bracha, Webster, Winters, Irwin, and Bloedel, 1994) or red nucleus (Bracha, Stewart, and Bloedel, 1993) reduces the amplitude of URs and can increase their latency, especially when a US equivalent to the CS in its force-generating ability is employed. However, a lesion of the anterior interpositus still has a greater effect on the CR than on the UR, even after equating the CS and US psychophysically.

An opposing view—that the cerebellum does not facilitate performance but only encodes associative memory—was proposed by Steinmetz, Lavond, Ivkovich, Logan, and Thompson (1992b). Based on a previous study by Disterhoft, Quinn, Weiss, and Shipley (1985), they proposed that if the cerebellum served to facilitate motor performance, it would be the UR rather than the CR that should be impaired more by cerebellar lesions (i.e., that the UR was the weaker and more fragile response). This hypothesis contradicted a century of research on conditioned reflexes (Pavlov, 1927) and more than two centuries of research on the cerebellum (see Welsh and Harvey, 1992; Bloedel and Bracha, 1995). Steinmetz et al. (1992b) reported that destruction of the primary motor nucleus for eyeball retraction, the accessory abducens nucleus, reduced the amplitude of the CR and UR to the same extent (i.e., to approximately 7 percent of normal amplitudes). However, with time there was a recovery of CR amplitude to 56 percent of prelesion values, but a nonsignificant recovery in UR amplitude to 23 percent of preoperative values (see figure 13 of Steinmetz et al., 1992b). Given that the preoperative values for the UR were 13.3 mm, we concluded that lesioned animals were demonstrating UR amplitudes of 3.1 mm after the lesion and that the lesions had not destroyed all the motoneurons in the accessory abducens nucleus (see Cegavske, Thompson, Patterson, and Gormezano, 1976; Marek, McMaster, Gormezano, and Harvey, 1984). A second consideration is based on the study of Delgado-Garcia, Evinger, Escudero, and Baker (1990). That study reported that the abducens nucleus could provide a second degree of freedom for CR expression that was not available to the UR. Nevertheless, the highly specific deficits produced by lesions of individual motor nuclei have little bearing on the function of the cerebellum, which obviously is more global and influences multiple pools of motor neurons. Consequently, the experiments of Steinmetz et al. (1992b) provided little insight into the cerebellar regulation of motoneurons responsible for the NM reflex.

Kinematic analysis of unconditioned NM responses (Welsh, 1992) suggested that the cerebellum regulates performance by facilitating, or perhaps by participating in, the longer-latency components of the eyeblink reflex circuit (figure 6.6). Indeed, after an anterior interpositus lesion, the UR evoked by an air puff US is performed with normal velocity until the amplitude of the

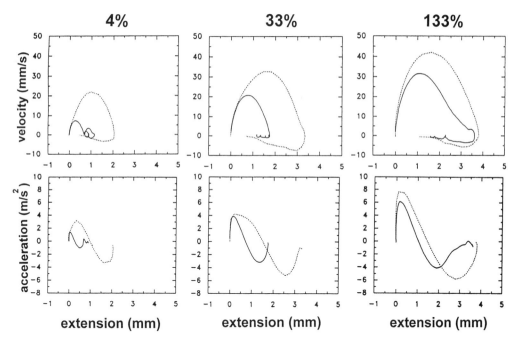

Figure 6.6 Effects of anterior interpositus lesions on the performance of the unconditioned NM response in the rabbit. Plots are shown for URs elicited by three intensities of a corneal air-puff US, and each intensity is expressed as a percentage (4%, 33%, and 133%) of the US intensity that was employed for conditioning. The conditioning intensity elicited a maximal UR amplitude (4–5 mm) and yielded an optimal rate of conditioning. In the top row, UR velocity is graphically represented as a function of UR extension for each of the US intensities. Filled curves represent the mean of seven rabbits with anterior interpositus lesions. Broken curves represent the mean of 10 normal rabbits. Note that (1) peak UR extension is impaired at the lower two intensities but not at the highest intensity after an anterior interpositus lesion; (2) peak UR velocity is reduced at all three intensities after an anterior interpositus lesion; and (3) UR velocity is normal through the first 0.5 mm of the UR but is thereafter impaired at all three US intensities. In the bottom row, UR acceleration is graphically represented as a function of UR extension. Note that there is an early cessation in the acceleration of URs of lesioned rabbits. The data demonstrate the importance of the anterior interpositus nucleus for allowing the long-latency components of the reflex to contribute to the ongoing performance of the UR. (Modified from Welsh, 1992.)

movement reaches about 0.5 mm, approximately 40 ms after UR initiation. At that moment, the NM cannot continue to accelerate, and the velocity is significantly reduced compared to normal URs. This difference was noted across a wide range of US intensities, including US intensities that elicited URs of maximal amplitude. These data suggested that the early disynaptic and the later polysynaptic components of the UR are differentially sensitive to anterior interpositus lesions, so that these lesions leave only the disynaptic contribution toward the UR. Indeed, this hypothesis has been verified by two independent laboratories. First, Gruart and Delgado-Garcia (1994) showed that the firing of identified neurons within the anterior interpositus nucleus does not occur before the initiation of the UR but rather at a latency consistent with an involvement in the longer-latency components of the reflex. Second, Hesslow (1994b) demonstrated that the anterior interpositus is not likely to modulate the early, disynaptic component of the UR phasically; unfortunately, he did not employ US intensities sufficient to elicit longer-latency components of the UR and could not evaluate the magnitude of the cerebellar contribution to the polysynaptic components of the reflex.

The previously cited evidence (indicating that the cerebellum does indeed regulate the motor performance of the UR) in turn makes it impossible to conclude that the impaired acquisition of CRs after interpositus lesions is due solely to a learning deficit. More importantly, recent experiments have provided additional evidence that the cerebellum regulates the performance of CRs in a manner that excludes any interpretation for its role in learning. First, measurement of eyelid responses with electromyography or magnetography have shown that CR latency is much shorter than had been previously thought, is nearly identical to the latency of the weak muscle response elicited by the CS prior to conditioning (Gruart, Blazquez, and Delgado-Garcia, 1994), and occurs before evoked activity within the anterior interpositus (Gruart and Delgado-Garcia, 1994). The latency data indicate that the essential sites of plasticity are located within brainstem pathways and not in a side loop to the cerebellum. Precisely what these pathways are is a matter of conjecture at this time, although anatomical and physiological studies have implicated the pontomedullary reticular formation as contributing to the long-latency component of the UR and as a site of multisensory convergence. CR expression via the polysynaptic pathways of the UR could help explain why cerebellar lesions produce such a devastating effect on CRs (as compared with URs) because cerebellar lesions that impair the polysynaptic component of the UR would necessarily impair the CR. Later components of the CR are even more dependent on normal cerebellar function, as some cerebellar lesions selectively abolish a second accelerative component in the CR but do not reduce CR frequency. Such lesions unarguably leave the memory intact but decrease performance by 30 percent (Welsh, 1992). These results demonstrate that complete specification of a behavior in terms of its kinematics and dynamics can aid in determining effects of a brain lesion on performance versus learning.

More controversial yet have been the conflicting reports of the effects of temporary inactivation of the cerebellum on learning versus performance of eyeblink conditioning. In the first study of this nature (Welsh and Harvey, 1991), we showed that reversible inactivation of the anterior interpositus with microinjections of lidocaine did not prevent eyeblink conditioning, whereas the performance of CRs was prevented (see figure 6.7 for a representative example of this study). However, Nordholm, Thompson, Kersarkissian, and Thompson (1993) obtained a learning deficit by injecting up to 24 times more lidocaine into the anterior interpositus nucleus. Quantitative measurement of diffusion after a 1-μl infusion of 4% lidocaine (see figure 6.7A) suggests that the far larger quantity of lidocaine employed by these investigators—19.2 μl of up to 32% lidocaine—would have produced a diffusion most likely not restricted to the cerebellum, much less the anterior interpositus nucleus, making interpretation of the results difficult.

A second study by Krupa, Thompson, and Thompson (1993) attempted to inactivate the anterior interpositus with muscimol. This experiment found that muscimol injected into either the red nucleus or the anterior interpositus blocked CR performance but that only inactivation of the anterior interpositus would prevent learning when performance was abolished. Krupa et al. (1993) concluded that associative memory is formed and stored in the anterior interpositus nucleus and is expressed via a serial pathway: from the cerebellum to the red nucleus to the motoneurons. However, there were several serious problems with this study. First of all, it employed an unusually high dose of muscimol, approximately 140 times the amount required to block the CR (Bracha et al., 1994; Bloedel and Bracha, 1995). Consequently, there was a large diffusion of muscimol throughout the cerebellar hemisphere, making highly problematic an interpretation about the role of the interpositus in the effects obtained. In addition, the conclusions of Krupa et al. (1993) were based on the arguable assumption that the red nucleus is the only brainstem structure whose input was blocked by a large inactivation of the deep nuclei. The anterior interpositus projects not just to the red nucleus but substantially to the ventrolateral complex of the thalamus, to the nucleus reticularis tegmentum pontis, and to the inferior olive, and likewise to many areas within the mesodiencephalic junction (including the zona incerta, the central gray, and the posterior and anterior pretectal nuclei; see Nieuwenhuys, Voogd, and Van Huijzen, 1991). The conclusion that the learning deficit produced by cerebellar inactivation was specifically due to inactivation of the site of memory storage is not compelling, because it relies on the extreme oversimplification that the anterior interpositus is connected only with the red nucleus. More importantly, it is difficult to interpret this negative outcome, because one cannot know whether learning was disrupted solely by the local effects of the inactivation or by the consequent disruption of the multitude of brainstem circuits receiving input from the region of inactivation.

Finally, the recent development of gene "knockout" animals reinforces the importance of distinguishing between changes in performance and changes in learning. For instance, mGluR1 mutant mice, which lack the metabotropic glutamate receptors normally located in Purkinje cells, have been developed, and their ability to demonstrate eyeblink conditioning has been assessed (Aiba et al., 1994). Both normal mice and mGluR1-deficient mice acquired eyeblink CRs to a tone paired with an eyeshock US. However, though the CR amplitude of normal mice increased over five conditioning sessions, the CRs of mutant mice reached a plateau after the second session and then remained approximately 30 percent below that of controls (see parts A and C of figure 10 in Aiba et al., 1994). This 30 percent reduction in CR amplitude in the absence of the mGluR1 gene is precisely that estimated to be the cerebellar

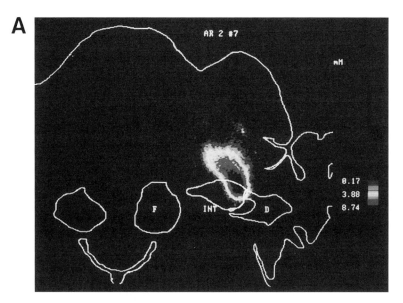

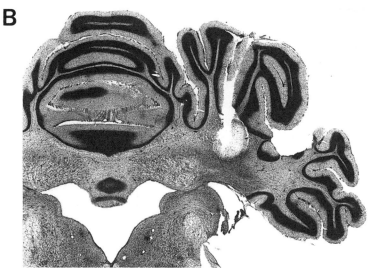

Figure 6.7 Anesthesia of the anterior interpositus nucleus reversibly impairs CRs, but not learning. A. Calibrated autoradiograph of the diffusion of 1 μl of 4% [³H]-lidocaine injected over 1 minute into the dorsolateral anterior interpositus nucleus, which severely impaired CRs. Calibration represents millimolar concentrations of [³H]-lidocaine at 7 minutes after the injection, when CRs were nearly abolished. The area inactivated by anesthetic concentrations of lidocaine (> 0.8 mM) extends 0.8 mm from the dorsolateral anterior interpositus nucleus to the light blue perimeter. Peak concentration within the interpositus was 10.1 mM. Black within the infusion center represents local concentrations exceeding 8.7 mM and not tissue damage. Lidocaine anesthetized the dorsolateral anterior interpositus and overlying white matter without diffusing into the cortex. D, dentate nucleus; INT, anterior interpositus nucleus; F, fastigial nucleus. B. A Nissl-stained section through the cerebellum of another rabbit showing the site in the dorsolateral anterior interpositus where lidocaine was continuously infused (0.1 μl/min) to abolish CRs to a visual CS for 70 minutes. C. The rabbit shown in part B, whose dorsolateral anterior interpositus was anesthetized with lidocaine, did not acquire CRs to a novel tone CS

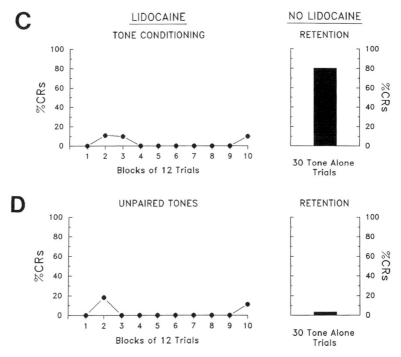

Figure 6.7 (continued)
during the anesthesia (line graph). After lidocaine was withdrawn and performance returned, the rabbit showed normal retention of learning to presentations of the tone alone (bar graph). D. A third rabbit whose dorsolateral anterior interpositus nucleus was anesthetized did not respond to tones presented in an explicitly unpaired manner with the US (line graph). After lidocaine was withdrawn, performance returned but the rabbit showed no CRs to the tone (bar graph). Thus, there was no evidence that retention in part C was due to some nonassociative contributors to responding. For further details, see Welsh and Harvey (1991).

contribution to the longer-latency CR component as determined by kinematic analysis after cerebellar lesions (Welsh, 1992). Thus, this mutant mouse reproduces the now-familiar outcome in that it demonstrated significant associative learning along with an impaired performance of the CR.

CONCLUSION

This review of the literature dealing with the role of the cerebellum in instrumental and classical conditioning has attempted to distinguish effects on performance from those on learning. As has been seen, the majority of studies employing destructive, reversible, and genetically determined lesions of the cerebellum or its circuitry have demonstrated that animals are still able to demonstrate a significant acquisition of CRs. In all these studies, there is a clear deficit in the topography of the CR and UR that represents the classic cerebellar deficits, which include an increased response latency and a decreased response amplitude. It is impossible to ascribe any differences in CR acquisition to a role for the cerebellum in learning, because both instrumental and classical conditioning paradigms have revealed a clear role for the cerebellum in the expression of optimal motor performance. Rather, these data strongly point to the importance of the cerebellum in supporting the optimal execution of motor acts in time and space.

ACKNOWLEDGMENTS

This work was supported by Merit award MH16841 from the National Institute of Mental Health to J. A. Harvey, and by grant NS31224 from the National Institute on Neurological Disorders and Stroke to J. P. Welsh.

REFERENCES

Aiba A, Kano M, Chen C, Stanton ME, Fox GD, Herrup K, Zwingman TA, Tonegawa S (1994). Deficient cerebellar long-term depression and impaired motor learning in mGluR1 mutant mice. Cell 79:377–388.

Albus JS (1971). A theory of cerebellar function. Math Biosci 10:25–61.

Auvray N, Caston J, Reber A, Stelz T (1989). Role of the cerebellum in the ontogenesis of the equilibrium behavior in the young rat: A behavioral study. Brain Res 505:291–301.

Bleek C, Peters M (1974). Learning performance of rats with cerebellar lesions. Acta Biol Med Germ 32:517–525.

Bloedel JR, Bracha V (1995). On the cerebellum, cutaneomuscular reflexes, movement control and the elusive engrams of memory. Behav Brain Res 68:1–44.

Bracha V, Stewart SL, Bloedel JR (1993). The temporary inactivation of the red nucleus affects performance of both conditioned and unconditioned nictitating membrane responses in the rabbit. Exp Brain Res 94:225–236.

Bracha V, Webster ML, Winters NK, Irwin KB, Bloedel JR (1994). Effects of muscimol inactivation of the cerebellar interposed-dentate nuclear complex on the performance of the nictitating membrane response in the rabbit. Exp Brain Res 100:453–468.

Buchtel HA (1970). Visual-learning deficits following cerebellar damage in rats. J Comp Physiol Psychol 72:296–305.

Cegavske CE, Thompson RF, Patterson MM, Gormezano I (1976). Mechanisms of efferent neuronal control of the reflex nictitating membrane response in the rabbit. J Comp Physiol Psychol 90:411–423.

Dahhaoui M, Caston J, Auvray N, Reber A (1990). Role of the cerebellum in an avoidance conditioning task in the rat. Physiol Behav 47:1175–1180.

Davis HN, Watkins GM, Angermeier WP, Rubia FJ (1970). The role of the cortical parts of the cerebellar hemispheres in discrimination learning of cats. Pflügers Arch 318:346–352.

Delgado-Garcia JM, Evinger C, Escudero M, Baker R (1990). Behavior of accessory abducens and abducens motoneurons during eye retraction and rotation in the alert cat. J Neurophysiol 64:413–421.

Denk H, Haider M, Kovac W, Studynka G (1968). Verhaltensänderung und neuropathologie bei der 3-acetylpyridinvergiftung der ratte. Acta Neuropathol 10:34–44.

Disterhoft JF, Quinn KJ, Weiss C, Shipley MT (1985). Accessory abducens nucleus and conditioned eye retraction nictitating membrane extension in rabbit. J Neurosci 5:941–950.

du Lac S, Raymond JL, Sejnowski TJ, Lisberger SG (1995). Learning and memory in the vestibulo-ocular reflex. Annu Rev Neurosci 18:409–441.

Fanardjian VV (1961). The influence of cerebellar ablation on conditioned motor reflexes in dogs (GG Champe transl). Zhurnal Vyshei Nervoi D'eyatel'njosti 11:920–926.

Fish BS, Baisden RH, Woodruff ML (1979). Cerebellar nuclear lesions in rats: Subsequent avoidance behavior and ascending anatomical connections. Brain Res 166:27–38.

Gambaryan LS (1960). Conditioned avoidance reflexes induced in dogs with cerebellar lesions. Physiol Bohemoslov 9:261–266.

Gruart A, Blazquez P, Delgado-Garcia JM (1994). Kinematic analyses of classically-conditioned eyelid movements in the cat suggest a brain stem site for motor learning. Neurosci Lett 175:81–84.

Gruart A, Delgado-Garcia JM (1994). Discharge of identified deep cerebellar nuclei neurons related to eye blinks in the alert cat. Neuroscience 61:665–681.

Harvey JA, Welsh JP, Yeo CH, Romano AG (1993). Recoverable and nonrecoverable deficits in conditioned responses after cerebellar cortical lesions. J Neurosci 13:1624–1635.

Hesslow G (1994a). Correspondence between climbing fibre input and motor output in eyeblink-related areas in cat cerebellar cortex. J Physiol (Lond) 476:229–244.

Hesslow G (1994b). Inhibition of classically conditioned eyeblink responses by stimulation of the cerebellar cortex in the decerebrate cat. J Physiol (Lond) 476:245–256.

Holmes GM (1917). The symptoms of acute cerebellar injuries due to gunshot injuries. Brain 40:461–535.

Holmes G (1939). The cerebellum of man. Brain 62:1–30.

Kennedy PR, Ross H-G, Brooks VB (1982). Participation of the principle olivary nucleus in neocerebellar motor control. Exp Brain Res 47:95–104.

Kirk WT, Berntson GG, Hothersall D (1982). Effects of paleocerebellar lesions on DRL performance in the albino rat. J Comp Physiol Psychol 96:348–360.

Krupa DJ, Thompson JK, Thompson RF (1993). Localization of a memory trace in the mammalian brain. Science 260:989–991.

Lalonde R (1994). Motor learning in lurcher mutant mice. Brain Res 639:351–353.

Lalonde R, Joyal CC, Cote C, Botex MI (1993). Simultaneous visual discrimination learning in lurcher mutant mice. Brain Res 618:19–22.

Lalonde R, Lamarre Y, Smith AM (1988). Does the mutant mouse lurcher have deficits in spatially oriented behaviors? Brain Res 455:24–30.

Langer R, Klingberg F (1969). Die ausarbeitung bedingter fluchtreflexe unter dem einfluss eines kobaltherdes im kleinhirn der ratte. Acta Biol Med Germ 22:819–820.

Lashley KS, McCarthy DA (1926). The survival of the maze habit after cerebellar injuries. J Comp Physiol Psychol 6:423–433.

Lavond DG, Steinmetz JE (1989). Acquisition of classical conditioning without cerebellar cortex. Behav Brain Res 33:113–164.

Lavond DG, Steinmetz JE, Yokaitis MH, Thompson RF (1987). Reacquisition of classical conditioning after removal of cerebellar cortex. Exp Brain Res 67:569–593.

Lincoln JS, McCormick DA, Thompson RF (1982). Ipsilateral cerebellar lesions prevent learning of the classically conditioned nictitating membrane/eyelid response. Brain Res 242:190–193.

Marek GJ, McMaster SE, Gormezano I, Harvey JA (1984). The role of the accessory abducens nucleus in the rabbit nictitating membrane response. Brain Res 299:215–229.

Marr D (1969). A theory of cerebellar cortex. J Physiol (Lond) 202:437–470.

McCormick DA, Thompson RF (1984). Cerebellum: Essential involvement in the classically conditioned eyelid response. Science 223:296–299.

Monjan AA, Peters MH (1970). Cerebellar lesions and task difficulty in pigeons. J Comp Physiol Psychol 72:171–176.

Munson JB, Monjan AA (1967). Cerebellar lesions and auditory thresholds in cat. Physiol Behav 2:161–165.

Nieuwenhuys R, Voogd J, Van Huijzen C (1991). The Human Central Nervous System: A Synopsis and Atlas, 3rd rev ed. Berlin: Springer-Verlag.

Nordholm AF, Thompson JK, Kersarkissian C, Thompson RF (1993). Lidocaine infusion in a critical region of cerebellum completely prevents learning of the conditioned eyeblink response. Behav Neurosci 107:882–886.

Pavlov IP (1927). Conditioned Reflexes (GV, Anrep trans). New York: Dover.

Popov NF (1929). The role of the cerebellum in the formation of conditioned motor reflexes. In DS Fursikov, MO Gurevich, AN Zalmanzon (eds), Vishaya N'Ervnaya D'Eyatel'Nost. Sbornik Trudov Instituta, vol 1, pp 140–148.

Rosenfield ME, Moore JW (1985). Red nucleus lesions impair acquisition of the classically conditioned nictitating membrane response but not eye-to-eye savings or unconditioned response amplitude. Behav Brain Res 17:77–81.

Rubia FJ, Angermeier WF, Davis HN, Watkins GM (1969). The effects of unilateral and bilateral cortical ablations of the cerebellar hemisphere upon learning and retention of an instrumental light-dark discrimination task in adult cats. Pflügers Arch 310:101–108.

Shimansky Y, Wang J-J, Bloedel JR, Bracha V (1994). Effects of inactivating the deep cerebellar nuclei on the learning of a complex forelimb movement. Soc Neurosci Abstr 20:21.

Soechting JF, Ranish NA, Palminteri R, Terzuolo CA (1976). Changes in a motor pattern following cerebellar and olivary lesions in the squirrel monkey. Brain Res 105:21–44.

Spidalieri G, Busby L, Lamarre Y (1983). Fast ballistic arm movements triggered by visual, auditory, and somesthetic stimuli in the monkey: II. Effects of unilateral dentate lesion on discharge of precentral cortical neurons and reaction time. J Neurophysiol 50:1359–1379.

Steinmetz JE, Lavond DG, Ivkovich D, Logan CG, Thompson RF (1992b). Disruption of classical eyelid conditioning after cerebellar lesions: Damage to a memory trace system or a simple performance deficit? J Neurosci 12:4403–4426.

Steinmetz JE, Logue SF, Miller DP (1993). Using signaled barpressing tasks to study the neural substrates of appetitive and aversive learning in rats: Behavioral manipulations and cerebellar lesions. Behav Neurosci 107:941–954.

Steinmetz JE, Logue SF, Steinmetz SS (1992a). Rabbit classically conditioned eyelid responses do not reappear after interpositus nucleus lesion and extensive post-lesion training. Behav Brain Res 51:103–114.

Steinmetz JE, Sears LL, Gabriel M, Kubota Y, Poremba A (1991). Cerebellar interpositus nucleus lesions disrupt classical nictitating membrane conditioning but not discriminative avoidance learning in rabbits. Behav Brain Res 45:71–80.

Thach WT, Goodkin HG, Keating JG (1992). The cerebellum and the adaptive coordination of movement. Annu Rev Neurosci 15:403–442.

Thompson RF (1986). The neurobiology of learning and memory. Science 233:941–947.

Thompson RF, Krupa DJ (1994). Organization of memory traces in the mammalian brain. Annu Rev Neurosci 17:519–549.

Timmann D, Shimansky Y, Larson PS, Wunderlich DA, Stelmach GE, Bloedel JR (1994). Visuomotor learning in cerebellar patients. Soc Neurosci Abstr 20:21.

Topka H, Valls-Solé J, Massaquoi SG, Hallett M (1993). Deficit in classical conditioning in patients with cerebellar degeneration. Brain 116:961–969.

Voneida TJ, Christie D, Bogdanski R, Chopko B (1990). Changes in instrumentally and classically conditioned limb-flexion responses following inferior olivary lesions and olivocerebellar tractotomy in the cat. J Neurosci 10:3583–3593.

Welsh JP (1992). Changes in the motor pattern of learned and unlearned responses following cerebellar lesions: A kinematic analysis of the nictitating membrane reflex. Neuroscience 47: 1–19.

Welsh JP (1994). Importance of the inferior olive in timing a skilled movement: A role for coherent complex spike activity. Soc Neurosci Abstr 20:21.

Welsh JP, Harvey JA (1989a). Modulation of conditioned and unconditioned reflexes. In P Strata (ed), The Olivocerebellar System in Motor Control. Berlin: Springer, vol 17, pp 374–379.

Welsh JP, Harvey JA (1989b). Cerebellar lesions and the nictitating membrane response: Performance deficits of the conditioned and unconditioned response. J Neurosci 9:299–311.

Welsh JP, Harvey JA (1991). Pavlovian conditioning in the rabbit during inactivation of the interpositus nucleus. J Physiol (Lond) 444:459–480.

Welsh JP, Harvey JA (1992). The role of the cerebellum in voluntary and reflexive movements: history and current status. In RR Llinás, C Sotelo (eds), The Cerebellum Revisited. New York: Springer, pp 301–334.

Yeo CH, Hardiman MJ (1992). Cerebellar cortex and eyeblink conditioning: A reexamination. Exp Brain Res 88:623–638.

Yeo CH, Hardiman MJ, Glickstein M (1985). Classical conditioning of the nictitating membrane response of the rabbit: I. Lesions of the cerebellar nuclei. Exp Brain Res 60:87–98.

7 Hippocampal Neuron Changes During Trace Eyeblink Conditioning in the Rabbit

John F. Disterhoft, Michelle A. Kronforst,
James R. Moyer, Jr., L. T. Thompson,
Eddy A. Van der Zee, and Craig Weiss

The hippocampus is thought to be required for the storage of most new cognitive memories in the human. Dramatic evidence for this came from the initial description of the profound amnesia exhibited by the patient HM after bilateral neurosurgical removal of most of the hippocampal formation, amygdala, and associated temporal cortex (Scoville and Milner, 1957). An important feature of temporal lobe amnesia is that patients (such as HM) suffering from it have intact recall of information that was learned and consolidated prior to the trauma to their temporal lobes. In addition, if allowed without distraction to rehearse material containing a limited number of bits of new information, patients can demonstrate recall successfully (Squire, 1987). Their difficulty is in transferring newly learned information from the immediate- or short-term store to long-term storage sites. Further important support for the role of the hippocampus in forming long-term memories came with the description of patient RB, who suffered neuropathologically confirmed bilateral destruction of only his hippocampal CA1 pyramidal neuron region after an ischemic episode (Zola-Morgan, Squire, and Amaral, 1986). RB showed the same type of amnesia as that shown by HM, although it was somewhat less severe, apparently owing to the fact that the neural damage was more limited.

There has been significant effort during the past 40 years (extensively reviewed elsewhere: Cohen and Eichenbaum, 1993; Squire, 1987) to use animal models to explore the mechanisms by which the hippocampal system stores new information in the mammalian brain. The literature covering this research is not only extensive but complicated, as many apparently contradictory results have been reported, but from it a few points may be distilled relevant to the material we will discuss here. First, the lesion method often has been used to determine whether the hippocampus is required for the learning of a particular task (i.e., if the task is hippocampally dependent). This method has the acknowledged limitation that a demonstration of the effect of a lesion on the ability of an animal to learn a task merely indicates that the region under study is a necessary component of the brain circuitry that mediates learning the task. A positive effect of a lesion cannot be interpreted necessarily as indicating that a brain region such as the hippocampus shows localized changes during learning. Second, the kinds of learning tasks sensitive to hippocampal lesions in animal studies are higher-order tasks requiring the animal to integrate spatial information (O'Keefe & Nadel, 1978), to use previously learned information in a flexible fashion (Sutherland and Rudy, 1989; Cohen and Eichenbaum, 1993), or to integrate information temporally (Solomon, 1979; Meck, Church, and Olton, 1984; Moyer, Deyo, and Disterhoft, 1990). Third, in several situations, the hippocampus has shown well-defined neurophysiological or neurochemical changes during learning, even in tasks that do not require the hippocampus for successful acquisition (Olds, Anderson, McPhie, Staten, and Alkon, 1989; Segal, 1973; Berger, Alger, and Thompson, 1976). This could reflect the fact that the hippocampus may store information as a parallel processor, even when it is not required for successful acquisition of a learned task being adequately handled by neural circuits in other brain regions.

Our laboratory has chosen eyeblink or nictitating membrane conditioning in the rabbit as a behavioral model system (Thompson, Berger, Cegavske, Patterson, Roemer, Teyler, and Young, 1976; Disterhoft, Kwan, and Lo, 1977) for exploring the cellular mechanisms by which hippocampal neurons become engaged during the learning process. The eyeblink conditioning model has several advantages for a program such as ours. Rabbits accept restraint readily, facilitating conditioned (CS) and unconditioned stimulus (US) application and measurement of behavioral responses (Akase, Thompson, and Disterhoft, 1994; Thompson et al., 1994a), intravenous or intraventricular drug application (Deyo, Straube, and Disterhoft, 1989; Thompson, Moskal, and Disterhoft, 1992), and single-neuron recording during and after conditioning (Kraus and Disterhoft, 1982; Disterhoft, Quinn, Weiss, and Shipley, 1985; Weiss, Kronforst, Thompson, and Disterhoft, 1993; Weiss, Kronforst, and Disterhoft, 1994). The behavioral parameters of eyeblink conditioning in the rabbit are low in variance and have been well characterized (Gormezano, Prokasy, and Thompson, 1987). Eyeblink conditioning was originally designed by experimental psychologists as a well-defined task for investigating the laws of learning in humans and was subsequently adapted for the rabbit (Gormezano, 1966). In recent years, we and other groups have begun to experiment with human subjects to evaluate hypotheses generated from the animal work (Woodruff-Pak, 1988; Solomon, Beal, and Pendlebury, 1988). Thus, we have considerable confidence that insights into the neurobiological substrates of learning possibly gained from experiments done in rabbits may be generalized to the human (e.g., McGlinchey-Berroth, Cermak, Carrillo, Armfield, Gabrieli, and Disterhoft, 1995; Gabrieli, McGlinchey-Berroth, Carrillo, Gluck, Cermak, and Disterhoft, 1995).

An issue of some relevance for us is our rationale for using the eyeblink conditioning paradigm to study the involvement of the hippocampus in associative learning. The crux of the issue is that, although hippocampal multiple and single neurons have been shown definitively to alter their activity in a conditioning-specific fashion during delay eyeblink conditioning (tone CS precedes and overlaps the air puff US: Berger, Alger, and Thompson, 1976; Berger, Rinaldi, Weisz, and Thompson, 1983), hippocampectomized rabbits can readily acquire this version of the task (Schmaltz and Theios, 1972; Akase, Alkon, and Disterhoft, 1989). In addition, lesions of the cerebellar dentate-interpositus will eliminate ipsilaterally conditioned eyeblink responses that have been acquired previously and make it impossible to acquire new eyeblink conditioned responses (CRs) on that side (Thompson, 1990; Steinmetz, Lavond, Ivkovich, Logan, and Thompson, 1992; however, see Welsh and Harvey, 1989, for a differing view). This has led some neuroscientists to view eyeblink conditioning as a cerebellar or brainstem-mediated task and not an appropriate behavioral model to use for investigating the involvement of forebrain structures such as the hippocampus in learning.

Our strategy for dealing with these issues has been to use a version of the eyeblink task that adds a temporal requirement to the behavioral association. A short tone CS is paired, after a 500-ms interval, with the air puff. Conceptually, the animal must retain a "stimulus trace" that the CS has occurred at a specific point so as to blink its eye at a time that minimizes the impact of the air puff on the cornea. This variant of eyeblink conditioning is termed *trace* conditioning, after the terminology of Pavlov (1927). Trace eyeblink conditioning has been demonstrated to be dependent on the hippocampus for acquisition in the rabbit with a 500-ms trace interval (Solomon, Vander Schaff, Thompson, and Weisz, 1986; Moyer, Deyo and Disterhoft, 1990). Our paradigm with a short CS (100 ms) is especially sensitive to hippocampal damage. We found that hippocampectomized rabbits did not acquire the trace eyeblink response even when trained for 25 successive 80-trial sessions (Moyer et al., 1990). These data indicate empirically that the addition of the long trace period (especially after a short CS, which makes it more difficult to time the CR successfully), makes the contribution of the hippocampus obligatory to form the association. This is consistent with the general concept that the hippocampus is required when animals are learning higher-order tasks that necessitate using information in a novel fashion or to form temporal maps of the environment (Solomon, 1979; Cohen and Eichenbaum, 1993).

In this chapter, we will review our recent experiments using the hippocampally dependent trace eyeblink conditioning task in the albino rabbit. These studies have focused on exploring how single hippocampal neurons change their firing patterns during and after trace conditioning with in vivo recording of single neurons in the behaving animal. They also have focused on determining the involvement of different isoforms of protein kinase C in neuronal changes during learning by using immunocytochemical and biochemical approaches. Finally, they have focused on characterizing the fashion in which postburst afterhyperpolarization (AHP) and spike-frequency accommodation both change in CA1 and CA3 pyramidal neurons during the time at which the trace eyeblink CR is being consolidated (Kim, Clark, and Thompson, 1995).

SINGLE-NEURON RECORDING STUDIES

A well-known series of multiple- and single-unit recording studies were done by Berger, Thompson, and their colleagues during and after delay eyeblink conditioning (Berger and Thompson, 1978; Thompson, Berger, Berry, Hoehler, Kettner, and Weisz, 1980; Berger and Weisz, 1987). They first demonstrated that multiple units in the hippocampus showed enhanced firing very early in the trial sequence, well before rabbits began to show eyeblink CRs (Berger et al., 1976). The altered firing occurred first during the unconditioned response (UR) period of the trial, then moved forward in time and began to occur as the CR was being elicited. In many multiple-unit recordings from CA1 and CA3 hippocampus, the overall shapes of the poststimulus time histogram and of the averaged behavioral response were very similar. Berger and Thompson demonstrated that this temporal modeling was especially prominent in the CA1 and CA3 output regions of the hippocampus. In a subsequent single-neuron study, this group demonstrated that the neural models in hippocampus occurred in pyramidal neurons in the CA1 and CA3 (Berger et al., 1983). They also reported that 83 percent of the hippocampal pyramidal neurons recorded after delay eyeblink conditioning demonstrated altered firing rates at some point within the trial period (i.e., during the CS or US periods).

Permeating the literature from the important series of studies by Berger and Thompson is an overall impression that the majority of neurons in the hippocampus change during eyeblink conditioning, even though this structure is not required for successful acquisition of this version of the task (Schmaltz and Theios, 1972; Berger and Orr, 1983; Akase et al., 1989). Because the "neural modeling" figures have been so widely reprinted, another impression exists: that a large number of neurons demonstrate such a dramatic response during eyeblink conditioning. We sought to reevaluate the percentage of single neurons showing this phenomenon. We were intrigued by the fact that almost all the alterations in pyramidal neurons reported by Berger and Thompson were excitatory, with a relatively small number of changes in the inhibitory direction reported. We also wanted to determine the pattern of single-neuron activity alterations when recordings were done during trace eyeblink conditioning, a hippocampally dependent version of the task. Finally, we set out to sample hippocampal single-neuron activity pattern changes with indwelling electrode arrays, which might record from a broader range of neurons than the sharpened tungsten electrodes inserted on the recording day by Berger et al. (1983) in their single-neuron recording study. This is particularly important given the high percentage of "silent" and slowly firing neurons which have been reported for the hippocampus (Berger et al., 1983; Thompson and Best, 1989).

Therefore, we undertook a series of studies using a moveable array of microwires for recording (Kubie, 1984). The DataWave (formerly Brain Wave) computerized waveform separation system was used to isolate single-neuron activity from the wires. The conditioning task involved pairing a brief tone CS (6 kHz, 100 ms, 85 dB, 5-ms rise and fall time) with an air puff US (150 ms, 3 psi), after a 500-ms stimulus-free trace period. The CS and US presentations were controlled, and the behavioral data was taken with a computerized data acquisition system (Akase et al., 1994; Thompson et al., 1994a). Conditioned rabbits were trained with paired presentations of tones and air puffs. Control rabbits were presented with randomly presented, unpaired tones and air puffs to ensure that the changes were associative and not related to pseudoconditioning or sensitization. The data we will summarize here were gathered during and after behavioral learning had occurred.

Our observations suggest that a smaller percentage of neurons are related to CRs during trace than during delay conditioning. We observed many well-isolated but slow firing "silent cells" that were engaged during trace eyeblink conditioning and that would have been difficult to study with previously used recording techniques. The same number of neurons exhibited decreased as exhibited increased firing rates during various temporal epochs of the conditioning trial. The most frequent response that we observed during the posttrial period (2-s window after a 500-ms UR period) was inhibition. This response appeared to be nonspecific, because it was equally likely to occur during conditioning as during pseudoconditioning. Finally, both excitatory and inhibitory neuron response changes during the trial period occurred.

We have recently completed recordings from 220 neurons in 11 conditioned rabbits (Weiss, Kronforst, Thompson, and Disterhoft, 1993, Weiss, Kronforst, and Disterhoft, 1994); 93 of those neurons were identified as CA1 pyramidal cells and 4 (plus 3 probable) were theta interneurons, based on the spike rate and width criteria accepted for use in these studies (Ranck, 1973; Berger et al., 1983). Surprisingly few theta cells were recorded in this sample, in agreement with Jung, Wiener, and McNaughton (1994) who recorded from rat hippocampus with similar techniques. Statistical criteria were used to define individual neurons as demonstrating excitation or inhibition during a set of trials (40 or 80 trials) as compared to neuronal firing rate during a comparable background period just before the time of CS onset. An analysis of the CA1 pyramidal cells indicated that 58 percent of the cells recorded from rabbits showing at least 60 percent CRs had significant changes in firing rate during the trial. Another 13 percent of the cells also had a significant change in their firing rate, but only during the posttrial period (2 s after a 500-ms UR period). Significant changes during the trial period occurred for all three periods (CS, trace, and UR). During the tone CS, 23 percent of the CA1 pyramidal neurons changed their firing rate. Excitation predominated, but inhibition did occur (14 percent versus 9 percent). During the trace period, 28 percent of the cells had a significant change in firing rate with both excitation and inhibition noted (11 percent versus 17 percent). During the UR period, excitation and inhibition were noted equally, with 47 percent of the cells showing a significant change in firing rate. Approximately

40 percent of the cells had a baseline firing rate of 0.5 Hz or less. Many of these silent CA1 pyramidal cells (N = 34) responded in 5 or fewer of the 20 bins within each analysis period. Those cells were analyzed with the nonparametric binomial test. During the trial period, 12 percent of those slow firing cells had a significant change in firing rate and another 8 percent changed their firing rate during the posttrial period. An approximately equal number of neurons responded both in the 2-s posttrial time period during conditioning and pseudoconditioning trials. This indicates that the posttrial responses, most of which were inhibitory, were not specific for learning the association between tone and air puff.

We did not see the pattern of responses we had anticipated based on the previously published data from delay conditioning (Thompson et al., 1980; Berger et al., 1983). As mentioned, the total number of neurons that changed during the trial period was 58 percent; this number increases to 85 percent if the silent cells are omitted from the analysis. Regardless of whether the silent cells are included, as many of the changes were excitatory as were inhibitory. Figure 7.1 shows as good an example of a "neural model" of the CR as we observed in our recordings during trace conditioning. Because these responses were relatively infrequent, we trained some rabbits in the short-delay paradigm, using a CS which overlapped and coterminated with the US after a 250-ms interstimulus interval as Berger et al. did (1983). As can be seen in figure 7.2, we observed robust neural modeling of the CRs and URs by CA1 pyramidal neurons similar to that which had been reported previously by Berger, Thompson, et al. in both multiple-unit and single-unit recording studies.

Our recordings were made from rabbits that showed at least 60 percent CRs during trace eyeblink conditioning sessions. When we compared activity patterns of the same neurons on trials in which rabbits exhibited CRs and on those where no CR was given, interesting differences were seen in the overall patterns of responses (figure 7.3). Pyramidal neurons simultaneously recorded from nearby electrodes showed a burst of activity during the trace interval and a second burst in correlation with the UR. These responses were distributed more evenly and were considerably larger (on average) across the trial period on CR trials than on interspersed trials in which no CR was present. It was clear that hippocampal neuron activity patterns differentiated CR from non-CR behavioral responses.

One other interesting response pattern might be mentioned. Some presumably inhibitory interneurons showed a temporal model of the CRs and URs sculpted from a high baseline firing rate (figure 7.4). These were termed *inhibitory theta cells* by Berger et al. (1983). The neuron illustrated had a relatively high background firing rate, then reduced its firing rate sharply at or shortly before the beginning of the CR and the UR.

In summary, comparisons of single-unit recordings from rabbits trained in a delay or trace eyeblink conditioning paradigm indicate that neurons recorded in the trace paradigm exhibit less robust but more diverse responses than

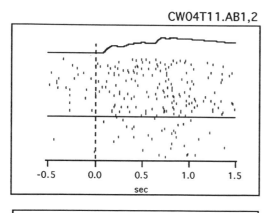

CW04T11.AB1,2

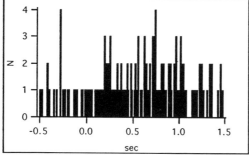

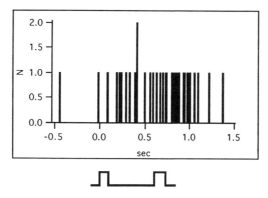

Figure 7.1 The top panel shows a raster display of activity for two single neurons recorded from the same stereotrode during a trace conditioning session with 93 percent of CRs. The rasters for the two neurons are separated by the horizontal line. A plot of the average behavioral data is shown by the top line in this panel. In each raster there are an equal number of trials (trials without activity are not shown). The timing and duration of the tone and airpuff are shown at the bottom of the figure. Histograms of the activity for each neuron are shown below the rasters.

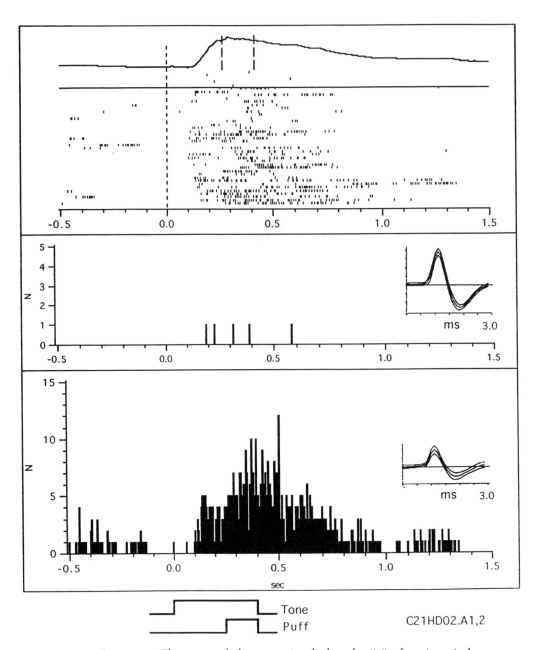

Figure 7.2 The top panel shows a raster display of activity from two single neurons recorded from the same microwire during a delay conditioning session with 97 percent of CRs. A plot of the average behavioral data is shown by the top line in this panel. The rasters for the two cells are separated by a horizontal line. (Note that the first cell responds during very few trials.) Histograms of the activity for each of the two cells are shown below the rasters with an inset which portrays the shape of the average action potential (± 1 standard deviation). The timing and duration of the tone and airpuff are indicated at the bottom of the figure.

150   Disterhoft et al.

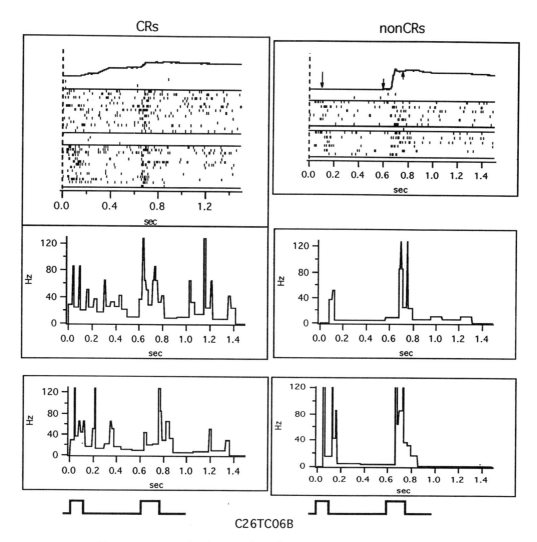

Figure 7.3 Example of activity from the same set of five neurons during a trace conditioning session with 70 percent of CRs. The data are separated into trials with and without CRs. Histograms from two of the five neurons are presented. The firing rate per 10-ms bin is indicated to equate for the difference in the number of trials: 20 CRs, 11 nonCRs. (Note the responses to the air puff during non-CR trials.) The responses have greater "signal to noise" during CR trials, especially during the trace period. Time of tone CS and air puff US presentation are indicated at the bottom.

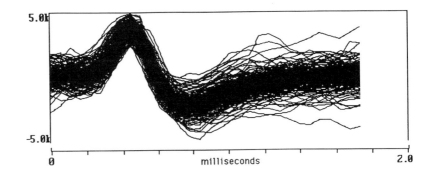

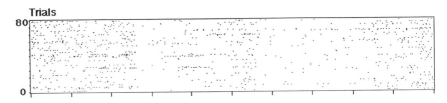

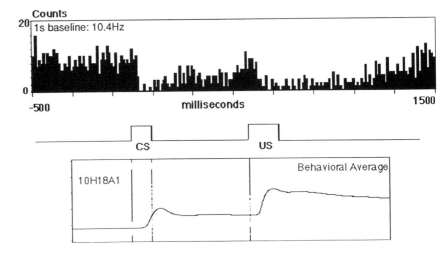

Figure 7.4 Data from an inhibitory interneuron recorded from CA1 during a trace conditioning session with 100 percent of CRs. The top panel shows several superimposed waveforms that characterize this cell. The second panel indicates a raster of the activity recorded from this cell in relation to the tone and air puff. A histogram of the summed activity in the raster is shown in the third panel just above the time-line for the tone CS and air puff US. Tick marks are every 200 ms, and time is measured from tone onset. The bottom panel shows the average behavioral response for this rabbit during the session. (Note the dramatic decrease in firing rate after tone onset with excitation superimposed on the inhibtion.) The inhibition persists for approximately 500 ms after US onset.

those recorded in the delay paradigm. This may reflect more complex processing by specific neurons in hippocampally dependent trace conditioning as compared to a generalized activation of most neurons`in the delay paradigm. The prolonged changes in the posttrial period may represent consolidation processes that occur during the intertrial interval or nonspecific changes, because similar changes were seen after both paired and unpaired trials. It will be necessary to record from single neurons over the course of trace conditioning to determine if the changes during and after the trial period occur as early in the trial sequence as they have been reported to occur in delay conditioning. It also will be of interest to determine if the percentage of neurons which are significantly related to different portions of the CR increases or decreases during training.

ALTERATIONS IN PROTEIN KINASE C$_\gamma$

The protein kinase C (PKC) family consists of at least 10 different isoforms, of which 4 (α, βI, βII, and γ) are calcium-dependent (Nishizuka, 1988). PKC is a cellular second messenger regulated protein involved in neuronal signal transduction pathways by which neurons increase their excitability in response to external inputs (Nishizuka, 1986). PKC activation may serve as a critical step in the chain of biologic events leading to memory formation. PKC activity has been shown to be translocated from the cytosol to the membrane 1 hr after the induction of long-term potentiation (Akers, Lovinger, Colley, Linden, and Routtenberg, 1986), but the data regarding translocation of total PKC from the cytosolic to the membrane fraction in hippocampus 24 hr after delay eyeblink conditioning are inconsistent (Bank, DeWeer, Kuzirian, Rasmussen, and Alkon, 1988; Sunayashiki, Lester, Schreurs, and Alkon, 1993). Evidence for a role of PKC in associative learning has been observed in the rabbit hippocampus after delay eyeblink conditioning (Olds et al., 1989) and in the rat hippocampus after swimming-maze learning (Olds, Golskie, McPhie, Olton, Mishkin, and Alkon, 1990). Increased immunoreactivity for PKC$_\gamma$ has been found in mouse hippocampus after learning a spatial food retrieval task (Van der Zee, Compaan, de Boer, and Luiten, 1992). It is known that application of phorbol esters onto hippocampal slices, which activates PKC, also increases excitability of hippocampal pyramidal neurons by reducing the postburst AHP (Baraban, Snyder, and Alger, 1985). Phorbol ester stimulation of brain slices mimics the increased immunoreactivity for PKC$_\gamma$ as observed after learning (Van der Zee, Strossberg, Bohus, and Luiten, 1993). As will be shown in a following section, hippocampal pyramidal neurons show increased excitability, as evidenced by reduced AHPs, after trace eyeblink conditioning. We sought to determine whether hippocampally dependent 500-ms trace eyeblink conditioning induced changes in the immunoreactivity for calcium-dependent PKC isoforms (Van der Zee, Kronforst, and Disterhoft, 1994). Such altered immunoreactivity could reflect cellular changes that modulate neuronal activity in the hippocampus during learning and memory processes.

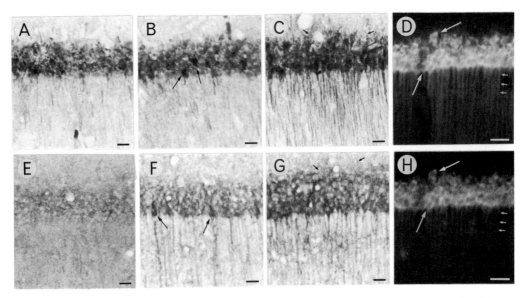

Figure 7.5 Photomicrographs depicting the changes in PKC_γ immunoreactivity (regulatory domain, A–D; catalytic domain, E–H) in the hippocampal CA1 pyramidal cells of naive (A, E), pseudoconditioned (B, F), and trace-conditioned (C, G) rabbits. A significant increase in staining intensity in the cell bodies and apical and basal (small arrows in C, G) dendrites was found only after trace conditioning, although a few cells showed enhanced staining for PKC_γ after pseudo-conditioning (large arrows in B, F). Fluorescence double-labeling demonstrated that the changes for both antibodies raised against different parts of the PKC_γ protein occurred within single cells at the same cellular compartments (arrows in D, H). Scale bar in A–C and E–G = 20 μm; in D and H = 30 μm.

Young adult rabbits were trained to a criterion of 80 percent of CRs in an 80-trial training session in the hippocampally dependent 500-ms trace eye-blink conditioning task as described above. The rabbits were sacrificed 24 hr after reaching behavioral criterion. Brain sections were prepared and immu-nostained with polyclonal antibodies raised against the catalytic subdomain of the calcium-dependent isoforms α, βI, βII, and γ, and a monoclonal anti-body raised against the regulatory subdomain of PKC_γ. The occurrence of translocation, splicing of PKC protein into the single catalytic and regulatory domain, and the total amount of PKC were determined by Western blotting. Hippocampal slices were prepared and stimulated with phorbol ester so as to study the relations among activated PKC, the degree of immunostaining, and Western blot results.

The immunoreactivity for PKC_γ was markedly enhanced in the hippo-campus after conditioning for both the catalytic and regulatory subdomain as compared to pseudoconditioning (unpaired presentations of the tone CS and air puff US) and naive control rabbits (see figure 7.5). Fluorescence double-labeling (figure 7.5 D–H) showed that the increase was found in individual neurons, supporting the assumption that the increase for both antibodies reflects changes in single PKC_γ molecules, both at the level of catalytic and

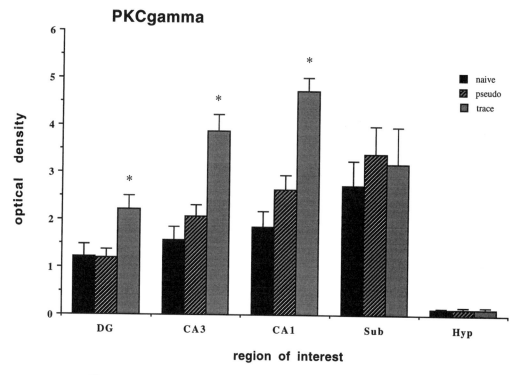

Figure 7.6 Optical density measures for PKC_γ immunoreactivity in the principle cells of the dentate gyrus (DG), CA3, CA1, subiculum (Sub), and hypothalamus (Hyp) of naive (n = 7), pseudoconditioned (n = 7), and trace-conditioned (n = 7) rabbits. A significant increase ($p <$ .05) in optical density was found in the DG, CA3, and CA1 in trace-conditioned as compared to naive and pseudoconditioned animals. No changes were found in the subiculum or hypothalamus.

regulatory subdomain. No gross changes were observed in immunoreactivity for PKC_α, βI, or βII in the three conditions. The optical density of the immunoreactivity for all PKC isoforms was determined, and conditioned animals revealed an approximate 2.5- and 1.8-fold increase in staining intensity in CA1 pyramidal cells for both PKC_γ antibodies over naive and pseudoconditioned animals, respectively (figure 7.6). The change for PKC_γ was found in all hippocampal subregions but the subiculum (figure 7.6). The hypothalamus, serving as a control region, showed no changes for any PKC isoform. Western blotting indicated that the total amount of PKC_γ (both catalytic and regulatory subdomain) did not change after conditioning; nor was there translocation or splicing of PKC_γ after conditioning as compared to the control conditions. An identical increase in PKC_γ immunoreactivity was seen in the phorbol ester–stimulated hippocampal slices as compared to nonstimulated slices. Western blots of such slices revealed translocation from the cytosol to the membrane for PKC_α, whereas no translocation occurred for PKC_γ.

Our data suggest that PKC_γ is the crucial calcium-dependent PKC isoform involved in the signal transduction pathways which alter cellular excitability in the hippocampus during learning. Translocation of PKC_γ seems not to be a crucial aspect of PKC_γ functioning, a finding in agreement with the literature (Oda, Shearman, and Nishizuka, 1991). Because the total amount of PKC_γ is unaltered and there is no detectable translocation or splicing of this PKC isoform, we conclude that a change in protein-protein interaction or a conformational change within the PKC_γ protein determines the degree of immunoreactivity which becomes evident after conditioning. This change must affect both subdomains of the PKC_γ molecule but leaves it intact from splicing. A corollary to this assumption is that this change in the protein could well be the critical cellular change that occurs during learning and contributes to the altered excitability which we observe both in vivo and in vitro after hippocampally dependent trace eyeblink conditioning.

POSTSYNAPTIC EXCITABILITY CHANGES AFTER LEARNING

Recordings of multiple and single neurons in the hippocampus during and after the eyeblink conditioning process show dramatic alterations in firing rate during and after learning. We have reviewed some of the experiments which demonstrate this in delay eyeblink conditioning (Berger et al., 1976, 1983), and we have demonstrated some of our own observations showing large firing rate changes in single CA1 pyramidal neurons after trace eyeblink conditioning (Weiss et al., 1993, 1994). During and after learning, hippocampal neurons increase their firing rate during the trial period (i.e., to the tone presentation) during the CS-US interstimulus interval, or after the air puff US presentation. In both delay and trace eyeblink conditioning, these firing rate alterations can be shown to be conditioning-specific, as they occur only occasionally to the tone CS or the air puff US when they are presented in a random, unpaired fashion during pseudoconditioning. Examination of the histograms shown in figures 7.1 to 7.4 indicate that a large percentage of hippocampal neurons exhibit substantial increases in excitability (evidenced by increased firing rates) during and after conditioning.

Our challenge is to begin to offer an explanation at the cellular or membrane level for these dramatic changes in firing rate which we can record with extracellular recording electrodes. A problem inherent in interpreting firing rate changes recorded in vivo, no matter how dramatic, is to localize the change to a specific set of cells. The interconnections between neurons in the brain are known to be substantial. In fact, there is such extensive interconnectivity within the brain that it is said that any one point is connected to all other points in the brain by some pathway or combination of pathways. Thus, it becomes extremely difficult to determine if an alteration in firing rate recorded from a CA1 pyramidal neuron is localized to that neuron (i.e., it is hard to know if the change in firing rate represents an alteration in the firing characteristics of the neuron under study or of the strength of synaptic weights onto that neuron). Serious consideration must be given to the possibility that the alteration in firing rate recorded from a single neuron in vivo may rather be projected from one of many other places in the brain and expressed secondarily by the CA1 neuron under study.

Localization of learning effects has been approached within in vivo recording situations with a detailed analysis of the timing of alterations between successive sites in a portion of the circuitry involved in the conditioned association (Olds, Disterhoft, Segal, Kornblith, and Hirsch, 1972; Woody, 1974). Our own approach has been somewhat different. We decided to train rabbits, then remove the hippocampus for in vitro analysis. We reasoned that any conditioning-specific alterations detected in this situation cannot be a secondary consequence of changes projected from elsewhere in the brain. Because all normal afferent and efferent connections are severed in the preparation of hippocampal slices, the alterations which are present must be a reflection of changes present within the hippocampus.

The most prominent alteration detected using this approach to date has been a postsynaptic excitability change within CA1 pyramidal neurons (i.e., a reduction in the postburst AHP (Disterhoft, Coulter, and Alkon, 1986). The reduction in the postburst AHP after learning has been shown to be conditioning-specific, to be dependent upon acquisition of the conditioned eyeblink response, and to be present in CA1 neurons even when sodium-dependent synaptic transmission was blocked by tetrodotoxin (TTX) and tetraethylammonium (TEA) (Disterhoft, Golden, Read, Coulter, and Alkon, 1988; Coulter, LoTurco, Kubota, Disterhoft, Moore, and Alkon, 1989; de Jonge Black, Deyo, and Disterhoft, 1990). The AHP has been well-characterized by others and is known to be a reflection of an outward potassium current which is activated by the influx of calcium into the neuron during the burst of action potentials (Hotson and Prince, 1980; Lancaster and Adams, 1986). The AHP is one postsynaptic mechanism to control a neuron's readiness to fire action potentials. A reduction in the AHP brings the membrane potential to a relative state of depolarization sooner after a burst of action potentials, thus allowing more activity to follow. We have suggested that a reduction in the AHP may be one mechanism contributing to the tendency for neurons to be more excitable (i.e., to fire more action potentials) during conditioning trials (Disterhoft et al., 1986).

The experiments we will summarize in this chapter have extended our earlier experiments in several ways. We have used the hippocampally dependent trace eyeblink conditioning paradigm, rather than delay conditioning, to train the rabbits. We have examined the time-course of retention of the excitability changes after rabbits reach a learning criterion, so as to determine how long-lasting the excitability changes are and to detect any potential relation of the excitability changes to the consolidation of the learned behavioral response that is occurring during the period after acquisition occurs. We have demonstrated an alteration in spike frequency accommodation, another measure of cellular excitability related to the postburst AHP, after conditioning. We have examined CA3 pyramidal neurons to determine if they are altered after conditioning in a fashion similar to that of changes observed in CA1 neurons.

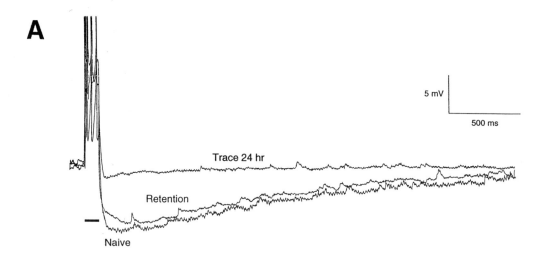

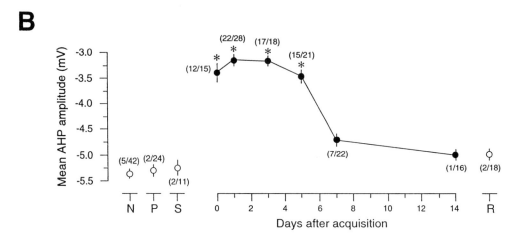

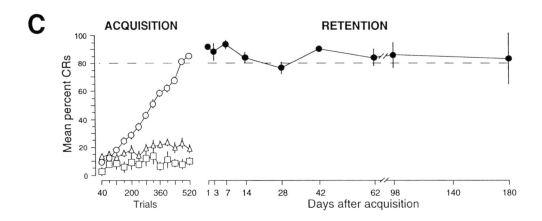

Rabbits were trained in the 500-ms trace eyeblink conditioning paradigm or served as pseudoconditioning controls (Moyer et al., 1990). Hippocampal slices were prepared at various intervals after learning to a criterion of 80 percent of CRs in a training session (Moyer, Thompson, Black, and Disterhoft, 1992). Intracellular current-clamp recordings were performed on more than 200 CA1 and 190 CA3 pyramidal neurons in slices taken from rabbits at time intervals ranging from 1 hr to 14 days after behavioral acquisition to criterion, so as to identify cellular changes occurring during memory consolidation. Strict neuronal stability criteria were used, including resting membrane potentials less than -60 mV and input resistance greater than 30 MΩ. Recordings were made at resting membrane potentials between -65 and -70 mV to control for voltage-dependent effects. Cells were injected with sufficient depolarizing current to elicit a burst of four action potentials for the purpose of studying hippocampal excitability. The amplitude, integrated area, and duration of the postburst AHP were measured.

Postburst AHPs were significantly reduced in both CA1 and CA3 neurons after acquisition of hippocampally dependent trace eyeblink conditioning (figures 7.7 and 7.8). The AHPs were significantly reduced in cells from slices prepared as early as 1 hr after learning (earliest interval tested), were maximally reduced by 24 hr after learning, and slowly decayed over a 1-week time period (figures 7.7 and 7.9). The effect was substantial, with more than 75

Figure 7.7 Acquisition of hippocampally dependent trace eyeblink conditioning transiently reduced the postburst AHP. A. Voltage trace shows an overlay of recordings of the postburst AHPs in CA1 neurons from a naive rabbit (Naive) and from trace-conditioned rabbits studied 24 hr after initial learning (Trace 24 hr) or 24 hr after receiving an additional training session given 14 days after initial learning (Retention). B. Learning-related reductions of the AHP amplitude were transient, lasting about 1 week in slices prepared at various times after learning (1 hr [0 days], 1 day, 3 days, 5 days, 7 days, or 14 days). Numbers in parentheses indicate the ratio of cells with reduced AHPs to number of cells studied (an AHP was considered reduced if its amplitude was more than 1 standard deviation less than the mean for all naive control CA1 cells). Similar numbers of cells were obtained per rabbit in both control and trace-conditioned rabbits, which were counterbalanced to minimize cohort effects. Asterisks indicate data significantly different from all three control groups. N, naive; P, pseudoconditioned; S, slow learners; R, retention; *, indicates $p < .001$. Slow learners were defined as rabbits that did not reach criterion within 15 training sessions and exhibited less than 30% conditioned responses on the last training session. Retention rabbits received an additional training session on the fourteenth day after initial learning. C. After learning, rabbits maintained the learned association. The left panel (acquisition) shows the normalized learning curves for trace-conditioned as compared with pseudoconditioned and slow-learning rabbits. Trace-conditioned rabbits (O, n = 46) required an average of 7.1 ± 0.6 sessions to learn the task. Neither the pseudoconditioned (Δ, n = 11) nor the slow-learning rabbits ($\square$, n = 3) showed significant improvement across sessions. Thus, the pseudoconditioned and slow-learning rabbits served as excellent controls for nonspecific effects of training unrelated to associative learning. The right panel (retention) shows the percent of CRs elicited during 20 paired CS-US trials delivered at various intervals after acquisition. (Note that when retention rabbits ($\bullet$, n = 10) received 20 paired CS-US conditioning trials at the indicated times after learning, they maintained their criterion performance.)

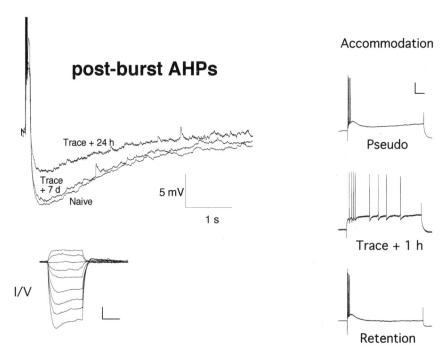

Figure 7.8 Intracellular postsynaptic measures from CA3 pyramidal neurons in hippocampal slices prepared at varying intervals after acquisition of hippocampally dependent 500-ms trace eyeblink conditioning. Evoked postburst AHPs, one measure of postsynaptic excitability, were markedly but transiently reduced after learning. Similarly, spike-frequency adaptation or accommodation was transiently reduced after learning. Other measures, including input resistance, were unaffected by conditioning. Calibration bars for accommodation and current-voltage (I/V) relationships: 20 mV, 100 ms.

percent of cells studied 24 hr after learning showing reduced AHPs (i.e., an AHP amplitude 1 standard deviation below the mean for all naive control cells). The AHPs remained reduced in cells studied up to 5 days after learning but by 14 days after learning, postburst AHPs were indistinguishable from controls, and reduced AHPs were seen in less than 15 percent of the cells studied. The results were the same when data from individual cells were pooled to obtain a mean CA1 or CA3 AHP amplitude value for each rabbit. Learning-related effects on the postburst AHP were not confined to reductions in the peak amplitude. Both the duration and the integrated area of the AHP also were significantly reduced in cells from conditioned rabbits. The reduced AHPs seen after learning were not due to differences in injected current, as the current required to fire a burst of four action potentials did not differ significantly between the groups. No statistically significant differences in resting membrane potential, apparent input resistance, action potential amplitude or action potential width were observed in cells from the trace-conditioned or control rabbits, indicating that the reduced AHPs seen after learning did not result from other voltage-dependent differences in CA1 or CA3.

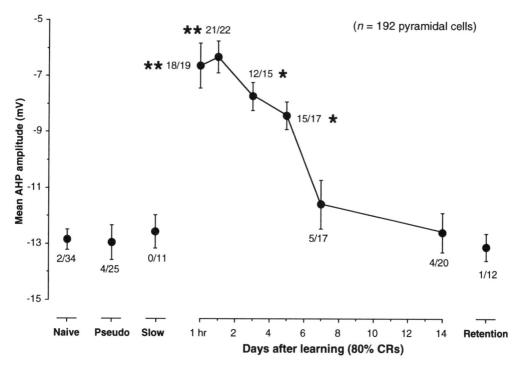

Figure 7.9 The postburst AHPs of CA3 pyramidal neurons were significantly reduced soon after successful acquisition of trace eyeblink conditioning. Neurons from pseudoconditioned or from unsuccesful (slow) learners showed no such change in postsynaptic excitability. The enhanced excitability was transient, sustained maximally for only 24 hr after learning. Over a time-course appropriate for consolidation of the new association, excitability was enhanced but slowly decayed to basal levels, taking approximately 7 days to return to normal. The enhancement was not retention-specific, as the excitability of neurons from rabbits exhibiting asymptotic behavioral retention 2 weeks after acquisition showed basal levels of excitability, quite different from that observed for similarly performing rabbits soon after acquisition.

Spike frequency adaptation or accommodation, another index of excitability, was also transiently reduced after associative learning (figures 7.8 and 7.10). Hippocampal CA1 and CA3 pyramidal neurons from naive, pseudo-conditioned, or slow-learning rabbits showed robust accommodation, which limited their within-burst firing frequencies. Reduced accommodation was apparent as early as 1 hr after learning but decayed quite rapidly (see figure 7.10A). The effect was still significant in CA1 neurons 3 days after learning but by 5 days after learning, accommodation had returned nearly to normal in both regions. Decreased accommodation suggests that hippocampal neurons would be more likely to fire action potentials to excitatory afferent inputs. This effect on accommodation was not previously observed after delay conditioning (Disterhoft, et al., 1986; Coulter et al., 1989), which is not hippo-campally dependent. Decreased accommodation in pyramidal neurons from trace-conditioned rabbits may reflect the added demand for hippocampal processing required for the acquisition or consolidation of the hippocampally

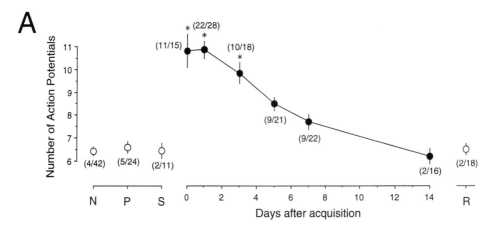

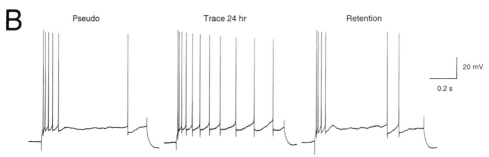

Figure 7.10 Trace eyeblink conditioning resulted in decreased spike frequency adaptation (accommodation) in CA1 neurons. A. The time-course of learning-related changes in accommodation of CA1 neurons was evaluated in the same cells as in figure 7.7, with the same depolarizing current intensity used to study the AHP. Neurons were depolarized for 800 ms and the number of action potentials (APs) was noted. Cells from slow-learning (S) or pseudo-conditioned (P) control rabbits showed no changes, as did cells from retention (R) rabbits that received an additional training session 14 days later. The ratio of cells with reduced accommodation versus the number of cells studied for each group is indicated in parentheses. A cell was classified as having reduced accommodation if the number of APs elicited was at least one standard deviation more than the mean for all naive (N) control cells. Asterisk indicates significant difference from all three control groups: $p < .001$. B. Examples of typical accommodation responses in CA1 pyramidal cells from rabbits after pseudoconditioning (Pseudo), 24 hr after learning (Trace 24 hr) and after receiving an additional training session 14 days after initial learning (Retention). (Note that although the cell from the trace-conditioned rabbit fired more action potentials, accommodation was certainly not abolished—as evidenced by the increase in interspike interval with time—but rather was significantly and transiently reduced after learning.

dependent form of the eyeblink conditioning task (Kim and Faneslow, 1992; Kim, Clark, and Thompson, 1995). Alterations in accommodation may be present in the time period after acquisition of the trace conditioning task during which the hippocampus serves an important function for consolidation of this learned behavior.

Previous multiple- and single-neuron recording studies in delay conditioning (as well as our own single-neuron recording studies with trace conditioning) indicate that CA1 and CA3 pyramidal neurons demonstrate functionally similar changes when recording in vivo in the behaving rabbit. We sought to determine what would occur with our brain-slice approach. The cellular excitability changes in CA3 neurons showed a qualitatively similar size and time-course as did those in CA1 (see figures 7.8 and 7.9). However, the baseline size of the postburst AHP and of the spike frequency accommodation were considerably larger in CA3 than in CA1 pyramidal neurons. This apparently reflects the fact that somatic calcium currents are much larger in CA3 neurons, resulting in larger AHPs and more spike frequency accommodation. The time-course of decay of the reduced spike frequency accommodation was somewhat more rapid than that for the reduced AHP. This suggests that the alterations in accommodation were determined by factors other than just the AHP.

The decay rate of learning-related changes in CA1 and CA3 neurons after trace conditioning was not an artifact related to differences in behavioral acquisition, as there was no difference in learning rate between the trace-conditioned rabbits studied at different intervals after learning. Alternatively, the decay rate could reflect a decrease in behavioral performance over time, as might occur with normal forgetting. To test this hypothesis, rabbits were trace-conditioned to a behavioral criterion of 80 percent of CRs, and CR retention (i.e., consistent performance of the CR) was tested using 20 paired CS-US conditioning trials presented at various intervals ranging from 1 to 128 days after initial acquisition. Their retention performance remained nearly asymptotic at all time intervals tested, evidence that the learned association was maintained or remembered (figure 7.7C). This suggests that the electrophysiological changes observed after learning were not directly related to performance or retention of the CR, as the physiological changes returned to baseline within 7 days, whereas animals maintained behavioral performance above criterion for months. Thus, increased excitability of CA1 and CA3 neurons was required transiently for long-term retention of the learned association.

One more manipulation was done to study more directly the time-dependent dissociation between behavioral retention and in vitro excitability changes. An additional group of rabbits was trained to criterion as described previously and returned to their cages for 14 days without additional training. On the fourteenth day, these rabbits received one 80-trial session of trace eyeblink conditioning. Hippocampal slices were prepared 24 hr later. No excitability increases were observed in CA1 or CA3 cells from this group (see figures 7.7B, 7.8A, and 7.10A), even though these rabbits retained the learned association near the behavioral criterion of 80 percent of CRs. In fact, rabbits that received an 80-trial trace conditioning session 14 days after initial learning performed in a manner indistinguishable from that seen on the day they reached criterion. This direct test, combined with the behavioral retention data cited, led to our conclusion that increased excitability of CA1 pyramidal neurons is related to consolidation (and possibly acquisition), but not to performance or to long-term memory of the learned association.

It is currently of great interest to determine how plastic changes are established during learning. Membrane conductance changes may represent one conserved mechanism used for learning. Such changes have been observed in both vertebrates (Disterhoft, et al., 1986; Coulter et al., 1989; Woody et al., 1991) and invertebrates (Alkon, 1984; Carew and Sahley, 1986). Cholinergic blockers such as scopolamine have been shown to impair classical conditioning in rabbits, but only when the hippocampus is intact (Solomon, Solomon, Vander Schaaf, and Perry, 1983), and acetylcholine application, like conditioning itself, decreases the AHP and blocks accommodation in hippocampal neurons in vitro (Madison and Nicoll, 1984). These data suggest involvement of the cholinergic system and activity of hippocampal neurons with associative learning. Varied other neurotransmitters modulate hippocampal membrane conductances (such as the slow AHP and spike frequency adaptation; Haas and Konnerth, 1983; Colino and Halliwell, 1987). Thus, changes in the release or uptake of neurotransmitters in vivo during learning may set up the excitability changes we observed in vitro after trace eyeblink conditioning. The prominent conductance underlying the postburst AHP is a calcium-activated potassium current, I_{AHP} (Lancaster and Adams, 1986; Storm, 1990). This current regulates excitability by clamping the membrane potential at hyperpolarized levels following a burst of action potentials. With smaller AHPs of shorter duration, CA1 and CA3 neurons can respond more readily to excitatory afferents. Such increased responsiveness could facilitate propagation of information through the hippocampal circuit to other cortical or subcortical regions involved in the trace-conditioned reflex arc (Thompson, 1990; Berger and Bassett, 1992).

The increased excitability that we observed after learning may be maintained by changes in second-messenger systems (e.g., kinases and phosphatases) which regulate the phosphorylation state of ion channels underlying the postburst AHP. Calcium imaging studies in hippocampal neurons have shown that acetylcholine and norepinephrine reduce the calcium-activated slow AHP directly, without reducing calcium influx (Knöpfel, Vranesic, Gähwiller, and Brown, 1990; Müller, Petrozzini, Griffith, Danho, and Connor, 1992). Muscarinic block of the AHP is mediated by increased activity of calcium-calmodulin-dependent protein kinase II (CaMKII; Müller et al., 1992), whereas norepinephrine and other monoamines modulate the AHP via increased activity of protein kinase A (PKA) (Pedarzani and Storm, 1993). Similarly, phorbol esters that directly activate PKC also reduce the AHP

(Baraban et al., 1985; Malenka, Madison, Andrade, and Nicoll, 1986), and altered PKC was reported in the CA1 region from classically conditioned rabbits (Bank et al., 1988; Olds et al., 1989; Sunayashiki-Kusuzaki et al., 1993). Immunoreactivity of PKC$_\gamma$ and of muscarinic receptor subunits is enhanced in hippocampal pyramidal cells after trace conditioning (Van der Zee et al., 1994), suggesting that phosphorylation participates in the regulation of hippocampal excitability and that acetylcholine may be pivotal in regulating the AHP during trace eyeblink conditioning. Because the slow AHP is generated by current through a calcium- and voltage-dependent potassium channel, phosphorylation of this channel during learning would decrease potassium efflux through the channel (and increase excitability), whereas dephosphorylation would leave the channel under the control of membrane potential and intracellular calcium levels (Molloy and Kennedy, 1991). Further study is required to determine whether the changes in hippocampal physiology that we have observed after learning reflect transient changes in various kinases or other second-messenger systems, to determine how these changes are regulated over the time-course of acquisition or consolidation of the trace-conditioned eyeblink response, and to determine whether or not these findings are a generalized feature common to other kinds of learning tasks.

The time-course of changes in hippocampal excitability which we observed are convergent with recent behavioral experiments from other laboratories. Rabbits receiving hippocampal lesions 1 day after acquisition of trace eyeblink conditioning did not retain the CR and could not relearn it, yet when lesions were performed 30 days after learning, retention of the CR was not affected (Kim et al., 1995). These data support our observations and suggest that the hippocampus is not the long-term storage site for this behavioral task. Rather, they indicate that the hippocampus is required temporarily to store information about the CS-US association during acquisition and during consolidation of the learned response, as neither occur if the hippocampus is removed before or shortly after training (Solomon et al., 1986; Moyer et al., 1990; Kim et al., 1995). Similar observations also have been noted in other hippocampally dependent learning tasks in other species. For example, contextual fear memory was abolished in rats that received hippocampal lesions 1 day after conditioned fear training, but not in rats that received lesions 7 to 28 days after training (Kim and Faneslow, 1992). Also, object discrimination learning revealed that monkeys with bilateral hippocampal lesions were severely impaired in their ability to remember recently learned objects, yet they showed normal memory for remotely learned objects (Zola-Morgan and Squire, 1990). The generality of these findings suggests that time-dependent memory consolidation is a conserved feature important for long-term storage of certain kinds of memories.

Finally, we should address the issue of the postsynaptic excitability changes we have described in CA1 and CA3 pyramidal neurons: Changes occur in a large number of pyramidal neurons in both hippocampal areas. In this particular set of data, by using a criterion of an AHP or accommodation change more than 1 standard deviation smaller than the mean of the naive group of neurons, we estimate that 70 to 80 percent of CA1 and CA3 neurons show excitability changes. The percentage of neurons showing an excitability change is much larger than one would expect to occur at random in a large population of neurons in the hippocampus. One might ask how such a postsynaptic excitability change, which would tend to alter the overall responsivity of a large number of neurons, could contribute to the specific patterns of synaptic change that might be anticipated to occur in a structure storing information during the process of associative learning. Conversely, if one considers the pattern of alterations in single-neuron firing rates described earlier in the chapter, how can a rather generalized enhancement in cellular excitability be congruent with the variable pattern of single-neuron firing rates which we have observed with in vivo recording techniques? This is especially paradoxical if one considers that a fairly large number of hippocampal pyramidal neurons (which we have recorded in vivo) are relatively silent or show *inhibitory* changes in response as compared to baseline firing levels.

Our answer to this paradox is a preliminary one at present. We would point out that a generalized postsynaptic alteration in excitability could be one component of the cellular mechanisms involved in setting the stage for more specific changes in synaptic excitability levels. A generalized excitability increase might make the neuron more able or more likely to store a pattern of inputs which were active during the time when the excitability change was being expressed (the period of consolidation of the memory?). Thus, the specificity in the information stored in hippocampal neurons during associative learning would be imposed on the system by the pattern of afferents activated during the learning trials. It seems theoretically possible for a generalized excitability change in the soma and proximal dendrites to contribute to the formation of a rather precise pattern of changes at specific synapses, as defined in a Hebbian fashion, by which afferents are activated by the learning situation. We should stress that while the AHP contributes to the overall tendency of neurons to fire, this one potential does not define totally the overall output firing of the neuron. Therefore, it seems reasonable to posit the theory that the AHP and accommodation changes are members of a family of cellular changes which occur during the learning process. The hippocampal neuron integrates all these changes in its information processing function and produces an individual pattern of firing by that neuron which contributes to the learned behavior.

CONCLUSIONS

We have reviewed recently gathered data with three approaches which describe different levels of neuronal change that occur in the hippocampus during learning and consolidation of an associative task. We assume that the alterations in PKC_γ, postsynaptic excitability, and firing patterns of neurons must be interrelated aspects of changes within the hippocampal system that contribute to the acquisition and performance of the eyeblink conditioned response. Because the variant of eyeblink conditioning that we have used is dependent upon the hippocampus for its acquisition, at least in the rabbit (Solomon et al., 1986; Moyer et al., 1990), we are confident that the conditioning-specific changes we have observed form an integral part of the neural alterations underlying the conditioned response.

The cellular integration of the immunocytochemical, biophysical, and neurophysiological changes we have seen is interesting, although the changes do not necessarily reflect successive steps in a cellular pathway of change. As mentioned in the section on the protein kinase C work, we examined the hippocampus for evidence of alteration in the calcium-dependent PKC isoforms. Our findings indicate that PKC_γ is the isoform most involved in the cellular mechanisms of change during eyeblink conditioning. This finding is consistent with suggestions of those studying PKC involvement in long-term potentiation and in other learning tasks (Akers et al., 1986; Olds et al., 1990; Van der Zee et al., 1992). It is known that phorbol ester activation of PKC pathways leads to reduction in the postburst AHP (Baraban et al., 1985; Malenka et al., 1986). Thus it is reasonable to find reductions in the AHP in the same hippocampal pyramidal cell populations in which PKC_γ is changed. Because the amount of spike frequency accommodation is dependent in large part on the size of the calcium-mediated potassium current underlying the AHP in hippocampal pyramidal neurons, it is reasonable that the two postsynaptic excitability changes we observed occurred together and in concert with PKC_γ changes. It should also be pointed out that the PKC_γ, the AHP, and the accommodation changes all involve calcium-activated cellular responses in an important fashion.

The alterations in single-neuron firing rate that we have observed in vivo are certainly dependent on or related in some important fashion to the immunocytochemical and membrane conductance changes during learning, which we have described in the hippocampus. However, the relationship is likely to be at a higher level. Both the alterations in PKC_γ and those in postsynaptic excitability occur in a large percentage (in fact, in the large majority) of hippocampal pyramidal neurons after learning. Yet the pattern of in vivo firing rate changes is much more complex—for example, there are as many inhibitory as excitatory changes observed, a large number of cells show no firing rate changes and, during the intertrial interval, there are a large number of inhibitory changes that are not conditioning-specific. We do not possess a complete understanding of the relationship between these rather generalized and much more specific patterns of change observed when different techniques are employed for observation. However, our working hypothesis (alluded to in discussing the brain-slice biophysical experiments) is that the generalized second messenger and membrane excitability changes act as facilitators or mediators of cellular change in a general fashion. The more specific pattern of neuronal changes, as defined by which synapses are altered, is defined by the particular pattern of inputs activated during a particular associative task. Thought of in another way, the cells are set up to change by the generalized mechanism. The pattern of change that actually occurs (and allows considerably more specificity of information storage during learning) depends on the population of active inputs as defined in a Hebbian fashion (Hebb, 1949). This conceptual approach is very reminiscent of that proposed by Woody in discussing the pattern of changes observed following eyeblink conditioning in the cat precruciate motor cortex (Woody, 1974).

Finally, we should touch briefly on the relation between alterations that occur in the hippocampus during eyeblink conditioning and other brain structures. The cerebellum is the other brain structure about which we know the most relating to rabbit eyeblink or nictitating membrane conditioning. Several groups agree that unilateral damage to the dentate-interpositus output nuclei leads to the elimination of delay eyeblink responses already acquired and make it impossible to form new CRs (Yeo, Hardimann, and Glickstein, 1984; Thompson, 1990; Steinmetz et al., 1993). In an interesting study combining multiple-unit recording and the lesion approaches, neural engrams in the hippocampus were shown to disappear when delay eyeblink CRs were eliminated by cerebellar deep nuclear damage (Clark, McCormick, Lavond, and Thompson, 1984; Sears and Steinmetz, 1990). Perrett, Ruiz, and Mauk (1993) have subsequently shown that lesions to the anterior cerebellar cortex cause interesting changes in the timing of eyeblink CRs very similar to those resulting from bilateral hippocampectomy. These studies indicated that there is an important relationship between alterations in the hippocampus and in the cerebellum during eyeblink conditioning.

The question of how the hippocampus and cerebellum may be interconnected must then be addressed. Berger and Bassett (1992) described an important multisynaptic pathway by which the hippocampus can affect the cerebellar sensorimotor program running from subiculum, to retrosplenial cortex, to dorsolateral pontine nuclei, and hence to the cerebellar cortex via mossy fibers. Our working assumption is that hippocampal neuron output, altered during conditioning in the ways that we have described, may have a profound effect on cerebellar output via this hippocampal-cerebellar pathway which traverses the retrosplenial cortex as it travels toward the brainstem. A reciprocal multisynaptic cerebellar-hippocampal pathway—from the cerebellar deep nuclei via the ventroanterior thalamus or directly to the frontal cortex and then back to hippocampus—is becoming better appreciated and could play an important role in mediating feedback from the cerebellum to the hippocampus (Larsell and Jansen, 1972; Goldman-Rakic, 1987; Kim, Ugurbil, and Strick, 1994; Middleton and Strick, 1994). In conclusion, the alterations in hippocampal output that we have observed have the potential to impact on the cerebellar circuitry, and thus the developing CR at the sensorimotor control level, via reciprocal pathways that are becoming better understood but remain relatively understudied, given their potential importance.

ACKNOWLEDGMENTS

The studies summarized here were supported by National Institutes of Health grants R01 AG08796, DA07633, and MH47340 (JF Disterhoft) and the Netherlands Organization for Scientific Research (NWO) (E Van der Zee).

REFERENCES

Akase E, Alkon DL, Disterhoft JF (1989). Hippocampal lesions impair memory of short-delay conditioned eye blink in rabbit. Behav Neurosci 103:935−943.

Akase E, Thompson LT, Disterhoft JF (1994). A system for quantitative analysis of associative learning: 2. Real-time software for MS-DOS microcomputers. J Neurosci Methods 54:119−130.

Akers RF, Lovinger DM, Colley PA, Linden DJ, Routtenberg A (1986). Translocation of protein kinase C activity may mediate hippocampal long-term potentiation. Science 231:587−689.

Alkon DL (1984). Calcium-mediated reduction of ionic currents: a biophysical memory trace. Science 226:1037−1045.

Bank B, DeWeer A, Kuzirian AM, Rasmussen H, Alkon DL (1988). Classical conditioning induces long-term translocation of protein kinase C in rabbit hippocampal CA1 cells. Proc Natl Acad Sci USA 85:1988−1992.

Baraban JM, Snyder SH, Alger BF (1985). Protein kinase C regulates ionic conductance in hippocampal pyramidal neurons: Electrophysiological effects of phorbol esters. Proc Natl Acad Sci USA 82:2538−2542.

Berger TW, Alger B, Thompson RF (1976). Neuronal substrate of classical conditioning in the hippocampus. Science 192:483−485.

Berger TW, Bassett JL (1992). System properties of the hippocampus In I Gormezano, EA Wasserman (eds), Learning and Memory: The Behavioral and Biological Substrates. Hillsdale, NJ: Lawrence Erlbaum Associates, pp 275−320.

Berger TW, Orr WB (1983). Hippocampectomy selectively disrupts discrimination reversal conditioning of the rabbit nictitating membrane response. Behav Brain Res 210:411−417.

Berger TW, Rinaldi PC, Weisz DJ, Thompson RF (1983). Single-unit analysis of different hippocampal cell types during classical conditioning of rabbit nictitating membrane response. J Neurophysiol 50:1197−1219.

Berger TW, Thompson RF (1978). Neuronal plasticity in the limbic system during classical conditioning of the rabbit nictitating membrane response: I. The hippocampus. Brain Res. 145:323−346.

Berger TW, Weisz, DJ (1987). Single unit analysis of hippocampal pyramidal and granule cells and their role in classical conditioning of the rabbit nictitating membrane response. In I Gormezano, WF Prokasy, RF Thompson (eds), Classical Conditioning, 3rd ed. Hillsdale, NJ: Lawrence Erlbaum Assoc.

Carew TJ, Sahley CL (1986). Invertebrate learning and memory: From behavior to molecules. Annu Rev Neurosci 9:435−487.

Clark GA, McCormick DA, Lavond DG, Thompson RF (1984). Effects of lesions of cerebellar nuclei on conditioned behavioral and hippocampal neuronal responses. Brain Res 291:125−136.

Cohen NJ, Eichenbaum H (1993). Memory, Amnesia, and the Hippocampal System. Cambridge, MA: MIT Press.

Colino A, Halliwell JV (1987). Differential modulation of three separate K-conductances in hippocampal CA1 neurons by serotonin. Nature 328:73–77.

Coulter DA, LoTurco JJ, Kubota M, Disterhoft JF, Moore JW, Alkon DL (1989). Classical conditioning reduces the amplitude and duration of the calcium-dependent afterhyperpolarization in rabbit hippocampal pyramidal cells. J Neurophysiol 61:971–981.

deJonge MC, Black J, Deyo RA, Disterhoft JF (1990). Learning-induced afterhyperpolarization reductions in hippocampus are specific for cell type and potassium conductance. Exp Brain Res 80:456–462.

Deyo RA, Straube K, Disterhoft JF (1989). Nimodipine facilitates associative learning in aging rabbits. Science 243:809–811.

Disterhoft JF, Coulter DA, Alkon DL (1986). Conditioning-specific membrane changes of rabbit hippocampal neurons measured *in vitro*. Proc Natl Acad Sci USA, 83:2733–2737.

Disterhoft JF, Golden DT, Read HR, Coulter DA, Alkon DL (1988). AHP reductions in rabbit hippocampal neurons during conditioning are correlated with acquisition of the learned response. Brain Res 462:118–125.

Disterhoft JF, Kwan HH, Lo WD (1977). Nictitating membrane conditioning to tone in the immobilized albino rabbit. Brain Res 137:127–143.

Disterhoft JF, Quinn KJ, Weiss C, Shipley MT (1985). Accessory abducens nucleus and conditioned eye retraction/nictitating membrane extension in rabbit. J Neurosci 5:941–950.

Gabrieli JDE, McGlinchey-Berroth R, Carrillo MC, Gluck MA, Cermak LS, Disterhoft JF (1995). Intact delay-eyeblink classical conditioning in amnesics. Behav Neurosci 109:819–827.

Goldman-Rakic PS (1987). Circuitry of primate prefrontal cortex and regulation of behavior by representational memory. In VB Mountcastle, F Plum, SR Geiger (eds), Higher Functions of the Brain, Handbook of Physiology. Bethesda, MD: American Physiological Society, vol 5, part 1, pp 373–417.

Gormezano I (1966). Classical conditioning. In JB Sidowski (ed), Experimental Methods and Instrumentation in Psychology. New York: McGraw-Hill, pp 385–420.

Gormezano I, Prokasy WF, Thompson RF (eds) (1987). Classical Conditioning. Hillsdale, NJ: Lawrence Erlbaum Associates.

Haas HL, Konnerth A (1983). Histamine and noradrenaline decrease calcium-activated potassium conductance in hippocampal pyramidal cells. Nature 302:432–434.

Hebb DO (1949). The Organization of Behavior: A Neurophysiological Theory. New York: Wiley.

Hotson JR, Prince DA (1980). A calcium-activated hyperpolarization follows repetitive firing in hippocampal neurons. J Neurophysiol 43:409–419.

Jung MW, Wiener SI, McNaughton BL (1994). Comparison of spatial firing characteristics of units in dorsal and ventral hippocampus of the rat. J Neurosci 14:7347–7356.

Kim JJ, Clark RE, Thompson RF (1995). Hippocampectomy impairs the memory of recently, but not remotely, acquired trace eyeblink conditioned responses. Behav Neurosci 109:195–203.

Kim JJ, Fanselow MS (1992). Modality-specific retrograde amnesia of fear. Science 256:675–677.

Kim SG, Ugurbil K, Strick PL (1994). Activation of a cerebellar output nucleus during cognitive processing. Science 265:949–951.

Knöpfel T, Vranesic I, Gähwiller BH, Brown DA (1990). Muscarinic and β-adrenergic depression of the slow Ca^{2+}-activated potassium conductance in hippocampal CA3 pyramidal cells is not mediated by a reduction of depolarization-induced cytosolic Ca^{2+} transients. Proc Natl Acad Sci USA 87:4083–4087.

Kraus N, Disterhoft JF (1982). Response plasticity of single neurons in rabbit auditory cortex during tone-signalled learning. Brain Res 246:205–215.

Kubie JL (1984). A driveable bundle of microwires for collecting single-unit data from freely moving rats. Physiol Behav 32:115–118.

Lancaster B, Adams PR (1986). Calcium-dependent current generating the afterhyperpolarization of hippocampal neurons. J Neurophysiol 55:1268–1282.

Larsell O, Jansen J (1972). The Comparative Anatomy and Histology of the Cerebellum. Minneapolis: University of Minnesota Press.

Madison DV, Nicoll RA (1984). Control of the repetitive discharge of rat CA1 pyramidal neurones in vitro. J Physiol (Lond) 354:319–331.

Madison D, Nicoll RA (1986). Actions of noradrenaline recorded intracellularly in rat hippocampal CA1 pyramidal neurones, in vitro. J Physiol (Lond) 372:221–244.

Malenka RC, Madison DV, Andrade R, Nicoll RA (1986). Phorbol esters mimic some cholinergic actions in hippocampal pyramidal neurons. J Neurosci 6:475–480.

McGlinchey-Berroth R, Cermak LS, Carrillo MC, Armfield S, Gabrieli JDE, Disterhoft JF (1995). Impaired delay eyeblink conditioning in amnesic Korsakoff's patients and recovered alcoholics. Alcoholism: Clin Exp Res 19:1127–1132.

Meck WH, Church RM, Olton DS (1984). Hippocampus, time, and memory. Behav Neurosci 98:3–22.

Middleton FA, Strick PL (1994). Anatomical evidence for cerebellar and basal ganglia involvement in higher cognitive function. Science 266:458–461.

Molloy SS, Kennedy MB (1991). Autophosphorylation of type II Ca/calmodulin-dependent protein kinase in cultures of postnatal rat hippocampal slices. Proc Natl Acad Sci USA 88: 4756–4760.

Moyer JR, Deyo RA, Disterhoft JF (1990). Hippocampal lesions impair trace eye-blink conditioning in rabbits. Behav Neurosci 104:243–252.

Moyer JR Jr, Thompson LT, Black JP, Disterhoft JF (1992). Nimodipine increases excitability of rabbit CA1 pyramidal neurons in an age- and concentration-dependent manner. J Neurophysiol 68:2100–2109.

Moyer JR Jr, Thompson LT, Disterhoft JF (1993). Hippocampally-dependent trace eye-blink conditioning increases excitability of rabbit CA1 neurons in vitro. Soc Neurosci Abstr 19:801.

Moyer JR Jr, Thompson LT, Disterhoft JF (1994). The hippocampus as an intermediate storage buffer after associative learning: In vitro evidence from rabbit CA1. Soc Neurosci Abstr 20:796.

Müller W, Petrozzino JJ, Griffith LC, Danho W, Connor JA (1992). Specific involvement of Ca^{2+}-calmodulin kinase II in cholinergic modulation of neuronal responsiveness. J Neurophysiol 68:2264–2269.

Nishizuka Y (1986). Studies and perspectives of protein kinase C. Science 233:305–312.

Nishizuka Y (1988). The molecular heterogeneity of protein kinase C and implications for cellular regulation. Nature 334:661–665.

Oda T, Shearman MS, Nishizuka Y (1991). Synaptosomal protein kinase C subspecies: B. Down-regulation promoted by phorbol ester and its effect on evoked norephinephrine release. J Neurochem 56:1263–1269.

O'Keefe J, Nadel L (1978). The Hippocampus as a Cognitive Map. Oxford: Oxford University Press.

Olds J, Disterhoft JF, Segal M, Kornblith CL, Hirsh R (1972). Learning centers of rat brain mapped by measuring latencies of conditioned unit responses. J Neurophysiol 35:202–219.

Olds JL, Anderson ML, McPhie DL, Staten LD, Alkon DL (1989). Imaging of memory-specific changes in the distribution of protein kinase C in the hippocampus. Science 245:866–869.

Olds JL, Golski S, McPhie DL, Olton D, Mishkin M, Alkon DL (1990). Discrimination learning alters the distribution of protein kinase C in the hippocampus of rats. J Neurosci 10:3707–3713.

Pavlov IP (1927). Conditioned Reflexes. An Investigation of the Physiological Activity of the Cerebral Cortex. London: Oxford University Press.

Pedarzani P, Storm JF (1993). PKA mediates the effects of monoamine transmitters on the K^+ current underlying slow spike frequency adaptation in hippocampal neurons. Neuron 11:1023–1035.

Perrett SP, Ruiz BP, Mauk MD (1993). Cerebellar cortex lesions disrupt learning-dependent timing of conditioned eyelid responses. J Neurosci 13:1708–1718.

Ranck JB, Jr (1973). Studies on single neurons in dorsal hippocampal formation and septum of unrestrained rats: I. Behavioral correlates and firing repertoires. Exp Neurol 41:461–555.

Sanchez-Andres JV, Alkon DL (1991). Voltage-clamp analysis of effects of classical conditioning on the hippocampus. J Neurophysiol 65:796–807.

Schmaltz LW, Theios J (1972). Acquisition and extinction of a classically conditioned response in hippocampectomized rabbits (Oryctolagus cuniculus). J Comp Physiol Psychol 79:328–333.

Schwindt P, Spain WJ, Crill WE (1992). Calcium-dependent potassium currents in neurons from cat sensorimotor cortex. J Neurophysiol 67:216–226.

Scoville WB, Milner B (1957). Loss of recent memory after bilateral hippocampal lesions. J Neurol Neurosurg Psychiatry 20:11–21.

Sears LL, Steinmetz JE (1990). Acquisition of classically conditioned-related activity in the hippocampus is affected by lesions of the cerebellar interpositus nucleus. Behav Neurosci 104:681–692.

Segal M (1973). Flow of conditioned responses in limbic telencephalic system of the rat. J Neurophysiol 36:840–854.

Solomon PR (1979). Temporal versus spatial information processing theories of hippocampal function. Psychol Bull 86:1272–1279.

Solomon PR, Beal MF, Pendlebury WW (1988). Age-related disruption of classical conditioning: A model systems approach to memory disorders. Neurobiol Aging 9:535–546.

Solomon PR, Solomon SD, Vander Schaaf EV, Perry HE (1983). Altered activity in the hippocampus is more detrimental to classical conditioning than removing the structure. Science 220:329–331.

Solomon PR, Vander Schaff E, Thompson RF, Weisz DJ (1986). Hippocampus and trace conditioning of the rabbit's classically conditioned nictitating membrane response. Behav Neurosci 100:729–744.

Squire LR (1987). Memory and Brain. New York: Oxford University Press.

Steinmetz JE, Lavond DG, Ivkovich D, Logan CG, Thompson RF (1992). Disruption of classical eyelid conditioning after cerebellar lesions: Damage to a memory trace system or a simple performance deficit? J Neurosci 12:4403–4426.

Storm JF (1990). Potassium currents in hippocampal pyramidal cells. Prog Brain Res 83:161–187.

Sunayashiki-Kusuzaki K, Lester DS, Schreurs BG, Alkon DL (1993). Associative learning potentiates protein kinase C activation in synaptosomes of the rabbit hippocampus. Proc Natl Acad Sci USA 90:4286–4289.

Sutherland RJ, Rudy JW (1989). Configural association theory: The role of the hippocampal formation in learning, memory, and amnesia. Psychobiology 17:129–144.

Thompson LT, Best PJ (1989). Place cells and silent cells in the hippocampus of freelybehaving rats. J Neurosci 9:2382–2390.

Thompson LT, Moskal JR, Disterhoft JF (1992). Hippocampus-dependent learning facilitated by a monoclonal antibody or D-cycloserine. Nature 359:638–641.

Thompson LT, Moyer JR Jr, Akase E, Disterhoft JF (1994a). A system for quantitative analysis of associative learning: 1. Hardware interfaces with cross-species applications. J Neurosci Methods 54:109–117.

Thompson LT, Moyer JR Jr, Disterhoft JF (1994b). Learning (not performance or memory) increases *in vitro* excitability of hippocampal CA3 neurons. Soc Neurosci Abstr 20:796.

Thompson LT, Moyer JR Jr, Trommer B, Disterhoft JF (1993). Hippocampally-dependent eyeblink conditioning also increases excitability of rabbit CA3 neurons *in vitro*. Soc Neurosci Abstr 19:801.

Thompson RF (1990). Neural mechanisms of classical conditioning in mammals. Phil Trans R Soc Lond B Biol Sci 329:161–170.

Thompson RF, Berger TW, Berry SD, Hoehler FK, Kettner RE, Weisz DJ (1980). Hippocampal substrate of classical conditioning. J Physiol Psychol 8:262–279.

Thompson RF, Berger TW, Cegavske CF, Patterson MM, Roemer RA, Teyler TA, Young RA (1976). The search for the engram. Am Psychol 31:209–227.

Van der Zee EA, Compaan JC, de Boer M, Luiten PGM (1992). Changes in PKCgamma-immunoreactivity in mouse hippocampus induced by spatial discrimination learning. J Neurosci 12:4808–4815.

Van der Zee EA, Kronforst MA, Disterhoft JF (1994). Hippocampally dependent trace eyeblink conditioning induces changes in the immunoreactivity for muscarinic receptors and PKC$_\gamma$ in the rabbit hippocampus. Soc Neurosci Abstr 20:1433.

Van der Zee EA, Strosberg AD, Bohus B, Luiten PGM (1993). Colocalization of muscarinic acetylcholine receptors and protein kinase C$_\gamma$ in rat parietal cortex. Mol Brain Res. 18:152–162.

Weiss C, Kronforst MA, Disterhoft JF (1994). Comparison of hippocampal single cell activity during hippocampal-dependent and hippocampal-independent eyeblink conditioning. Soc Neurosci Abstr 20:796.

Weiss C, Kronforst MA, Thompson LT, Disterhoft JF (1993). Electrophysiological characterization of hippocampal neurons during trace eyeblink conditioning in the rabbit. Soc Neurosci Abstr 19:801.

Welsh JP, Harvey JA (1989). Cerebellar lesions and the nictitating membrane reflex: Performance deficits of the conditioned and unconditioned response. J Neurosci 9:299–311.

Woodruff-Pak DS (1988). Aging and classical conditioning: Parallel studies in rabbits and humans. Neurobiol Aging 9:511–522.

Woody CD (1974). Aspects of the electrophysiology of cortical processes related to the development and performance of learned motor responses. Physiologist 17:49–69.

Woody CD, Gruen E, Birt D (1991). Changes in membrane currents during Pavlovian conditioning of single cortical neurons. Brain Res 539:76–84.

Yeo CH, Hardiman MJ, Glickstein M (1984). Discrete lesions of the cerebellar cortex abolish the classically conditioned nictitating membrane response of the rabbit. Behav Brain Res 13:261–266.

Zola-Morgan SM, Squire LR (1990). The primate hippocampal formation: Evidence for a time-limited role in memory storage. Science 250:288–290.

Zola-Morgan SM, Squire LR, Amaral DG (1986). Human amnesia and the medial temporal region: Enduring memory impairment following a bilateral lesion limited to field CA1 of the hippocampus. J Neurosci 6:2960–2967.

8 The Multiple-Pathway Model of Circuits Subserving the Classical Conditioning of Withdrawal Reflexes

Vlastislav Bracha and James R. Bloedel

The fundamental question facing investigators in the neurophysiology of learning and memory is the nature of functional or structural changes in the nervous system subserving individual experience-induced, long-lasting changes of behavior. It is generally assumed that the basic changes responsible for the storage of memory or for the consolidation of new forms of behavior occur at the cellular level. Based on this, several other important questions arise: At which subpopulations of central nervous system (CNS) neurons do the learning-induced plastic changes occur? Where are these cells located? Are they distributed over circuits subserving the studied behavior or are they concentrated in specialized sites restricted to a few or even a single anatomical structure? These questions have motivated extensive research efforts attempting to localize where the learning occurs, because a study of the cellular mechanisms of behavioral plasticity in vertebrates first requires the identification of sites among the 10^{10} cells in the CNS where the "learning" neurons are located.

Perhaps the most common strategy to localize neural substrates of learning uses systematic permanent lesions or temporary inactivation methods (chapter 6). One of the basic assumptions of this approach is that one can, by means of exclusion, demonstrate which brain systems are not directly involved in the given form of learning and then deduce which circuits are essential for the learning to occur and to be maintained. The method of exclusion has as its complement the method of inclusion. The latter assumes that lesions producing marked deficits in the acquisition or execution of the learned behavior indicate that the lesioned structure is an integral part of the system subserving the given form of learning. Systematic use of the exclusion and inclusion methods has led to proposals of essential systems involved in the learning of several different behaviors (e.g., the conditioned taste aversion [Garcia, Hankins, and Rusiniak, 1974; Tassoni, Bucherelli, and Bures, 1992], adaptation of the vestibuloocular reflex [du Lac, Raymond, Sejnowski, and Lisberger, 1995], or classical conditioning of the nictitating membrane response [Thompson and Krupa, 1994]).

In this chapter, we will analyze existing approaches used to localize more specifically sites of plastic changes within systems subserving the classical conditioning of withdrawal reflexes. The examination will concentrate on the model of the classically conditioned nictitating membrane eyeblink response in the rabbit. We will argue that the current notion that considers the cerebellar nucleus interpositus and the cerebellar cortex to be an "essential and sufficient" site of plastic changes related to the classical conditioning of the eyeblink reflex is a product of an oversimplified model of the circuits involved in the control of conditioned and unconditioned responses. The alternative we suggest is a new, more realistic schematic of involved circuits—the multiple-pathway model. This model incorporates known connectivity within cerebellar systems and between the cerebellum and brainstem eyeblink circuits, and it includes interactions between the brainstem and the cerebrum. Considering the complexity of the multiple-pathway model, we will discuss available experimental approaches used to localize specific sites of plastic changes subserving the classical conditioning of the nictitating membrane response in the rabbit. We will demonstrate that available experimental evidence favors the concept of distributed sites of neural plasticity.

A fundamental question in the physiology of both motor control and learning and memory is the issue of specialization and multifunctionality of control circuits. Are the concepts of the intermediate cerebellar function emerging from the studies of the classically conditioned eyeblink response applicable to conditioned responses in other effector systems? How is the intermediate cerebellar involvement in classically conditioned reflexes related to its involvement in other cutaneomuscular reflexive systems? These questions will be addressed in the second part of this chapter, summarizing our current studies of the cerebellar involvement in the cutaneomuscular limb reflexes in the cat.

SYSTEMS "ESSENTIAL" FOR THE EXPRESSION OF THE CLASSICALLY CONDITIONED NICTITATING MEMBRANE RESPONSE IN THE RABBIT

The eyeblink nictitating membrane reflex is a response elicited to protect the eye following the activation of trigeminal afferents. This reflex usually is evoked by tactile or nociceptive stimulation of the periocular region or the surface of the eye. The function of the eyeblink is to provide protection of the eye against mechanical agents and to moisturize periodically the corneal surface. The eyeblink represents the synchronized action of the orbicularis oculi and lavator palpebrae muscles along with the extraocular muscles. In species possessing a developed third eyelid, the nictitating membrane (NM), the act of blinking also involves the extension of this structure. NM extension in the rabbit is a passive consequence of the eyeball's retraction inside the orbit. The brainstem contains the basic circuitry subserving the unconditioned eyeblink, a system that consists of a basic three-neuron arc (neurons in the semilunar ganglion of the trigeminal nerve, spinal trigeminal nucleus, and motor nuclei) in addition to a multitude of polysynaptic pathways. The basic features of eyeblink behavior have been studied and reviewed by Evinger, Pellegrini, and Manning (1989), and its neuronal circuitry has been investigated by Hiraoka and Shimamura (1977); Harvey, Land, and McMaster (1984); Cegavske, Harrison, and Torigoe (1987); and Holstege (1990), among others.

The unconditioned eyeblink can be conditioned in the Pavlovian classical conditioning paradigm. In the typical experimental arrangement, an originally irrelevant conditioning stimulus (CS)—for example, a tone or flash of light —is paired with (followed by) the presentation of an unconditioned stimulus (US)—for example, a corneal air puff—which reliably elicits an unconditioned response (UR). After several hundred presentations of the CS and US, the rabbit starts to respond to the CS with the eyeblink conditioned response (CR) in expectation of the forthcoming US. In the rabbit, the CR consists of the synchronous movement of the external eyelids and the NM (McCormick, Lavond, and Thompson, 1982). Consequently, the terms *eyeblink* and *nictitating membrane response* (NMR) will be used as synonyms in this context. Because of the relative simplicity of circuits controlling the unconditioned eyeblink and because this paradigm can be easily controlled, the classically conditioned NMR in the rabbit has become one of the most investigated models of associative memory in mammals.

Delineation of Circuits Subserving the CR by the Method of Exclusion

Permanent lesions of the cerebral cortex (Oakley and Russell, 1972, 1977) do not prevent acquisition or retention of the classically conditioned NMR. The eyeblink can be successfully conditioned and retained in the decerebrate preparation (Norman, Buchwald, and Villablanca, 1977; Mauk and Thompson, 1987; Kelly, Zuo, and Bloedel, 1990; Yeo, 1991). Studies by Kelly et al. (1990) and Norman et al. (1977) indicate that not even the cerebellum or the red nucleus is required for the expression of the conditioned eyeblinks in the decerebrate preparation.

Though the preceding data suggest that circuits contained in the brainstem have the capacity to support the classically conditioned NMR, they do not prove that the lesioned structures do not participate in the acquisition and expression of the CR in an intact animal. One of the major drawbacks of the lesioning approach is that it addresses the function of the lesioned structure only indirectly. By lesioning a given structure, one actually studies the functional capacity of the remainder of the system. Deficits induced by the lesion can represent either the lack of a specific function normally supplied by the lesioned structure or a nonspecific functional modification of the remainder of the system. Similarly, the persistence of normal function following a specific lesion can indicate an absence of involvement of the structure in the studied behavior, can reflect parallel and redundant organization of the system, or can simply be a consequence of failing to monitor the parameter which the structure normally controls.

There are substantial data suggesting cerebral, hippocampal, cerebellar, and rubral involvement in normal NMR conditioning (for review, see Bloedel and Bracha, 1995). For example, temporary functional cerebral decortication blocks expression of the CR (Papsdorf, Longman, and Gormezano, 1965; Gutmann, Brozek, and Bures, 1972; Megirian, 1973). Permanent lesions of the hippocampus prevent the acquisition of CRs when a short trace interval separates the CS from the US (Solomon, Vander Schaaf, Thompson, and Weisz, 1986; Moyer, Deyo, and Disterhoft, 1990). Permanent destruction of the red nucleus (Rosenfield and Moore, 1983, 1985) or the cerebellar nucleus interpositus (Lavond, Lincoln, McCormick, and Thompson, 1984) in otherwise intact animals blocks both retention and acquisition of the conditioned NMRs. These data indicate that demarcation of systems essential for NMR conditioning by the method of exclusion has only a relative character because the results of these experiments depend on the extent of the lesions, on a particular combination of lesioned structures, and on the complexity and nuances of the behavioral tests. The complete model of the systems participating in the eyeblink conditioning should include the brainstem, cerebellum, hippocampus, and cerebral cortex.

Delineation of Circuits Based on the Method of Inclusion

In contrast to the relatively moderate extent of deficits induced by permanent lesions of structures above the level of the thalamus, lesions of several brainstem and cerebellar regions produce severe and permanent deficits in the acquisition and retention of the classically conditioned NMR. The CR expression is permanently abolished following lesions of the inferior olives (Yeo, Hardiman, and Glickstein 1986), the dentate, anterior interposed cerebellar nuclear region (Lavond et al., 1984), the red nucleus (Rosenfield and Moore, 1983), and the middle cerebellar peduncle (Lewis, Lo Turco, and Solomon, 1987). This set of observations, together with data from exclusion experiments, led to a proposal of an "essential and sufficient" circuit for the acquisition and retention of the classically conditioned nictitating membrane response in the rabbit (Thompson, 1986; Thompson and Krupa, 1994) (figure 8.1). For purposes of this chapter, we will refer to the circuit advocated by Thompson et al. as the *single-pathway model*.

Single-Pathway Model

The single-pathway circuit is built around the logical skeleton of a modified Albus-Marr hypothesis (chapters 2, 10, 11, and 20), which originally proposed that the cerebellar cortex operates as a substrate for learning by virtue of the interaction of parallel fibers and climbing fibers on the dendritic tree of Purkinje cells. It is assumed that the information concerning the CS enters the circuit through the pontine nuclei, whereas the US signals are conveyed via the trigeminal nuclei and inferior olives. Because lesions of the cerebellar

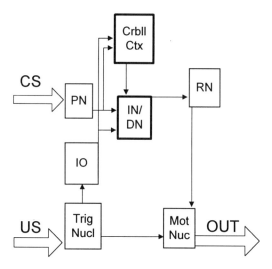

Figure 8.1 Schematic of the single-pathway model of circuits involved in the control of the classically conditioned NMR in the rabbit. CS, conditioned stimulus input; Crbll Ctx, cerebellar cortex; IN/DN, cerebellar interposed and dentate nuclei; IO, inferior olive; Mot Nuc, motor nuclei subserving the eyeblink/NMR response; PN, pontine nuclei; RN, red nucleus; Trig Nucl, trigeminal sensory nuclei; US, unconditioned stimulus input; boldly framed boxes, putative sites of plasticity related to the NMR conditioning. (Adapted from Thompson, 1986, and Thompson and Krupa, 1994.)

cortex do not seem to completely eliminate a rabbit's capacity to produce conditioned eyeblinks (Harvey, Welsh, Yeo, and Romano 1993; Woodruff-Pak, Lavond, Logan, Steinmetz, and Thompson 1993), it has been suggested that the major interaction between inputs from the pontine nuclei and the inferior olive occurs at the level of the cerebellar nucleus interpositus (Thompson, 1986). Critical to this view, the cerebellar nuclei (and possibly also the cerebellar cortex) is considered in the single-pathway model to be the only site of interaction of the CS and US. At the output of the cerebellum, the nucleus interpositus starts the CR pathway, which consists of the interposed nucleus, red nucleus, and motor nuclei. The interconnection of the cerebellar systems with the unconditioned reflex pathways follows the blueprint of the metasystematic hypothesis, which considers the cerebellum to be part of a multisynaptic side-loop of the basic reflex arc (e.g., MacKay and Murphy, 1979; Ito, 1984).

The single-CR-pathway model is distinguished by four key features: (1) it assumes a mostly serial, unidirectional flow of information; (2) it emphasizes phasic rather than tonic interactions between involved structures (e.g., Chapman, Steinmetz, Sears, and Thompson, 1990); (3) it postulates that single anatomical and functional pathways are essential and sufficient for mediating separately each of the critical inputs and responses (the CS, US, and CR) during normal eyeblink conditioning; and (4) it postulates that the single essential and sufficient site of plastic changes during eyeblink conditioning is located at a restricted region of the interposed nucleus (Thompson, 1986). The most recent incorporation in the model suggests that perhaps the site also may be within the overlying cerebellar cortex (Thompson and Krupa, 1994). It should be pointed out that feature 4 is a consequence of postulates 1, 2, and 3. The function of the circuit can be described as follows: During learning, the nucleus interpositus and cerebellar cortex receive concomitant input signaling the CS and US. As a consequence of yet-unspecified cellular mechanisms, the interaction of mossy and climbing fiber inputs induces a long-lasting modification in the responsiveness of nuclear cells (and maybe also of cortical Purkinje cells) to the mossy-fiber pontine (CS) input. This process results in increased responses of interposed nuclear cells that cause the generation of the CR.

The physiological feasibility of the single-pathway model has been studied extensively using mostly electrophysiological and lesioning or inactivation methods (for review, see Thompson, 1986; Yeo, 1991; Thompson and Krupa, 1994; Bloedel and Bracha, 1995). Though it is generally agreed that the intermediate cerebellum and red nucleus are structures critical for expression of the classically conditioned NMR in the rabbit, the point of contention is the physiological explanation of this peculiar dependency of the CR on cerebellar integrity. Two major classes of interpretations were considered: The single-pathway model indicates that the CRs are affected simply because lesions of the cerebellum or its inputs interrupt either the site at which the CR "engram" is stored, or they interrupt the CS, US, or CR pathways. The alternative interpretation suggests that deficits of the conditioned responding following lesions within cerebellar systems are due to the altered performance of the brainstem circuits subserving the CR acquisition and expression (Welsh and Harvey, 1989; Kelly et al., 1990). The last ten years have revealed how difficult, if not impossible, it is to dissociate these two interpretations experimentally.

The authors of the single-pathway model (Thompson and Krupa, 1994) acknowledge its most problematic aspect: that it represents only a subset of the structures involved in the control of the CRs and URs and that, within this subset, only a part of the known neuroanatomical connectivity is considered. As will be demonstrated later, this feature seriously limits its capacity to explain all of the known experimental findings. Knowledge of the functional and neuroanatomical incompleteness of the single-pathway model led us to propose an alternate schematic of the cerebellum-related circuits involved in the control of the conditioned and unconditioned NMR in the rabbit. For purposes of this manuscript, this model will be termed the *multiple-pathway model*.

Multiple-Pathway Model

Two principles were chosen for the construction of the multiple-pathway model (figure 8.2). First, the model attempts to include most of the known

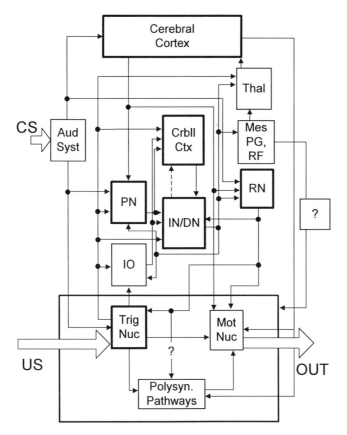

Figure 8.2 Schematic of the multiple-pathway model of circuits involved in the control of the classically conditioned NMR. Aud Syst, auditory system; Mes PG, RF, mesencephalic periaqueductal gray and reticular formation; Polysyn. Pathways, medullary polysynaptic UR pathways; Thal, thalamus; ?, projections not yet documented; boldly framed small boxes, putative sites of plasticity underlying the eyeblink conditioning. Other abbreviations are the same as in figure 8.1. The large bold box on the bottom of the figure segregates medullar UR circuits.

neuroanatomical connectivity. Second, it reflects most of the accumulated functional (lesioning and electrophysiological) data pertinent to NMR conditioning.

Four neuroanatomical features distinguish the multiple-pathway model from the previously described single-pathway circuit. First, the multiple-pathway model includes multiple efferent targets for the interposed nucleus. It has long been known that anterior interposed nucleus projections include the ventrolateral thalamus, the mesencephalic and bulbar reticular formation, the basilar pons, the reticulotegmental nucleus, and the inferior olive (for review, see Chan-Palay, 1977; Voogd, 1995). Because of the scarcity of available data regarding connectivity of the interposed nucleus in the rabbit, we examined projections of the functionally defined subregions of this structure (Bartholomew, Webster, Bloedel, and Bracha, 1994). For this purpose, the interposed nucleus of rabbits pretrained in the eyeblink conditioning paradigm was systematically mapped in our laboratory with nanoinjections of the gamma aminobutyric acid ($GABA_A$) agonist muscimol (each injection contained 20 ng of muscimol dissolved in 50 nl of vehicle). Nuclear sites producing maximal behavioral effects (immediate and complete abolition of CRs) were injected with either Phaseolus vulgaris-leucoagglutinin (PHA-L) or the cholera toxin B subunit as tracers of nuclear afferent and efferent projections, respectively. The histological analysis injected anterograde tracer distribution revealed consistent projections to the red nucleus, the ventrolateral thalamus, the mesencephalic reticular formation, the dorsolateral pontine nuclei, the reticulotegmental nucleus, and the dorsal accessory olive. This finding has important implications for the interpretation of lesion or inactivation experiments. Among other concerns, the interaction of the interposed nucleus with the eyeblink circuits cannot be restricted to the interpositorubral pathway. At least three of the interposed nuclei's projections (red nucleus, thalamus, and mesencephalic reticular formation) can mediate effects of the nucleus interpositus manipulations on the eyeblink response. The first is the red nucleus through its direct projections to the trigeminal nucleus and to the motor nuclei. The second is the thalamus, through its projections to the cerebral cortex and cerebrobulbar projections. Finally, the interposed nuclear interactions with the unconditioned reflex circuits can be mediated through the mesencephalic reticular formation, which was shown to be involved in the control of other types of withdrawal reflexes (Zemlan and Behbehani, 1988).

Second, several major connections of the interposed nucleus are reciprocal. One of the features of the cerebellar connectivity is its reciprocal character. Perhaps the best known is the olivo-cerebello-olivary projection. The inferior olive has a topographically organized projection to the cerebellar cortex and cerebellar nuclei (for review, see Voogd, 1995). The anterior interposed nucleus receives olivary input mostly from the dorsal accessory olive. In turn, the anterior interposed nucleus sends projections to the dorsal accessory olive (for review see Ruigrok and Cella, 1995). Our studies have confirmed the presence of this pattern in the rabbit. We have observed a similar reciprocal pattern of interposed nuclear connections with the dorsolateral pontine nuclei, reticulotegmental nucleus, and red nucleus (figure 8.3). Though it is not yet known whether the reciprocal connections of the interposed nucleus form closed or open loops, their presence should be included in the interpretations of experimental data. For example, inactivation of the interposed nucleus should affect, through these reciprocal connections, activity at several locations from which nuclear afferents originate: the cerebellar cortex, the red nucleus, the inferior olive, the pontine nuclei (Gohl, Clark, and Lavond, 1993), and (in some species), in the trigeminal nuclei. Conversely, besides its traditionally considered output targets, inactivation of the red nucleus can affect the origin of one of its major inputs—the cerebellar nuclei (Keifer, 1994).

Third, there are several pathways conveying the US to the cerebellum. Besides the trigemino-olivary-cerebellar pathway, the US can reach the cere-

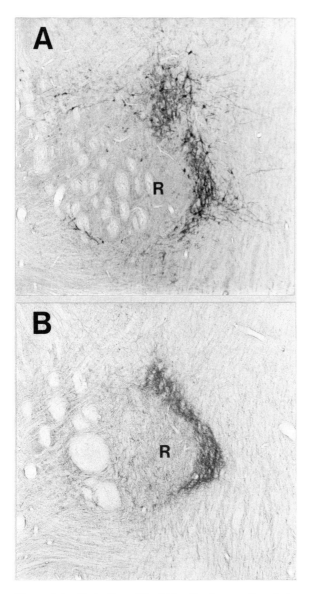

Figure 8.3 Illustration of the bidirectional connections between structures involved in the multiple-pathway recurrent model. A. Labeled cells in the red nucleus following the retrograde transport of CTB injected in the interposed nucleus area. B. The terminal field of the interposed nucleus projections to the red nucleus. Terminals are visualized using biocytin, which was anterogradely transported following the injection in the contralateral nucleus interpositus. R = red nucleus. A and B illustrate that the red nucleus and intermediate cerebellum are both afferent sources and efferent targets of each other.

bellum by two additional routes: The first is a direct trigeminocerebellar pathway (van Ham and Yeo, 1992; Bartholomew et al., 1994). The second is the trigeminopontocerebellar projection (van Ham and Yeo, 1992). Consequently, the cerebellar cortex and nuclei receive US information through both mossy *and* climbing fibers. The physiological implications of this neuroanatomical circumstance are not yet known.

Fourth, the model includes the cerebrum. As was indicated earlier, supramesencephalic structures often have been excluded as essential circuits participating in the eyeblink conditioning based on the results of experiments employing the exclusion methodology. Several other studies, however, implicated the cerebral cortex in the normal expression of the conditioned NMR (Papsdorf et al., 1965; Gutmann et al., 1972; Megirian, 1973) in addition to the unconditioned eyeblink (Kimura, 1974). Spreading depression temporarily blocks the execution of the CR. Interestingly, temporal inactivation of both the auditory cortex (when a tone was used as a CS) and the motor cortex affects the performance of the CR. These data indicate that in an intact rabbit, the cerebral cortex participates in the CR expression. This notion is supported further by findings of changes in the regional blood flow in the cerebral cortex of human subjects during classical conditioning of the eyeblink response (Molchan, Sutherland, McIntosh, Herscovitch, and Schreurs, 1994). In our opinion, the fact that decerebrate animals are able to be conditioned (Mauk and Thompson, 1987) reflects the hierarchical organization of the nervous system, as do the experiments in decerebrate-decerebellate animals (Kelly et al., 1990) and the studies on the conditionability of the flexion reflex in spinalized animals (Durkovic, 1975; Beggs, Steinmetz, Romano, and Patterson, 1983). Each level of the system possesses plastic features reflected by its ability to modify the behavior. However, the fact that lower levels of the organizational hierarchy exhibit the capacity to learn by no means implies that, during learning in an intact animal, all learning occurs at lower stages of the control systems. Most probably, parallel plastic changes at all system levels contribute to the adaptability of behavior in general and to the classical conditioning of the eyeblink reflex in particular.

The wiring diagram of the multiple-pathway model (figure 8.2) is centered around the possible involvement of cerebellar systems in the control of conditioned eyeblink responses. Though it is appreciably more complete than the single-pathway schematic, it is still sketchy regarding other possible CR-related inputs to the UR control system. (For a recent review of neural substrates involved in the control of the unconditioned eyeblink response, see Holstege, Blok, and Ter Horst, 1995).

One additional aspect of the multiple-pathway model is highly significant. The operation of the system represents a delicate balance of tonic and phasic interactions. The tonic interactions are emphasized when contrasting the present circuit with the previously described single-pathway model. The physiological importance of tonic interactions was demonstrated by Benedetti, Montarolo, Strata, and Tempia (1983); Batini, Billard, and Daniel (1985), and Billard, Batini, and Daniel (1988), who showed that lesion to one of the cerebellar afferent sources, the inferior olive, leads to long-lasting, aberrant spontaneous activity at several subsequent stages of the system (cerebellar cortex to cerebellar nuclei to red nucleus). Similarly, pharmacological tonic activation of the cerebellar interposed nucleus leads to a tonic inhibition of the inferior olive (KM Horn, TJH Ruigrok, and AR Gibson, personal communication). A practical implication of these findings is that they provide an empirical basis for the performance hypothesis. More specifically, they remind us that the outcomes of manipulating one of the circuit components do not necessarily reflect its function, because the same experimental intervention most probably also affects the basic operation of several subsequent parts of the system.

Comparison of the single-pathway (see figure 8.1) and multiple-pathway (see figure 8.2) models reveals several principal differences: First, the single-pathway model represents a subset of the multiple-pathway system. Second, whereas in the single-pathway model the cerebellum is the only postulated site of the CS and US interaction, the multiple-pathway model proposes at least six such locations: the trigeminal nucleus, the pontine nuclei, the red nucleus, the cerebellar cortex, the cerebellar nuclei, and the cerebral cortex. This suggestion is based on the fact that the lesion or inactivation of each of these structures affects CR performance (Megirian, 1973; Rosenfield and Moore, 1983; Lavond, Lincoln, McCormick, and Thompson, 1984; Yeo, Hardiman, and Glickstein, 1985; Knowlton and Thompson, 1988; Bracha, Wu, Cartwright, and Bloedel, 1991) and that electrophysiological studies at each of these sites demonstrated neuronal activity correlated with the CS, US, and CR (Berthier and Moore, 1986; Desmond and Moore, 1991; Richards, Ricciardi, and Moore, 1991; Woody and Birt, 1992; Yang and Weisz, 1992; Gohl, Clark, and Lavond, 1993). Other structures not specifically considered in our model also could undergo learning-related functional changes even when they do not fulfill the criterion of receiving information related to both CS and US. One of them could be the cochlear nuclei, which were documented to undergo changes in conditioning-related responsiveness to auditory CSs (Woody, Wang, and Gruen, 1994). Third, because of the complex pattern of connectivity in the multiple-pathway model (the number of parallel connections transmitting the CS and US, and the presence of multiple recurrent connections), the traditional terminology related to the serial and unidirectional connectivity within the single-pathway model (CS, US, CR, and UR pathways) is inadequate for describing the operation of the multiple-pathway model. For example, the output of the cerebellar nuclei at which the CR pathway originates in the single-pathway model can, in the multiple-pathway model, also exert its influence on the motor nuclei, but this action can occur through several parallel pathways: the red nucleus, the mesencephalic reticular formation, and the cerebellothalamocorticobulbar loop. In addition to this connection with the motor output, the cerebellar output also has access to inputs of the system (the trigeminal nucleus, the inferior olives, and the pontine nuclei) either by direct projections or through the red nucleus, cerebrum, and (potentially) via the mesencephalic reticular formation. Consequently, a structure assigned to be part of the CR pathway also could be part of a loop superimposed on CS and US pathways. If so, the terms of CS, US, and CR pathways are losing their separate morphological and functional substantiation.

LOCALIZATION OF PLASTIC CHANGES UNDERLYING THE CLASSICAL CONDITIONING OF THE NMR

The complexity of the wiring diagram of the multiple-pathway model makes it extremely difficult to analyze specific functions of its multiply interrelated components. Just as difficult is the analysis of the contribution of the individual structures to any of the functions of the system as a whole. Where in this system are the modifiable neural elements causal to the eyeblink conditioning located? Are they distributed over the system in such a manner that the behavioral plasticity becomes an emergent property of the whole control system, or are they located in some functionally "dedicated," spatially restricted, and definable part of the circuit? In the following sections, we will continue to argue in favor of the concept of distributed substrates of the eyeblink conditioning. This argument is based on indications of plastic modifications at several involved structures and on the absence of evidence which would suggest a single "learning" structure. At this point, definite answers to the preceding questions are not available. Their resolution will depend on a node-to-node examination of the eyeblink system using the best of the available experimental strategies.

There is a limit to the experimental tools that effectively address the localization of behaviorally causal plastic changes. Traditional lesion or inactivation methods are useful for delineation of involved systems but are useless in revealing sites of learning because of the uncertainty regarding their specific effects on the performance of the system. Single-unit recording methods are useful for indicating whether a specific structure is related to the examined behavior or whether it receives inputs required for learning to occur, but they cannot identify the origin of observed components of the neuronal responses. The lesion and extracellular recording methods epitomize the difficulty of dealing with correlational tools while searching for causal relationships. The most productive methods employed so far use one of the four following experimental strategies: (1) mapping of the functional changes accompanying the learning; (2) comparison of the timing of learned behavioral components with correlated neural activity; (3) separation of the process of response acquisition from response execution; and (4) selective manipulations of putative molecular mechanisms of learning.

Mapping of Functional Changes Accompanying CR Acquisition

The application of this method is based mostly on electrophysiological measurements of changes in the responsiveness of specific subpopulations of neurons involved in CR control. Although this approach has not been used extensively in the rabbit NMR delay conditioning model, it has been implemented systematically in closely related paradigms: the classical conditioning of the eyeblink reflex in the cat and the classical conditioning of the cat limb withdrawal response using intracranial electrical stimulation as the CS. The classical conditioning of cat eyeblinks leads to long-term excitability changes of neurons in the facial nucleus (Matsumura and Woody, 1986) and in the motor cortex (Aou, Woody, and Birt, 1992). Classical conditioning of the forelimb withdrawal reflex is accompanied by changes in the responsiveness of red nucleus neurons when stimulation of the cerebral peduncles (Murakami, Oda, and Tsukahara, 1988; Ito and Oda, 1994) or the cerebellar output (Pananceau, Meftah, and Rispal-Padel, 1994) was used as the conditioned stimulus. In addition, in the last model parallel changes also occur in the cerebello-thalamo-cortical pathway (Rispal-Padel and Meftah, 1992). These data argue in favor of distributed plasticity, because they demonstrate that the classical conditioning–related functional changes can occur at multiple locations within circuits involved in the learned response execution.

Comparison of Latencies of Learned Behavior and Correlated Neuronal Activity

The complexity of circuits involved in the control of the classically conditioned NMR together with widely overlapping timing of neuronal correlates of CRs in different structures (Berger and Thompson, 1982; Berthier and Moore, 1986; Desmond and Moore, 1991; Richards et al., 1991; White et al., 1994) makes it extremely difficult to define the location of primary plastic changes. This effect applies specifically to later components of learned responses, which occur at the time of or after the onset of correlated cellular discharges. However, some protocols permit the exclusion of specific structures from the causal link of structures involved in generating the learned behavior by testing temporal relationships between the earliest behavioral and cellular responses. This approach has been used successfully in the study of the adaptation of the vestibuloocular reflex (Pastor, De la Cruz, and Baker, 1994). Experiments conducted by De la Cruz and Baker (1994) demonstrated that the timing of discharges of cerebellar Purkinje cells does not permit their participation in the earliest components of the modified vestibuloocular reflex (see chapter 2). These data directly indicate that brainstem plasticity is involved in the adaptation of this reflex response.

A similar strategy has been employed in the eyeblink conditioning model. Gruart, Blázquez, and Delgado-Garcia, (1994) demonstrated that the earliest components of the classically conditioned eyeblink response in the cat occur too early to be under cerebellar control. This provides additional evidence for participation of brainstem plasticity in the classical conditioning of the eyeblink reflex.

Separation of the Process of the Response Acquisition from the Response Execution

Perhaps the most investigated putative sites of plastic changes subserving the classical conditioning of the NMR have been the cerebellar nucleus interpositus and the cerebellar cortex. Notwithstanding the views of some investigators (Thompson, 1986), early experiments failed to provide direct evidence proving the central hypothesis of the single-pathway model. These studies were not capable of dissociating learning and performance explanations of the deficits induced by lesions of the cerebellum or its inputs and outputs (for a detailed discussion of this topic and the comparison of different interpretations, see Yeo, 1991; Welsh and Harvey, 1992; Thompson and Krupa, 1994; Bloedel and Bracha, 1995). As indicated in the foregoing section describing the multiple-pathway model, available data indicate that lesions within different parts of the cerebellar system result in long-lasting disturbances in the functionality of the remainder of the system. Moreover, it is reasonable to assume that the same circuits participating in the learning are also involved in the expression of the learned response. If so, the sharing of the same substrates for regulating tonic and phasic interactions and for the learning and expression of the response pose a particular challange to dissociating any of these processes.

Though it is difficult spatially to separate the learning and performance functions of the involved circuits, it is possible to dissociate the response acquisition from the response expression in the time domain. The strategy of temporal dissociation between response acquisition and expression was implemented in studies inactivating different parts of the circuit during the response acquisition (Welsh and Harvey, 1991; Clark, Zhang, and Lavond, 1992; Krupa, Thompson, and Thompson, 1993). The feasibility of these experiments is based on a remarkable feature of the classical conditioning process: for the rabbit to learn the CR, it does not have to be able to express it during learning. The major advantage of the inactivation-during-learning approach is that whereas the training occurs in the temporarily lesioned animal, the testing for retention of the CR is done after recovery from the lesion. Consequently, the retention test should reveal specific learning deficits (if any) because at the time of the retention test, the examined animal is intact and free of any possible sensory or motor disturbances. The major disadvantage of this approach is, however, that it fails to distinguish whether the incapacity to learn while the particular structure is inactivated should be ascribed to an effect on local mechanisms of learning or to the disturbance of learning mechanisms at some remote part of the system.

To overcome this inherent deficiency of the method, Clark et al. (1992), Clark and Lavond (1993), and Thompson and Krupa (1994) recently performed experiments in which they compared effects of temporary inactivation of the cerebellar nucleus interpositus and the red nucleus during CR acquisition. These authors reported that though the inactivation of the red nucleus did not block CR acquisition, the inactivation of the interposed nuclear region interrupted the learning. Based on these data, the authors concluded that the interposed cerebellar nuclear region is a site of "essential and sufficient" plastic changes subserving CR acquisition. Putting aside inconsistencies in basic findings (cf. chapter 6 and Krupa et al., 1993), this conclusion is possible only under the oversimplified assumptions of the single-pathway model in which the red nucleus is the only relay of the cerebellar output to the brainstem eyeblink circuits. The more realistic multiple-pathway model does not allow such direct comparison of cerebellar and red nuclear lesions because they affect different sets of circuit elements and operations.

The "Ideal" Experiment for Dissociating Learning from Performance

The preceding sections illustrate how the complexity of the "building plan" of circuits involved in the control of the classically conditioned eyeblink responses effectively limits access to the information characterizing plastic changes subserving the CRs. Though it is possible to exclude participation of particular structures in the learning process or to characterize functional changes accompanying the learning, the study of the causal relationship between local plasticity and systematic (behavioral) expressions of learning is extremely difficult. The major obstacle in this effort is the mnemonic an executive duality of the function of studied circuits. Could one design and ideal experiment to dissociate learning from performance and, in this way, address the possible behavioral causality of local plasticity? The answer to this fundamental question is: theoretically yes, assuming that one would be able to manipulate the cellular mechanism related to the establishment of plastic changes without affecting the on-line operation of the involved circuits. This postulate creates a paradoxical situation. We started by assuming that to study the cellular mechanisms of learning and memory, we first must find where learning occurs. We have argued thus far that to search effectively for locations of plasticity, we have to know the cellular mechanisms of learning.

The circular character of the foregoing reasoning indicates that the search for the sites of plasticity and its cellular mechanisms is not serial but comprises parallel and asymptotic processes. If not the best, then certainly the most pragmatic answer to the aforementioned dilemma is to combine the latest knowledge of possible cellular mechanisms of learning with the latest information from localization studies in the design of experiments targeting relationships between the local cellular plasticity and learning on the behavioral level.

Recently, we adapted this approach to experiments performed in our laboratory. We assumed that classical conditioning of the eyeblink reflex is a form of long-term memory and as such is highly likely to be dependent on the synthesis of new proteins. In the first experiments, we mapped the learning-induced expression of the *c-fos* immediate-early gene, expecting to see an elevated expression of the gene in structures in which the learning induces synthesis of new proteins (Irwin, Craig, Bracha, and Bloedel, 1992). The comparison of the distribution of the immunolabeled *c-fos* product between the groups of conditioned and pseudoconditioned animals failed to detect any learning-induced activation of this immediate-early gene in structures conventionally considered to be putative sites of plasticity subserving the NMR conditioning. The main finding of this study was that the conditioning-induced changes of *c-fos* expression were observed in the raphé nuclei and in the ventrolateral medulla (the A5 and A9 neuronal groups). Our neuroanatomical studies indicate that both the A5 noradrenergic group and raphé nuclei project to the cerebellar interposed nucleus in the rabbit. These data indicate possible involvement of neuromodulatory inputs in the cascade of events leading to CR acquisition.

The absence of learning-specific expression of the *c-fos* gene in other parts of the circuit does not exclude the possible involvement of other immediate-early genes. Because of the uncertainly in determining which of the other members of the ever-growing family of immediate-early genes could be instrumental in the induction of protein synthesis in the rabbit conditioning model, we adapted an alternate strategy in which we locally inhibit protein synthesis during learning, using microinjections of the protein synthesis inhibitor anisomycin. Anisomycin, an inhibitor of peptidyltransferase, was chosen from among other protein synthesis inhibitors because it causes fewer physiological side effects (Bull, Ferrera, and Orrego, 1976) and its intracranial application lacks any substantial metabolic and physiological (e.g., aversive) effects not related to the inhibition of protein synthesis at dosages used for obtaining the latter effect (Rosenblum, Meiri, and Dudai, 1993). Furthermore, it does not affect electrical brain activity significantly (Otani, Marshall, Tate, Goodard, and Abraham, 1989). The prediction for such experiments is that if the protein synthesis-dependent and behaviorally relevant plasticity occurs at a particular structure, local injections of anisomycin in this location during learning should affect the process of CR acquisition. In the first series of these experiments, we applied this method at the most discussed node of the multiple-pathway model—the cerebellar nucleus interpositus.

Effects of Anisomycin Microinjections in the Interposed Nucleus on the Acquisition of the Classically Conditioned NMR

Guide cannulae were implanted bilaterally near the rabbits' cerebellar nucleus interpositus. After the rabbits' recovery from surgery, a protein synthesis inhibitor, anisomycin was injected bilaterally in the interposed nuclei, and 30 min after the drug infusion, the nictitating membrane reflex was conditioned in the classical conditioning delay paradigm. This procedure was repeated in three consecutive training sessions, each consisting of 100 paired presentations of conditioned and unconditioned stimuli. On the next day, no drug was injected, and animals were tested for the retention of CRs possibly acquired in the previous anisomycin infusion sessions. The retention test consisted of trials in which only the CS was presented. Next, all animals were conditioned for an additional 3 to 6 days, during which no anisomycin was injected. The purpose of this test was to determine whether the previous drug treatment produced any irreversible cerebellar nuclei damage that would impair normal acquisition of CRs. The animals that achieved a learning criterion of 90 percent of CRs per training session were further tested in three more experiments. In each of these sessions, the interposed nuclei were injected either with vehicle, anisomycin, or muscimol. The purpose of the anisomycin injections was to test its effect on the normal operation of the interposed nuclei as measured by the behavioral performance of conditioned eyeblinks. The muscimol injections served as a functional test of the injection site location. It was expected that if the drugs were injected directly into (or in the vicinity of) the anterior nucleus interpositus, the muscimol would block the expression of CRs (Bracha, Webster, Winters, Irwin, and Bloedel, 1994). The vehicle injections served as the within-subject control for muscimol and anisomycin experiments. The control group of animals was subjected to a treatment identical to that of the experimental group, with the sole exception of substituting anisomycin with vehicle during the initial 3 days of training.

The retention tests demonstrated that infusions of the protein synthesis inhibitor in to the interposed nuclei prevented normal acquisition of CRs (figure 8.4A). When compared to the control animals, rabbits injected with anisomycin during training exhibited significantly fewer CRs in the retention test. The anisomycin application did not permanently affect the functional integrity of the cerebellar nuclear region, as revealed by the fast learning following the discontinuation of the drug (see figure 8.4). Interestingly, the application of the protein synthesis inhibitor did not block the expression of CRs during training sessions (see figure 8.4A) and had negligible effects on the incidence of previously acquired CRs when tested at the end of experiments (see figure 8.4B). This suggests that anisomycin has relatively few immediate effects on the CR expression-related functionality of the cerebellar nuclei. The reduced incidence of CRs during the retention tests along with the reduced *but not abolished* occurrence of CRs during initial training sessions indicate that the blockade of protein synthesis in the cerebellar nuclear region affected the process of the CR consolidation.

The foregoing data are the first experimental evidence suggesting that the formation of plastic changes underlying the classical conditioning of the nictitating membrane response in the rabbit is dependent on protein synthesis at the cerebellar nuclear region. Although this finding is consistent with the possibility of protein synthesis-dependent plasticity at the cerebellar nuclei,

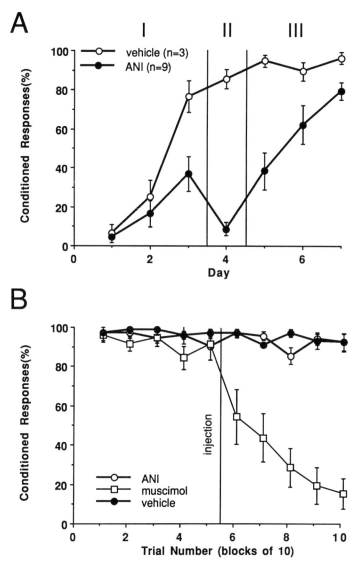

Figure 8.4 Effects of the protein synthesis inhibitor anisomycin (ANI) injected into the interposed nucleus on the acquisition (A) and retention (B) of the classically conditioned NMR in the rabbit. A. Incidence of conditioned responses in anisomycin and control (vehicle) experiments. I, initial 3 days of training performed with anisomycin injected before each training session; II, retention test (no injections, the day delineated by two vertical lines); III, additional 3 training days (no injections); n, number of animals included in the corresponding plot. B. Effects of the anisomycin, muscimol, and vehicle injections in the interposed nucleus on the incidence of the CRs in subjects from the ANI group represented in plot A. The drugs were injected following training phase III at the sites infused with anisomycin during the initial training (phase I).

several additional considerations have to be clarified before this conclusion can be made. First, it should be remembered that it is not certain whether the method of local protein synthesis inhibition affects the operation of structures related to the cerebellar nuclei. The local application of anisomycin clearly has a smaller effect on the performance of cerebellar circuits then those agents traditionally used to inhibit cellular firing. This point is reflected in the capacity of anisomycin-injected animals to express behavioral CRs. It is possible, however, that the drug affects subtle learning processes located elsewhere, which do not affect the immediate CR expression. Second, it is possible that the putative learning-induced synthesis of new proteins at the interposed nucleus is instrumental in inducing plastic changes occurring elsewhere. If so, the observed results do not reflect as much the localization of plastic changes as they illustrate the distributed cascade of events leading to the CR acquisition. Third (and relevant to the discussion of the distributed versus localized engrams of memory), it is not clear if the inhibition of protein synthesis at other segments of the conditioned reflex circuitry would affect the CR acquisition as well. Additional experiments are necessary to clarify these issues.

CEREBELLAR INVOLVEMENT IN THE CONTROL OF CONDITIONED AND UNCONDITIONED NMRs

One of the most discussed topics related to classical conditioning of the NMR in the rabbit is the issue of *learning* versus *performance*. As indicated earlier, the CR deficits induced by the interposed cerebellar lesions were originally interpreted either as a consequence of damage to the physical site of underlying plastic changes (Thompson, 1986) or as a result of the general NMR performance impairment induced by the lesion (Welsh and Harvey, 1989; Welsh, 1992; chapter 6). The learning-versus-performance argument has been centered around interpretations of the effects of cerebellar lesions on URs. The performance hypothesis is supported by findings of deficits in the late components of URs caused by permanent cerebellar nuclear lesions (Welsh, 1992). On the other hand, the learning concept is supported by a differential recovery of conditioned and unconditioned NMRs following permanent cerebellar interposed lesions (Steinmetz, Lavond, Ivkovich, Logan, and Thompson, 1992).

Studies performed in our laboratory demonstrated that, in contrast to permanent lesions, the temporary inactivation of the red nucleus (Bracha, Stewart, and Bloedel, 1993) or the interposed nucleus (Bracha et al., 1994) not only disrupts CRs, but in parallel it also severely reduces the amplitude of URs. The data from these inactivation experiments led to the conclusion that in the intact rabbit, the intermediate cerebellum influences expression of both CRs and URs. After permanent lesions, the UR performance significantly recovers, and the expression of CRs remains permanently disrupted. These data argue against the notion of the selective involvement of the intermediate cerebellum in the control of the conditioned NMR (Steinmetz et al., 1992). However, the same data do not prove or disprove either the learning or the performance hypothesis (for discussion, see Bracha et al., 1994, and Bloedel and Bracha, 1995). The data acquired in studies of UR performance cannot be used to localize sites of plastic changes subserving NMR conditioning, because they simply reflect—but cannot conclusively dissociate between—the parallel involvement of overlapping circuits in both the learning and expression of the learned and unlearned response (see previous section).

The operation of the intermediate cerebellum is not limited to the control of the eyeblink response. Earlier studies indicated that cerebellar ablations affect performance of other types of conditioned withdrawal reflexes (Popov, 1929) and of several types of postural cutaneomuscular reflexes (Amassian, Weiner, and Rosenblum 1972; Chambers and Sprague, 1955a, b). To further analyze the involvement of the intermediate cerebellum in reflex control, we recently investigated the effects of interposed nucleus inactivation on the performance of conditioned and unconditioned limb withdrawal responses in the cat (Kolb, Irwin, Winters, Bloedel, and Bracha, 1994). The limb withdrawal model offers several advantages over the eyeblink preparation, the most important of which are that the limb effector system has more degrees of freedom and that it is functionally more diverse than the highly specialized facial eyeblink reflex. These features of the limb withdrawal model allow a detailed analysis of the effects of cerebellar manipulations on withdrawal reflex operation along with comparisons of the effects of these manipulations on the performance of other cutaneomuscular reflexes.

EXPERIMENTS EXAMINING THE CEREBELLAR INVOLVEMENT IN THE LIMB CUTANEOMUSCULAR REFLEXES

Food-motivated cats were rewarded for standing quietly on four elevated platforms. After acquisition of the operantly conditioned quiet stance, the eyeblink, forelimb, and hindlimb withdrawal reflexes were classically conditioned in each animal. Cats were conditioned in the delay-conditioning paradigm, using a 550-ms-long CS (tone for the eyeblink, air puff to the shoulder for the forelimb, and air puff to the hip area for the hindlimb) and a 100-ms US (air puff for the eyeblink and electrical stimulation of the skin at the distal part of the corresponding extremity for the forelimb and hindlimb). The interstimulus interval was 450 ms. After the cats learned to respond to each CS by the withdrawal in the corresponding effector system, we analyzed the influence of the interposed nucleus inactivation on the performance of the conditioned and unconditioned withdrawal reflexes. For that purpose, the region of the interposed nucleus was injected with 1 μl (800 ng) of the GABA$_A$ agonist muscimol or with 1 μl of saline (control experiments) during each experiment. In each session, the effects of the interposed nucleus inactivation on the performance of several other cutaneomuscular reflexes (the tactile contact placing response, the hopping response, and the magnet response) were also examined.

The inactivation of the interposed nucleus affected the performance of CRs in all three effector systems (Kolb et al., 1994). The conditioned eyeblink responses were completely abolished in several experiments. This finding closely resembles the effects of nucleus interpositus inactivation on the conditioned NMR in the rabbit (Bracha et al., 1994). The conditioned forelimb and hindlimb responses were affected in a qualitatively different fashion. The conditioned limb withdrawal response consists of three main components: a postural adjustment followed by the flexion and lifting-up of the limb and concluding with the extension of the limb and its placement back on the supporting platform. At the most effective injection sites, the CR limb flexion component was abolished soon after the infusion of muscimol (figure 8.5B, C). The early postural component of the CR was more resistent to this treatment (figure 8.5A) and in most experiments it was present to the end of behavioral testing (approximately 60 min. after the muscimol infusion). Interestingly, one of the most dramatic effects of interposed nucleus inactivation was observed during the placement of the limb on the platform. Following muscimol infusions at the most effective injection sites, cats frequently failed to place the limb correctly back on the support and this usually elicited several corrective postural responses. The corrective responses were hypermetric, and this deficit frequently resulted in large-amplitude limb oscillations. In the most severe cases, the animal failed to place the limb on the platform and had to be assisted by the experimenter to complete the experiment.

Similar to results from our eyeblink studies in the rabbit (Bracha et al., 1994), the interposed nucleus inactivation in the cat severely reduced the amplitude of unconditioned withdrawal responses in the limb both in trials with paired presentation of stimuli and in the US alone trials (figures 8.5B and C and 8.6B and C). Frequently, the interposed inactivation altered direction and trajectory of the wrist during the UR. Parallelling the effects on the conditioned and unconditioned withrawal reflexes, the injections of muscimol in the interposed nucleus also affected other cutaneomuscular reflexes. All the tested postural responses were down regulated. Their threshold increased, and placing and hopping responses in the limb ipsilateral to the injection were hypermetric. At the most effective injection sites, all three postural responses (placing, hopping, and magnet responses) were abolished.

The incapacity of cats with inactivated interposed nuclei to generate the classically conditioned forelimb and hindlimb flexion confirms previous reports of similar findings from experiments lesioning the inferior olive (Voneida, Christie, Bogdanski, and Chopko, 1990) or the red nucleus (Smith, 1970) in the cat. This set of observations indicates that components of the system involved in the classical conditioning of the NMR also participate in execution of conditioned limb flexion. The similarities between the CR and UR deficits of the eyeblink in the rabbit and those of the limb withdrawal

A

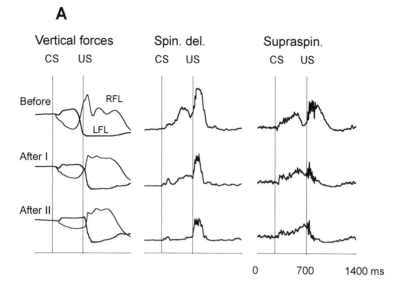

Vertical forces   Spin. del.   Supraspin.

CS   US   CS   US   CS   US

Before   RFL

LFL

After I

After II

0   700   1400 ms

B

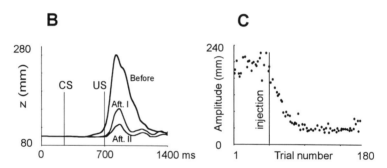

280

N (mm)

CS   US   Before

Aft. I

80   Aft. II

0   700   1400 ms

C

240

Amplitude (mm)

injection

0

1   Trial number   180

Figure 8.5   Example of effects of the left interposed nucleus inactivation on the performance of the classically conditioned withdrawal response in the left forelimb. A. Vertical forces recorded on platforms supporting the left forelimb (LFL) and right forelimb (RFL) and integrated and rectified EMG activity recorded in the spinal deltoideus (Spin. del.) and supraspinatus (Supraspin.) muscles in the left forelimb. Before, 25 trials before muscimol injection; After I (Aft. I), first 25 trials after injection; After II (Aft. II), next 25 trials following the inactivation. B. Vertical component (z) of the wrist withdrawal trajectory before and after muscimol injections. C. Changes of the amplitude of wrist movement during the withdrawal reaction as a function of trial number. The amplitude of the response was calculated in a three-dimensional space. CS, time of the conditioned stimulus onset; US, the unconditioned stimulus onset. Each trace in A and B represents averages of 25 trials. Each 25-trial period corresponds approximately to 25 minutes. In A, note the disappearance of the postural component (the rapid unloading [downward deflection] of the LFL just before the US onset) of the CR following the muscimol injection. The other postural component of the CR (the increase of the loading force in the LFL shortly after the CS onset) is preserved after the injection. The EMG activity in both proximal muscles during the CR interval is diminished but was not abolished following the injection. In B, note the disappearance of the conditioned limb flexion following the injection. Both B and C illustrate a decrease of the withdrawal amplitude induced by the interposed inactivation.

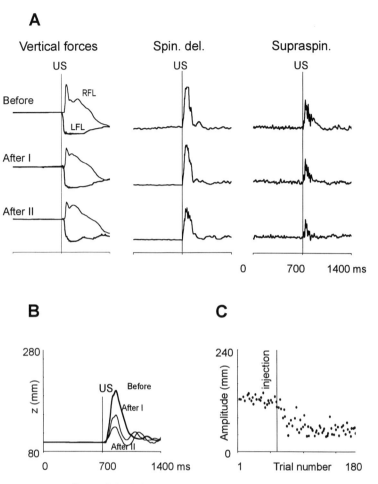

Figure 8.6 Effects of the left interposed nucleus inactivation on the performance of the unconditioned withdrawal response in the left forelimb. The data were acquired during trials consisting of the presentation of the US alone in the same experiment illustrated in figure 8.5. A. Vertical forces generated by both forelegs and the EMG activity in the spinal deltoideus and supraspinatus muscles in the left forelimb. B. Vertical component of the wrist trajectory during withdrawal before and after nuclear inactivation. C. Wrist withdrawal amplitude as a function of the trial number. For explanation of abbreviations see the legend of figure 8.5. Note the reduction of the duration of the left forelimb platform unloading and amplitudes of EMG responses following muscimol injection (A). The limb flexion was also affected by muscimol as illustrated by the reduction of the wrist withdrawal amplitude in B and C.

in the cat reported in this chapter further support the notion of general involvement of the intermediate cerebellum-related circuits in the control of withdrawal responses in multiple effector systems (Bracha et al., 1994; Bloedel and Bracha, 1995). However, the analogy between the eyeblink and limb withdrawal is not absolute. First, our experiments revealed important differences in the cerebellar inactivation-induced deficits in these two response systems. The most significant among them is the relative insensitivity of the postural preparation for the limb withdrawal to the interposed inactivation. (The implications of this finding will be discussed further.) Second, whereas the conditioned eyeblink is consistently found to be critically dependent on the intermediate cerebellum in all studied mammalian species, the interspecies comparisons of the cerebellar involvement in the conditioned limb flexion are more disparate. The inactivation of the interposed nucleus in the cat (see the foregoing), or permanent lesions of this structure in the rabbit (Donegan and Thompson, 1991), disable the execution of the flexion component of the conditioned limb withdrawal. In the mouse, however, permanent lesions of the interposed nuclei prevent acquisition of the conditioned limb flexion but do not block expression of the previously acquired CRs (Marchetti-Gauthier, Meziane, Devigne, and Soumireau-Mourat, 1990). In the dog, cerebellar ablations were reported ineffective in preventing either acquisition or retention of the conditioned limb withdrawal (Gambaryan, 1960, and Fanardjian, 1961). These data seem to indicate that the eyeblink reflex system is evolutionarily more conservative than the limb-withdrawal reflex and that it relies on circuits critically dependent on the cerebellar function. The limb flexion system shares components of the same circuits as the eyeblink but, because it is integrated in the phylogenetically more flexible (and functionally more versatile) locomotor system, it can use other circuits not available for the eyeblink control.

The relative persistence of the postural preparation for the limb withdrawal following interposed inactivation sheds a new light on the possible participation of the cerebellum in CR control. The persistence of postural components of the CR after the phasic flexion of the withdrawal was abolished by interposed inactivation indicates that the intermediate cerebellum is preferentially involved in generating a specific part of the CR—namely, the limb flexion response. It is not clear whether this perseverance of the CR postural component following interposed inactivation reflects its independence from the intermediate cerebellum or if this response would be abolished after larger inactivations of cerebellar nuclei. Data from previous studies seem to support the first alternative. Popov (1929) reported that cerebellectomy in the dog did not abolish signalized avoidance conditioned limb withdrawals, but it changed their direction: Lesioned animals had a tendency to produce limb extension instead of limb flexion. Interestingly, the prominent component of the postural preparation for the conditioned withdrawal in the cat is a loading of the limb to be subsequently withdrawn. Persistence of this CR component following interposed inactivation closely resembles Popov's original reports. These observations, together with deficits in unconditioned withdrawal responses, indicate that the CR impairment following the interposed inactivation reflects an incapacity to produce adequate limb flexion rather than a disturbance of substrates related to the CS-US association.

The effects of interposed nucleus inactivation on the tactile placing and hopping responses in the cat are in agreement with earlier observations in the monkey and in the cat (Amassian et al., 1972; Goldberger and Growdon,

1973; Chambers and Sprague, 1955a, b), which described similar deficits following permanent cerebellar lesions. These data, together with deficits in the execution of withdrawal responses, indicate general involvement of the intermediate cerebellum in the regulation of a group of cutaneomuscular reflexes. Interestingly, the described deficits in the withdrawal and other cutaneomuscular reflexes share several common features: modified amplitude of the flexion movements, scaling of movements requiring precision placement of the distal part of the limb, and increased irregularity of their spatiotemporal patterns. At this point, it is not clear whether the deficits in several different cutaneomuscular reflexes reflect the separate and unique participation of the intermediate cerebellum in each of these responses, a disruption of an unknown cerebellar operation shared among these reflexes, or a malfunction of other CNS components related to the cerebellum.

CONCLUSIONS

The preceding overview of data from our, and others', laboratories illustrates that circuits involved in the control of the classically conditioned nictitating membrane in the rabbit are represented more adequately in the multiple-pathway model than in the more traditional single-pathway model. The complex architecture of the multiple-pathway model and the multiple interactions between its components illustrate the basis for the difficulty in dissociating between learning and the on-line operation of the circuit. These features of the multiple-pathway model, together with data documenting plasticity at several of its components and at several levels of the circuit hierarchy, lead to the working hypothesis that the plastic changes subserving the acquisition and retention of the classically conditioned NMR in the rabbit are distributed across at least several structures (see chapter 2). Furthermore, the operation of the intermediate cerebellum in regulating reflexes is not specific to the conditioned eyeblink reflex. The output of the nucleus interpositus is also involved in the control of unconditioned eyeblinks, of conditioned and unconditioned withdrawal reflexes in other effector systems, and in several other cutaneomuscular reflexes. The pattern of deficits induced by inactivating the cerebellar interposed nucleus indicates multifunctional involvement of this structure in the control of automatic movements. The complex functions dependent on the operation of the intermediate cerebellum include the amplitude of flexion movements, the scaling of movements requiring precision placement of distal parts of the limb, and the temporal and spatial consistency of automatic movements.

ACKNOWLEDGMENTS

We thank ML Webster, KB Irwin, and NK Winters for their assistance in conducting experiments and in preparation of this manuscript. The research included in this paper was supported by National Institutes of Health grants NS 30013-04 and NS 21958.

REFERENCES

Amassian VE, Weiner H, Rosenblum M (1972). Neural systems subserving the tactile placing reaction: A model for the study of higher level control of movement. Brain Res 40:171–178.

Aou S, Woody CD, Birt D (1992). Increases in excitability of neurons of the motor cortex of cats after rapid acquisition of eye blink conditioning. J Neurosci 12:560–569.

Bartholomew SA, Webster ML, Bloedel JR, Bracha V (1994). Functional localization and neuro-anatomical connectivity of neural substrates within the anterior interposed nucleus involved in expression of the nictitating membrane reflex. Soc Neurosci Abstr 20:1011.

Batini C, Billard JM, Daniel H (1985). Long-term modification of cerebellar inhibition after inferior olive degeneration. Exp Brain Res 59:404–409.

Beggs AL, Steinmetz JE, Romano AG, Patterson MM (1983). Extinction and retention of a classically conditioned flexor nerve response in acute spinal cat. Behav Neurosci 97:530–540.

Benedetti F, Montarolo PG, Strata P, Tempia F (1983). Inferior olive inactivation decreases the excitability of the intracerebellar and lateral nuclei in the rat. J Physiol (Lond) 340:195–208.

Berger TW, Thompson RF (1982). Hippocampal cellular plasticity during extinction of classically conditoned nictitating membrane behavior. Behav Brain Res 4:63–76.

Berthier NE, Moore JW (1986). Cerebellar Purkinje cell activity related to the classically conditioned nictitating membrane response. Exp Brain Res 63:341–350.

Billard JM, Batini C, Daniel H (1988). The red nucleus activity in rats deprived of the inferior olivary complex. Behav Brain Res 28:127–130.

Bloedel JR, Bracha V (1995). On the cerebellum, cutaneomuscular reflexes, movement control and the elusive engrams of memory. Behav Brain Res 68:1–44.

Bracha V, Stewart SL, Bloedel JR (1993). The temporary inactivation of the red nucleus affects performance of both conditioned and unconditioned nictitating membrane responses in the rabbit. Exp Brain Res 94:225–236.

Bracha V, Webster ML, Winters NK, Irwin KB, Bloedel JR (1994). Effects of muscimol inactivation of the cerebellar interposed-dentate nuclear complex on the performance of the nictitating membrane response. Exp Brain Res 100:453–468.

Bracha V, Wu JZ, Cartwright S, Bloedel JR (1991). Selective involvement of the spinal trigeminal nucleus in the conditioned nictitating membrane reflex of the rabbit. Brain Res 556:317–320.

Bull R, Ferrera E, Orrego F (1976). Effects of anisomycin on brain protein synthesis and passive avoidance learning in newborn chicks. J Neurobiol 7:37–49.

Cegavske CF, Harrison TA, Torigoe Y (1987). Identification of the substrates of the unconditioned response in the classically conditioned, rabbit, nictitating-membrane preparation. In I Gormezano, WF Prokasy, RF Thompson (eds), Classical Conditioning, 3rd ed. Hillsdale, NJ: Lawrence Erlbaum Associates, pp 65–91.

Chambers WW, Sprague JM (1955a). Functional localization in the cerebellum: II. Somatic organization in cortex and nuclei. Arch Neurol Psychiatry 74:653–680.

Chambers WW, Sprague JM (1955b). Functional localization in the cerebellum: I. Organization in longitudinal corto-nuclear zones and their contribution to the control of posture, both extrapyramidal and pyramidal. J Comp Neurol 103:105–129.

Chan-Palay V (1977). Cerebellar Dentate Nucleus: Organization, Cytology and Transmitters. Berlin: Springer Verlag.

Chapman PF, Steinmetz JE, Sears LL, Thompson RF (1990). Effects of lidocaine injection in the interpositus nucleus and red nucleus on conditioned behavioral and neural responses. Brain Res 537:149–156.

Clark RE, Lavond DG (1993). Reversible lesions of the red nucleus during acquisition and retention of a classically conditioned behavior in rabbits. Behav Neurosci 107:264–270.

Clark RE, Zhang AA, Lavond DG (1992). Reversible lesions of the cerebellar interpositus nucleus during acquisition and retention of a classically conditioned behavior. Behav Neurosci 106:879–888.

Desmond JE, Moore JW (1991). Single-unit activity in red nucleus during the classically conditioned rabbit nictitating membrane response. Neurosci Res 10:260–279.

Donegan NH, Thompson RF (1991). The search for engram. In JL Martinez, Jr, RP Kesner (eds), Learning and Memory. A Biological View. San Diego: Academic Press, pp 3–58.

Du Lac S, Raymond JL, Sejnowski TJ, Lisberger SG (1995). Learning and memory in the vestibulo-ocular reflex. Annu Rev Neurosci 18:409–41.

Durkovic RG (1975). Classical conditioning, sensitization and habituation in the spinal cat. Physiol Behav 14:297–304.

Evinger C (1988). Extraocular motor nuclei: Location, morphology and afferents. Revi Oculomot Res 2:81–117.

Evinger C, Pellegrini JJ, Manning KA (1989). Adaptive gain modification of the blink reflex. A model system for investigating the physiologic bases of motor learning. Ann NY Acad Sci 563:87–100.

Fanardjian VV (1961). Influence of the cerebellum ablation on motor conditioned reflexes in dogs [in Russian]. Zh Vyssh Nerv Deiat Im I P Pavlova 11:920–926.

Gambaryan LS (1960). Conditioned avoidance reflexes induced in dogs with cerebellar lesions. Physiol Bohemoslov 9:261–266.

Garcia J, Hankins WG, Rusiniak KW (1974). Behavioral regulations of the milieu interne in man and rat. Science 185:824–831.

Gohl EB, Clark RE, Lavond DG (1993). Learning related unit activity in the lateral pontine nuclei is abolished with reversible inactivation of the interpositus nucleus. Soc Neurosci Abstr 19:999.

Goldberger ME, Growdon JH (1973). Pattern of recovery following cerebellar deep nuclear lesions in monkeys. Exp Neurol 39:307–322.

Gruart A, Blázquez P, Delgado-Garcia JM (1994). Kinematic analyses of classically-conditioned eyelid movements in the cat suggest a brain stem site for motor learning. Neurosci Lett 175:81–94.

Gutmann W, Brozek G, Bures J (1972). Cortical representation of conditioned eye blink in the rabbit studied by a functional ablation technique. Brain Res 40:203–213.

Harvey JA, Welsh JP, Yeo CH, Romano AG (1993). Recoverable and nonrecoverable deficits in conditioned responses after cerebellar lesions. J Neurosci 13:1624–1635.

Harvey JA, Land T, McMaster SE (1984). Anatomical study of the rabbit's corneal-VI nerve reflex: Connections between cornea, trigeminal sensory complex, and the abducens and accessory abducens nuclei. Brain Res 301:307–321.

Hiraoka M, Shimamura M (1977). Neural mechanisms of the corneal blinking reflex in cats. Brain Res 125:265–275.

Holstege G (1990). Neuronal organization of the blink reflex. In G Paxinos (ed), The Human Nervous System. San Diego: Academic Press, pp 287–296.

Holstege G, Blok BFM, Ter Horst GJ (1995). Brain stem systems involved in the blink reflex, feeding mechanisms, and micturition. In G Paxinos (ed), The Rat Nervous System. San Diego: Academic Press, pp 257–276.

Irwin KB, Craig AD, Bracha V, Bloedel JR (1992). Distribution of c-fos expression in brainstem neurons associated with conditioning and pseudo-conditioning of the rabbit nictitating membrane reflex. Neurosci Lett 148:71–75.

Ito M (1984). The Cerebellum and Neural Control. New York: Raven Press.

Ito M, Oda Y (1994). Electrophysiological evidence for formation of new corticorubral synapses associated with classical conditioning in the cat. Exp Brain Res 99:277–288.

Keifer J (1994). Inactivation of red nucleus blocks bursting in deep cerebellar nucleus: Evidence for a positive feedback circuit. Soc Neurosci Abstr 20:1744.

Kelly TM, Zuo CC, Bloedel JR (1990). Classical conditioning of the eyeblink reflex in the decerebrate-decerebellate rabbit. Behav Brain Res 38:7–18.

Kimura J (1974). Effect of hemispheric lesions on the contralateral blink reflex. Neurology 24:168–174.

Knowlton BJ, Thompson RF (1988). Microinjections of local anesthetic into the pontine nuclei reduce the amplitude of the classically conditioned eyelid response. Physiol Behav 43:855–857.

Kolb FP, Irwin KB, Winters NK, Bloedel JR, Bracha V (1994). Involvement of the cat cerebellar interposed nucleus in the control of conditioned and unconditioned withdrawal reflexes. Soc Neurosci Abstr 20:1746.

Krupa DJ, Thompson JK, Thompson RF (1993). Localization of a memory trace in the mammalian brain. Science 260:989–991.

Lavond DG, Lincoln JS, McCormick DA, Thompson RF (1984). Effect of bilateral lesions of the dentate and interpositus cerebellar nuclei on conditioning of heart-rate and nictitating membrane/eyelid responses in the rabbit. Brain Res 305:323–330.

Lewis JL, Lo Turco JJ, Solomon PR (1987). Lesions of the middle cerebellar peduncle disrupt acquisition and retention of the rabbit's classically conditioned nictitating membrane response. Behav Neurosci 101:151–157.

MacKay WA, Murphy JT (1979). Cerebellar modulation of reflex gain. Prog Neurobiol 13: 361–417.

Marchetti-Gauthier E, Meziane H, Devigne C, Soumireau-Mourat B (1990). Effects of bilateral lesions of the cerebellar interpositus nucleus on the conditioned forelimb flexion reflex in mice. Neurosci Lett 120:34–37.

Matsumura M, Woody CD (1986). Long-term increases in excitability of facial motoneurons and other neurons in and near the facial nuclei after presentations of stimuli leading to acquisition of a Pavlovian conditioned facial movement. Neurosci Res 3:568–589.

Mauk MD, Thompson RF (1987). Retention of classically conditioned eyelid responses following acute decerebration. Brain Res 403:89–95.

McCormick DA, Lavond DG, Thompson RF (1982). Concomitant classical conditioning of the rabbit nictitating membrane and eyelid responses: Correlations and implications. Physiol Behav 28:769–775.

Megirian D (1973). Unilateral cortical spreading depression and conditioned eye blink responses in rabbits. Acta Neurobiol Exp (Warsz) 33:699–710.

Molchan SE, Sunderland T, McIntosh AR, Herscovitch P, Schreurs BG (1994). A functional anatomical study of associative learning in humans. Proc Natl Acad Sci USA 91:8122–8126.

Moyer JR Jr, Deyo RA, Disterhoft JF (1990). Hippocampectomy disrupts trace eye-blink conditioning in rabbits. Behav Neurosci 104:243–252.

Murakami F, Oda Y, Tsukahara N (1988). Synaptic plasticity in the red nucleus and learning. Behav Brain Res 28:175–179.

Norman RJ, Buchwald JS, Villablanca JR (1977). Classical conditioning with auditory discrimination of the eyeblink in decerebrate cats. Science 196:551–553.

Oakley DA, Russell IS (1972). Neocortical lesions and Pavlovian conditioning. Physiol Behav 8:915–926.

Oakley DA, Russell IS (1977). Subcortical storage of Pavlovian conditioning in the rabbit. Physiol Behav 18:931–937.

Otani S, Marshall CJ, Tate WP, Goodard GV, Abraham WC (1989). Maintenance of long-term potentiation in rat dentate gyrus requires protein synthesis but not messenger RNA synthesis immediately post-tetanization. Neuroscience 28:519–526.

Pananceau M, Meftah EM, Rispal-Padel L (1994). Plasticity of the cerebello-rubral synapses during the conditioning of a forelimb motor response. Soc Neurosci Abstr 20:786.

Papsdorf JD, Longman D, Gormezano I (1965). Spreading depression: Effects of applying KC1 to the dura of the rabbit on the conditioned nictitating membrane response. Bull Psychon Sci 2:125–126.

Pastor AM, De la Cruz RR, Baker R (1994). Cerebellar role in adaptation of the goldfish vestibuloocular reflex. J Neurophysiol 72:1383–1394.

Popov NF (1929). The role of the cerebellum in the formation of conditioned motor reflexes. In DS Fursikov, MO Gurevich, AN Zalmanzon (eds), Vishaya N'ervnaya D'eyatel'nost': Sbornik Trudov Instituta. Moscow: Komunisticheskaya Akademiya, Institut Vyshey N'ervnoy D'eyatel'nosti, pp 140–148.

Richards WG, Ricciardi TN, Moore JW (1991). Activity of spinal trigeminal pars oralis and adjacent reticular formation units during differential conditioning of the rabbit nictitating membrane response. Behav Brain Res 44:194–204.

Rispal-Padel L, Meftah E (1992). Changes in motor responses induced by cerebellar stimulation during classical forelimb flexion conditioning in cat. J Neurophysiol 68:908–926.

Rosenblum K, Meiri N, Dudai Y (1993). Taste memory: The role of protein synthesis in gustatory cortex. Behav Neurol Biol 59:49–56.

Rosenfield ME, Moore JW (1983). Red nucleus lesions disrupt the classically conditioned nictitating membrane response in rabbits. Behav Brain Res 10:393–398.

Rosenfield ME, Moore JW (1985). Red nucleus lesions impair acquisition of the classically conditioned nictitating membrane response but not eye-to-eye savings or unconditioned response amplitude. Behav Brain Res 17:77–81.

Ruigrok TJH, Cella F (1995). Precerebellar nuclei and red nucleus. In G Paxinos (ed), The Rat Nervous System. San Diego: Academic Press, pp 277–308.

Smith AM (1970). The effects of rubral lesions and stimulation on conditioned forelimb flexion responses in the cat. Physiol Behav 5:1121–1126.

Solomon PR, Vander Schaaf ER, Thompson RF, Weisz DJ (1986). Hippocampus and trace conditioning of the rabbit's classically conditioned nictitating membrane response. Behav Neurosci 100:729–744.

Steinmetz JE, Lavond DG, Ivkovich D, Logan CG, Thompson RF (1992). Disruption of classical eyelid conditioning after cerebellar lesions: Damage to a memory trace system or a simple performance deficit? J Neurosci 12:4403–4426.

Tassoni G, Bucherelli C, Bures J (1992). Lateralized contributions of the cerebral cortex, parabrachial nucleus, and amygdala to acquisition and retrieval of passive avoidance reaction in rats: A functional ablation study. Behav Neurosci 106:933–939.

Thompson RF (1986). The neurobiology of learning and memory. Science 233:941–947.

Thompson RF, Krupa DJ (1994). Organization of memory traces in the mammalian brain. Annu Rev Neurosci 17:519–549.

van Ham JJ, Yeo CH (1992). Somatosensory trigeminal projections to the inferior olive, cerebellum and other precerebellar nuclei in rabbits. Eur J Neurosci 4:302–317.

Voneida TJ, Christie D, Bogdanski R, Chopko B (1990). Changes in instrumentally and classically conditioned limb-flexion responses following inferior olivary lesions and olivocerebellar tractotomy in the cat. J Neurosci 10:3583–3593.

Voogd J (1995). Cerebellum. In G Paxinos (ed), The Rat Nervous System. San Diego: Academic Press, pp 309–352.

Welsh JP (1992). Changes in the motor pattern of learned and unlearned responses following cerebellar lesions: A kinematic analysis of the nictitating membrane reflex. Neuroscience 47:1–19.

Welsh JP, Harvey JA (1989). Cerebellar lesions and the nictitating membrane reflex: performance deficits of the conditioned and unconditioned response. J Neurosci 9:299–311.

Welsh JP, Harvey JA (1991). Pavlovian conditioning in the rabbit during inactivation of the interpositus nucleus. J Physiol (Lond) 444:459–480.

Welsh JP, Harvey JA (1992). The role of the cerebellum in voluntary and reflexive movements: history and current status. In RR Llinas, C Sotelo (eds), The Cerebellum Revisited. New York: Springer-Verlag, pp 301–334.

White IM, Miller DP, White W, Dike GL, Rebec GV, Steinmetz JE (1994). Neuronal activity in rabbit neostriatum during classical eyelid conditioning. Exp Brain Res 99:179–190.

Woodruff-Pak DS, Lavond DG, Logan CG, Steinmetz JE, Thompson RF (1993). Cerebellar cortical lesions and reacquisition in classical conditioning of the nictitating membrane response in rabbits. Brain Res 608:67–77.

Woody CD, Birt D (1992). Changes in the activity of units of the cat motor cortex with rapid conditioning and extinction of a compound eye blink movement. J Neurosci 12:549–559.

Woody CD, Wang XF, Gruen E (1994). Response to acoustic stimuli increases in the ventral cochlear nucleus after stimulus pairing. Neuroreport 5:513–515.

Yang BY, Weisz DJ (1992). An auditory conditioned stimulus modulates unconditioned stimulus-elicited neuronal activity in the cerebellar anterior interpositus and dentate nuclei during nictitating membrane response conditioning. Behav Neurosci 106:889–899.

Yeo CH (1991). Cerebellum and classical conditioning of motor responses. Ann NY Acad Sci 627:292–304.

Yeo CH, Hardiman MJ, Glickstein M (1985). Classical conditioning of the nictitating membrane response of the rabbit: II. Lesions of the cerebellar cortex. Exp Brain Res 60:99–113.

Yeo CH, Hardiman MJ, Glickstein M (1986). Classical conditioning of the nictitating membrane response of the rabbit: IV. Lesions of the inferior olive Exp Brain Res 63:81–92.

Zemlan FP, Behbehani MM (1988). Nucleus cuneiformis and pain modulation: Anatomy and behavioral pharmacology. Brain Res 453:89–102.

9 Control of Motor Behavior Acquisition by Cortical Activity Potentiated by Decreases in a Potassium A-Current that Increase Neural Excitability

Charles D. Woody

After Pavlovian conditioning of an eyeblink response to a click conditioned stimulus (CS), the probability of discharge evoked by the CS in neurons of the motor (pericruciate) cortex of cats is increased, as is the excitability of the neurons to intracellularly injected depolarizing current (Woody, Vassilevsky, and Engel, 1970; Woody and Black-Cleworth, 1973). The increased excitability and probability of discharge occur selectively in cells that project polysynaptically through motoneurons to the target muscles of the CR. These increases are found in cells of the appropriate motor projection for performing the motor tasks when different conditioned responses (CRs) are learned (Woody and Engel, 1972). The conjoint changes in membrane/firing properties support initiation of the specific conditioned motor response, and thus represent a putative neural basis for this aspect of motor learning.

Motor learning can be defined in many ways. The definition that we prefer is based on recognition of the primacy of the circuitry and adaptive mechanisms that serve the relevant input-output transfer functions (Woody, 1982). Though broad, it allows definition of motor (output line–labeled) behavior on the basis of the complex reflexive processes (with and without feedback) from which the behavior arises (Woody, 1987). The behavior itself can generate feedback from the environment.

In the absence of the motor cortex, the short-latency blink CR that is normally established by pairing click as a CS with glabella-tap as an unconditioned stimulus (US) is not learned (Woody, Yarowsky, Owens, Black-Cleworth, and Crow, 1974). Once learned, the CR is not expressed when cortical spreading depression is induced by application of KCl (Woody and Brozek, 1969b). Direct electrical stimulation of the motor cortex is a satisfactory stimulus for acquisition of this CR in animals missing the posterior cortex (Woody and Yarowsky, 1972). Development of the CR depends on the order and interval of CS-US pairing, and the CR is elicited preferentially by forward-paired CSs. Thus, the CR is associative and discriminative (Engel and Woody, 1972; Hirano et al., 1987) and depends on the motor cortex.

The increases in neural excitability of the pericruciate cortex (increases that support acquisition of motor behavior) are effected, in large part, by decreases in a potassium A-current in layer V pyramidal (PT) cells (Sakai and Woody,

1980; Woody, Gruen, and Birt, 1991a). Postsynaptic decreases in this depolarization-dependent potassium current will cause increases in the size of excitatory postsynaptic potentials (EPSPs) along appropriate regions of the cable space of the cell (Holmes and Woody, 1989) and will facilitate elicitation of spike discharges by stimuli such as the CS. This facilitation can be measured by introducing depolarizing pulses intracellularly (Woody and Black-Cleworth, 1973) or by applying microstimulation extracellularly (Woody et al., 1970; Woody and Engel, 1972).

BLINK CONDITIONING AS A MODEL OF MOTOR LEARNING

Conditioned eye blinking provides a useful model system for investigating neural mechanisms underlying motor learning (Woody et al., 1970; Woody and Black-Cleworth, 1973, 1978; McCormick and Thompson, 1984; Berthier and Moore, 1986, 1990; Disterhoft, Coulter, and Alkon, 1986; Desmond and Moore, 1986, 1991; Sanchez-Andres and Alkon, 1991; Woody, Swartz, and Gruen, and Woody et al., 1991a). When considered from onset to termination, the conditioned eyeblink is a complex behavioral response containing several motor components of different onset latencies. Discriminative conditioning of short-and long-latency-blink CRs can be established rapidly within 21 or fewer pairings of electrical stimulation of the hypothalamus (HS) with click CS and glabella-tap US (Hirano et al, 1987; Aou, Woody, and Birt, 1992a). The different motor components of these conditioned blink responses can be separated and characterized according to their occurrence latencies. Four are associated with an increase in electromyogram (EMG) activity elicited by the CS in the orbicularis oculi muscles (16–48 ms, $alpha_1$; 56–80 ms, $alpha_2$; 88–120 ms, beta; > 128 ms, gamma). An example of a unit recorded from the motor cortex of an awake, conditioned cat together with the concurrently recorded EMG of the blink CR is shown in figure 9.1. The appearance of different components depends on the sensitivity of the apparatus used to measure the response. (We use averages of EMG recordings, as shown in figure 9.1.)

Many areas of the brain are involved in producing conditioned behavior, and different features of the blink CR are sensitive to ablation of different central regions. As noted in more detail in other chapters (e.g., chapter 5), long-latency components of blink or nictitating membrane CRs are particularly sensitive to ablation of the red nucleus (Rosenfield and Moore, 1983), the interpositus nucleus (McCormick, Guyer, and Thompson, 1982; Steinmetz et al., 1991), and various regions of the cerebellum (Yeo, Hardiman, and Glickstein, 1984; Thompson, 1992). Trace-conditioned responses of long latencies are particularly sensitive to lesions of the hippocampus (Moyer, Deyo, and Disterhoft, 1990; chapter 7). Short-latency components are sensitive to lesions of the motor cortex (Woody et al., 1974). The variability of these sensitivities depends in part on the amount of tissue removed. (Lashley noted years ago that more than 90 percent of some regions had to be removed

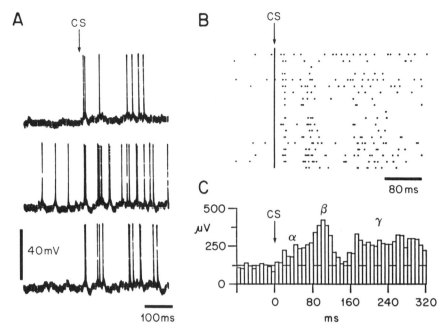

Figure 9.1 A. Intracellular recordings of activity from a unit of the motor cortex of a cat conditioned to eyeblink. B. A dot raster showing spike occurrences during sequential presentations (top to bottom) of the CS, the occurrence of which is indicated by the solid vertical line (and arrow under CS, as in A and C). Increased periods of spike discharge were correlated with alpha, beta, and gamma periods of increased EMG activity shown in the histogram average below C. Time and voltage calibrations are as indicated. Data in A and B were obtained from the same unit. The EMG data in C were obtained while recording from this unit. (Redrawn from Aou et al,, 1992a.)

before certain deficits appeared.) Some types of CRs can be acquired after complete removal of the cortex and diencephalon (Norman, Villablanca, Brown, Sckwafel, and Buchwald, 1974) or of the cerebellum (Llinas, Walton, Hillmon, and Sotelo, 1975; cf. Bloedel, 1992; Welsh, 1992). Note that on the basis of lesion studies alone, it is difficult to exclude the possibility that the lesion disrupted a tonic facilitatory pathway that gated transmission through another, adaptive pathway rather than disrupting the primary adaptive pathway itself (see chapter 15).

ROLE OF THE MOTOR CORTEX

Development of short-latency-blink CRs depends on a functionally intact rostral cortex. If 25% KCl is applied to the rostral cortex to produce spreading depression in conditioned animals, the short-latency blink CR is abolished reversibly, returning later after recovery, whereas the unconditioned blink response to glabella-tap is maintained throughout (Woody and Brozek, 1969b). This occurs in rabbits as well as in cats (Gutmann, Brozek, and Bures, 1972). As shown in figure 9.2, bilateral ablation of the rostral cortex prevents

gK$_A^+$, Neural Excitability, and Motor Control

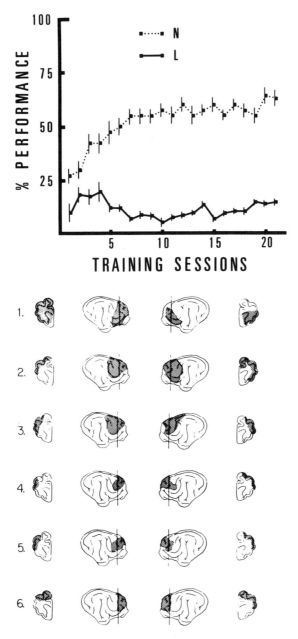

Figure 9.2 (Left) Mean performance levels of normal cats (N) and lesioned cats (L), with regions of rostral cortex removed (as shown to right) during training of classically conditioned eyeblink responses. Group averages and standard deviations (bars) were compiled from averages of response performance by each animal for the respective training session. Each session consisted of 150 trials of paired click CS and glabella-tap US. The CS-US interval was 400 ms; the intertrial interval was 10 s. (Redrawn from Woody et al., 1974.)

acquisition of short-latency conditioned blinking (Woody et al., 1974). The impairment persists despite extensive training for a period of 3 months after surgery. Control lesions of comparable size at more caudal regions fail to produce such deficits. The efferent pathway for mediation of the short-latency conditioned blink reflex runs from the motor cortex (by a possible interneuron) to the facial nucleus and finally to the orbicularis oculi muscles, where the blink CR is performed with an onset latency of 20 ms measured electromyographically.

Pyramidal tract (PT) cells of the motor cortex preferentially mediate transmission of short-latency auditory messages comparable to those used as the CS in our model of eyeblink conditioning (Sakai and Woody, 1980). Layer V PT cells of the rostral (pericruciate) cortex respond to click and hiss stimuli at latencies (8–10 ms) as short as those of the primary auditory cortex. On the basis of response latency, these cells constitute an "auditory-receptive cortex" within the cat motor cortex. Many of these cells show regular patterns of spike discharge to intracellularly applied depolarizing currents. This is of interest because four classes of neurons in area 4 gamma of the motor cortex of awake cats can be distinguished by their firing responses to depolarizing current: (1) inactivating bursting neurons, (2) noninactivating bursting neurons, (3) fast-spiking neurons, and (4) regularly spiking neurons. A recent study (Baranyi, Szeute, and Woody, 1993a,b) characterized the different classes by their antidromic and synaptic responses to stimulation of the pyramidal tract and ventrolateral (VL) thalamus. Cells of class 1 contained no cells with fast antidromic responses, class 2 had no cells with slow antidromic responses, class 3 had no antidromic responsive cells, and class 4 contained cells with both fast and slow antidromic responses. VL stimulation evoked responses in all cells with fast antidromic responses to PT stimulation. Fast-spiking neurons had a high frequency, nonaccommodative firing pattern and very brief action potentials of 0.25 ms at half amplitude. Regularly spiking neurons were the most commonly encountered (69 percent) type of cell. Average values of membrane potential, action potentials, and firing threshold did not differ significantly between classes. Input resistance was lower in cells with fast antidromic responses to peduncular stimulation (8.4 ± 1.2 MΩ) than in fast-spiking cells (20.9 ± 3.9 MΩ) and revealed correspondingly differing amounts of depolarizing current required to induce discharges.

MOVEMENT ENCODED BY INCREASED EXCITABILITY IN NEURONS OF THE MOTOR CORTEX

Development of the classically conditioned, short-latency eyeblink response to click in cats depends on neural adaptations in which stimulus-evoked neural activity and excitability are increased (Woody et al., 1970). The adaptations that have been found in cortical motor areas control performance of the learned motor response. The evidence for this arises from a series of experiments.

The first experiments established that increases in unit activity after conditioning were recorded preferentially at cortical motor areas that projected interneuronally to the target muscles of the conditioned response (Woody et al., 1970).

Then the changes in CS-evoked unit activity were found to be associated with reduction in the level of extracellular, electrical stimulation (at nA levels and greater) required to produce an EMG response in the target muscles of the CR (Woody and Engel, 1972). Results from activity-threshold studies of three different CRs are summarized in figure 9.3.

In awake, blink-trained cats, significantly less intracellularly injected current was required to initiate action potentials in units of the coronal-pericruciate cortex projecting ultimately to blink musculature than was required in adja-

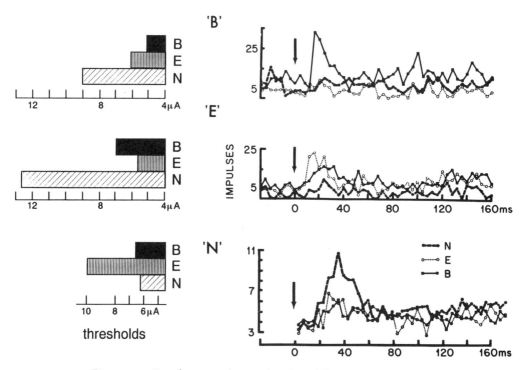

Figure 9.3 Data from animals trained to three different conditioned movements. B = both an eyeblink and a nose twitch; E = eyeblink alone; N = nose twitch alone. To the right are histogram averages of spike activity to click CS (delivered at arrows) obtained from the coronal-pericruciate cortex of cats in each behavioral state. Each histogram shows separate averages from units in areas projecting through facial nucleus to nose twitch muscles (N), eyeblink muscles (E), or both muscle groups (B). (Projection was determined by stimulating the recording location after every unit's spike activity was studied and then averaging the peripheral EMG from levator oris and orbicularis muscles.) To the left are shown the averaged currents required for cortical microstimulation to elicit detectable responses in the peripheral muscles. As can be seen, neural activity and excitability changed with the type of motor response that was learned, being greatest in the cells and areas that projected to the target muscles that performed the particular motor response. Further information may be found in Woody and Engel (1972) and Woody (1982).

cent units projecting elsewhere (Woody and Black-Cleworth, 1973). This indicated that the excitability changes were expressed postsynaptically, directly in the studied units.

In cats trained to a different movement involving both eyeblink and nose twitch muscles, Brons and Woody (1980) confirmed the observation that less intracellular current was required to discharge cortical units of target CR-musculature projection. Cortical neural excitability also increased in comparison with levels in naive animals after conditioning short- and long-latency-blink CRs with pairing of click CS, tap, and hypothalamic stimulation (HS) (see figure 9.4). The increases persisted with learnings savings through an extinction procedure (Aou et al., 1992b). Comparable increases in neural excitability were found in facial motoneurons after conditioning an eyeblink with click CS and tap US (Matsumura and Woody, 1986).

Earlier investigators have observed changes in cortical excitability related to motor performance (Graham-Brown and Sherrington, 1912; Graham-Brown, 1915; Ukhtomsky, 1926; Loucks, 1933; Doty and Giurgea, 1961). Our intracellular studies have advanced their observations by demonstrating directly (at the level of single cells) that the cortical excitability changes are coded according to the projection of the neurons in which they should appear for

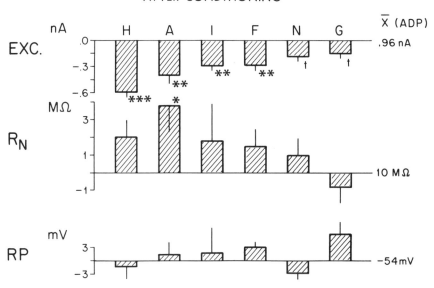

Figure 9.4 Differences between pre- and post-conditioning states in mean values of neural excitability (EXC.), input resistance (R_N), and resting potential (RP) obtained from cortical units of six cats trained to blink (CR) by pairing click CS, glabella-tap, and electrical stimulation of the lateral hypothalamus. Thin vertical bars show standard errors of the means. Letters identify cats. After conditioning, excitability increased and less intracellularly applied current was required for spike initiation (*$p \leq .05$; **$p \leq .01$; ***$p \leq .001$; '$p \leq .10$). Means for pre-conditioning values are shown to right, under $\overline{X}$ (ADP). (Redrawn from Aou et al., 1992b.)

gK_A^+, Neural Excitability, and Motor Control

the motor behavior to be performed (Woody and Black-Cleworth, 1973). The changes can be induced nonassociatively by serial presentations of tap USs alone but are more robust and enduring when induced by associative pairing of a CS and US (Brons and Woody, 1980).

BLINK CONDITIONING AS A MODEL FOR INVESTIGATING ELECTROPHYSIOLOGICAL CONSEQUENCES OF STIMULUS ASSOCIATIONS

Conditioned eye blinking provides a particularly useful model system for investigating electrophysiological consequences of stimulus associations that produce neural adaptations serving behavioral changes. Besides the unexpectedly broad scope of motor behavior investigation made possible by this model, there are several other reasons why it is extremely useful.

First, considerable attention has been devoted to placing conditioned eyeblink responses of both short and long latency within the behavioral context of traditional psychological descriptions of associative conditioning (Grant, 1943; Grant and Norris, 1947; Kimble and Dufort, 1956; Kimble, 1961; Gormezano and Moore, 1969; Woody, 1982; Gormezano, Prokasky, and Thompson, 1987). Studies that have incorporated sufficiently sensitive measures of EMG and unit activity have detected coincidental features of sensitization, habituation, and sensory preconditioning. They have been distinguished from those of conditioning on the basis of specificity of eliciting stimuli, latency, specificity and time-course of development, and extinction of the conditioned blink response (Woody, 1984).

Though latent facilitation can play a role in inducing some of the neural changes (Brons and Woody, 1980; Berthier and Woody, 1984), there is ample evidence (Kim, Woody, and Berthier, 1983; Hirano et al., 1987; Aou et al., 1992a) to indicate that rapidly acquired blink conditioning is behaviorally associative and does not represent simply a nonspecific sensitization or arousal effect of stimulating the hypothalamus. Extensive behavioral studies also have shown that the short, alpha-latency-blink CR formed by pairing click CS with glabella-tap US without HS is an associatively conditioned discriminative response (Engel and Woody, 1972; Woody, Kmispel, Crow, and Black-Cleworth, 1976). Both short- and long-latency components of blink CRs are acquired *pari passu* in the course of rapid associative conditioning with HS (Aou et al., 1992a,b). Thus, the different components appear to reflect common features of classical conditioning. The acquisition and expression of different components depends on temporal and other parameters of the paired stimuli (Woody and Brozek, 1969a; Woody, 1982; Kim, Woody and Bertier, 1983; Woody, Kim, and Bertier, 1983; Hirano et al., 1987). Gruart, Blazquez, and Delgado-Garcia (1994) have found 50-ms onset CRs after pairing 200-ms tones with an ocular air puff in cats. Kim et al. (1983) found late- but not early-onset blink CRs when a 340-ms interstimulus interval (ISI) was used instead of a 570-ms ISI for pairing click, tap, and HS (the latter producing early and late components; Hirano et al., 1987). Mayer et al.'s trace conditioning effects (1990) involved comparable differences in ISIs.

Second, the short-onset latencies of EMG and unit activation have proved advantageous in investigating the anatomical circuitry underlying production of the conditioned and unconditioned response (Kugelberg, 1952; Rushworth, 1962; Woody and Brozek, 1969a,b; Woody et al., 1970 cf.). We have traced the acoustic CS pathway electrophysiologically from dorsal and ventral cochlear nuclei (Woody, Wang, Gruen, and Landeira-Fernandez, 1992, Woody, Wang, and Gruen, 1994) to dentate nucleus (Wang, Woody, Chizhevsky, Gruen, and Landeira-Fernandez, 1991), rostral thalamus (Woody, Gruen, Melamed, and Chizhevsky, 1991b), and motor cortex (Sakai and Woody, 1980). The CR can be learned in the absence of the classical auditory cortex (Woody et al., 1974).

Third, significant advances have been made with this model system in measuring changes in the membrane properties of central neurons in vitro (Disterhoft et al., 1986, and Sanchez-Andres and Alkon, 1991) and in vivo in awake animals as a function of behavioral state and various experimental procedures (Woody and Black-Cleworth, 1973; Woody et al., 1978, 1991a; Baranyi, Szente, and Woody, 1991). Detailed findings will be described separately.

Fourth, an opportunity to study the neural basis of different rates of conditioning is provided by the ability to obtain discriminatively conditioned blink responses within a few minutes by adding HS associatively to 10 to 20 presentations of click CS and tap US. Voronin, Gerstein, Kudryashov, and Ioffe (1975) first established that pairing electrical stimulation of the lateral hypothalamus with a CS and US could reduce the number of pairings required to produce a conditioned foreleg movement in rabbits. They also showed that CR acquisition depended on the associative order of stimulus presentation. We confirmed that this could be done with blink CRs in cats (Kim et al., 1983; Hirano et al., 1987).

GLUTAMATE AS A SUBSTITUTE FOR HS IN PRODUCING CELLULAR CONDITIONING IN MOTOR CORTEX UNITS

Local iontophoretic application of glutamate has been found to be a successful substitute for HS to produce rapid conditioning of increases in CS-evoked activity in motor cortex cells (Woody et al., 1991a). Learning this cellular CR (which closely resembles the activity increase after behavioral conditioning) occurs after pairing glutamate with the same CS and US used behaviorally. The order of pairing of glutamate for successful cellular conditioning is similar to the order of pairing of HS required for increasing the rate of behavioral conditioning (having to come after rather than before the paired CS and US).

The finding of order dependence is significant because other investigators (Storozhuk, Ivanova, and Sanzharovski, 1992a) have shown that iontophoretic application of glutamate can potentiate responses to the CS of some cortical units in behaviorally conditioned animals when given just before the CS. That potentiation appears to reflect direct, transient interactions between glutamate and acetylcholine (Tremblay, Warren, and Dykes, 1990; Storozhuk, Ivanova, and Stezhka, 1992b). Long-lasting potentiation of the type observed in our conditioned animals may develop more rapidly if glutamate follows rather than precedes the release of acetylcholine (Woody and Gruen, 1993).

DECREASED POTASSIUM A-CURRENT IN CONDITIONED CELLS

While conditioning increases in activity to click CS in neurons of the motor cortex of awake cats, using glabella-tap and glutamate applied locally after the CS, the membrane currents of the neurons were evaluated using the single-electrode voltage clamp approach. The glutamate was applied through a fine micropipette attached to the recording electrode. The excitability and apparent input resistance (R_n) of the neurons were also measured sequentially in bridge mode recordings, by switching back and forth from voltage clamp to bridge mode, thus allowing measurement of changes in spike activity, excitability, and R_n after conditioning. Electrodes passed steady, hyperpolarizing and depolarizing currents of greater than 10 nA prior to insertion and did not show rectification with pulse currents of ± 1 nA in vivo. The headstage output was monitored during voltage clamp operation and showed satisfactory settling times for the electrodes at switching frequencies up to 5000 Hz using a duty cycle of 50 percent.

Though the entire space of the cells could not be clamped, changes in net currents could be measured with holding currents ranging from -70 to -80 mV and command steps of ± 10 to 40 mV. Of 19 units that developed a conditioned spike discharge in response to a click CS after pairing the click with glabella-tap and local iontophoretic application of glutamate, 16 showed reductions of an early outward current induced by depolarizing commands or by return to holding potentials after hyperpolarizing commands (Woody et al., 1991a; see figure 9.5). Of 15 units that failed to develop a conditioned response, none showed these changes. Changes in later currents also were found in cells that developed CRs, as were increases in neural excitability and input resistance. The identities of the later currents were not established by these investigations. The changes in neural excitability and input resistance were comparable to those that occurred after behavioral conditioning and after applications of acetylcholine or cyclic guanosine monophosphate (GMP; Woody and Gruen, 1988). The decrease in the outward current after conditioning resembled that found after local application of acetylcholine or cyclic GMP-dependent protein kinase (Woody and Gruen, 1987).

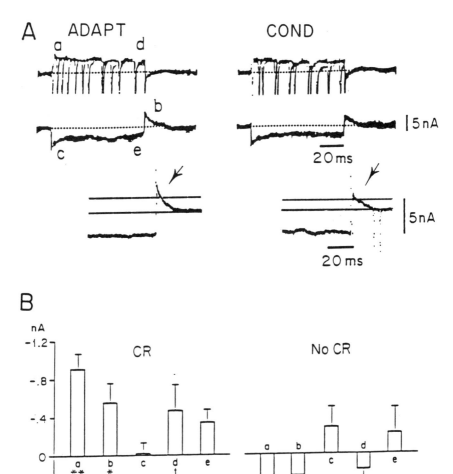

Figure 9.5 A. Single-electrode voltage clamp records from a unit before (ADAPT) and after (COND) development of a conditioned spike response to click CS after pairing the CS with tap US and iontophoresis of glutamate. Traces (two superimposed recordings each) show currents elicited by +20-mV and −20-mV commands and (below) averages of responses at point b to the offset of −20-mV commands. Conditioning produced a decrease in the outward deinactivation current (arrows). B. Averages ± standard errors of changes of currents found after conditioning in cells with and without development of CRs. (The latter include cells given a backward conditioning paradigm.) Currents were measured at times a to e, as shown in A. The statistical significance values shown (*$p < .01$; **$p < .0001$; $^t p = .10$) are results of comparing changes in currents at these times among groups of cells with and without CRs. (Redrawn from Woody et al., 1991a.)

215   gK_A^+, Neural Excitability, and Motor Control

Sensitivity to 4-Aminopyridine

The early outward current was determined to be an aminopyridine-sensitive current. Cells given pressure injection of 3- or 4-aminopyridine showed a reduction of the current (Woody et al., 1989).

The current increased with increasing, positive step voltage commands from holding potentials set between -60 and -80 mV. Preceding depolarizing pulses reduced this change whereas preceding hyperpolarizing pulses potentiated it. The current was thus identified as one of the family of potassium A-currents with a voltage dependence resembling that found in vitro in cortical cells (Gustafsson, Galvan, Grafe, and Wigstrom, 1982; Andreasen and Hablitz, 1994).

How the A-Current Works

In the awake cat, levels of baseline synaptic activity produce levels of depolarization sufficient for the A-current (I_A) to be activated. Given fluctuations in patterns of ongoing synaptic activity, complete inactivation of the A-current from sustained depolarization apparently does not occur. A partial, steady-state reduction of the remaining steady-state activation of I_A could contribute to the steady-state increase in input resistance and to the increased excitability to depolarizing inputs found after conditioning. Use of cable equations to simulate the cable properties of layer V cortical PT cells (Holmes and Woody, 1989) has shown that regional increases in membrane resistance can magnify selectively the spread of synaptic currents from the dendrites to the sites of spike initiation in or near the cell soma. An increase in resistance would contribute "passively" to the increased excitability of these cells, after conditioning, that underlies the increased probability of CS-evoked spike discharge, which controls production of the specific conditioned movement and the motor learning that it represents.

The early component of the outward current has a more "active" mode of functioning. Activation increases when presentation of a CS introduces a depolarizing EPSP into the cell. The increased potassium conductance counteracts the depolarizing effect of the EPSP. When conditioning causes a reduction in this conductance, the depolarizing effect of the EPSP is potentiated, and the probability that the EPSP will elicit spike activity is increased. Also increased is the likelihood that an intracellularly (or large, extracellularly) applied depolarizing current pulse will elicit spike discharge. This is exactly what was observed in these cells after behavioral conditioning. Thus, we suggest that postsynaptic conductance changes of this type constitute one of the prototypical cortical engrams needed for some forms of motor learning.

ACKNOWLEDGMENT

This work was supported in part by HD05958. I acknowledge with particular pleasure the contributions to this research made by the coinvestigators in the publications cited in the references.

REFERENCES

Andreasen M, Hablitz JJ (1992). Kinetic properties of a transient outward current in rat neocortical neurons. J Neurophysiol 68:1133–1142.

Aou S, Woody CD, Birt D (1992a). Changes in the activity of units of the cat motor cortex with rapid conditioning and extinction of a compound eye blink movement. J Neurosci 12: 549–559.

Aou S, Woody CD, Birt D (1992b). Increases in excitability of neurons of the motor cortex of cats after rapid acquisition of eye blink conditioning. J Neurosci 12:560–569.

Baranyi A, Szente MB, Woody CD (1991). Properties of associative long-lasting potentiation induced by cellular conditioning in the motor cortex of conscious cats. Neuroscience 42:321–334.

Baranyi A, Szente MB, Woody CD (1993a). Electrophysiological characterization of different types of neurons recorded in vivo in the motor cortex of the cat: I. Patterns of firing activity and synaptic responses. J Neurophysiol 69:1850–1864.

Baranyi A, Szente MB, Woody CD (1993b). Electrophysiological characterization of different types of neurons recorded in vivo in the motor cortex of the cat: II. Membrane parameters, action potentials, current-induced voltage responses and electrotonic structures. J Neurophysiol 69:1865–1879.

Berthier NE, Moore JW (1986). Cerebellar Purkinje cell activity related to the classically conditioned nictitating membrane response. Exp Brain Res 63:341–350.

Berthier NE, Moore JW (1990). Activity of deep cerebellar nuclear cells during classical conditioning of the nictitating membrane response in rabbits. Exp Brain Res 83:44–54.

Bloedel JR (1992). Functional heterogeneity with structural hoimogeneity: How does the cerebellum operate? Behav Brain Sci 15:666–678.

Brons JF, Woody CD (1980). Long-term changes in excitability of cortical neurons after Pavlovian conditioning and extinction. J Neurophysiol 44:605–615.

Desmond JE, Moore JW (1986). Dorsolateral pontine tegmentum and the classically conditioned nictitating membrane response: Analysis of CR-related single-unit activity. Exp Brain Res 65:59–74.

Desmond JE, Moore JW (1991). Single-unit activity in red nucleus during the classically conditioned rabbit nictitating membrane response. Neurosci Res 10:260–279.

Disterhoft JF, Coulter DA, Alkon DA (1986). Conditioning-specific membrane changes of rabbit hippocampal neurons measured in vitro. Proc Natl Acad Sci USA 83:2733–2737.

Doty RW, Giurgea C (1961). Conditioned reflex established by coupling electrical excitability of two cortical areas. In J Delafresnaye (ed), Brain Mechanisms and Learning. Oxford. Blackwell, pp 133–151.

Engel J, Woody CD (1972). Effects of character and significance of stimulus on unit activity at coronal-pericruciate cortex of cat during performance of conditioned motor response. J Neurophysiol 35:220–229.

Gormezano I, Moore JW (1969). Classical conditioning. In MH Marx (ed), Learning: Processes, part III. New York: MacMillan, pp 120–203.

Gormezano I, Prokasy WF, Thompson RF (1987). Classical Conditioning. Hillsdale, NJ: Lawrence Erlbaum Associates.

Graham-Brown T (1915). Studies in the physiology of the nervous system: 23. On the phenomenon of facilitation: Its occurrence in response to subliminal cortical stimuli in monkeys. Q J Exp Physiol 9:101–116.

Graham-Brown T, Sherrington CS (1912). On the instability of a cortical point. Proc R Soc Lond B Biol Sci 85:250–277.

Grant DA (1943). Sensitization and association in eyelid conditioning. J Exp Psychol 32: 201–212.

Grant DA, Norris EB (1947). Eyelid conditioning as influenced by the presence of sensitized beta-responses. J Exp Psychol 37:423–433.

Gruart A, Blazquez P, Delgado-Garcia JM (1994). Kinematic analyses of classically-conditioned eyelid movements in the cat suggests a brain stem site for motor learning. Neurosci Lett 175:81–84.

Gustafsson B, Galvan M, Grafe P, Wigstrom H (1982). A transient outward current in a mammalian central neurone blocked by 4-aminopyridine. Nature 344:240–242.

Gutmann W, Brozek G, Bures J (1972). Cortical representation of conditioned eyeblink in the rabbit studied by a functional ablation technique. Brain Res 40:203–213.

Hirano T, Woody C, Birt D, Aou S, Miyake J, Nenov, V (1987). Pavlovian conditioning of discriminatively elicited eyeblink responses with short onset latency attributable to lengthened interstimulus intervals. Brain Res 400:171–175.

Holmes WR, Woody CD (1989). Effects of uniform and non-uniform synaptic "activation-distributions" on the cable properties of modeled cortical pyramidal neurons. Brain Res, 505: 12–22.

Kim EH-J, Woody CD, Berthier NE (1983). Rapid acquisition of conditioned eye blink responses in cats following pairing of an auditory CS with glabella tap US and hypothalamic stimulation. J Neurophysiol 49:767–779.

Kimble GA (1961). Hilgard and Marquis' Conditioning and Learning. 2nd ed. New York: Appleton-Century-Crofts.

Kimble GA, Dufort RH (1956). The associative factor in eyelid conditioning. J Exp Psychol 52:386–391.

Kugelberg E (1952). Facial reflexes. Brain 75:385–396.

Llinas R, Walton K, Hillman ED, Sotelo C (1975). Inferior olive: Its role in motor learning. Science 190:1230–1231.

Loucks RB (1933). Preliminary report of a technique for stimulation or destruction of tissues beneath the integument and the establishment of conditioned reactions with faradization of the cerebral cortex. J Comp Psychol 16:439–444.

Matsumura M, Woody CD (1986). Long-term increases in excitability of facial motoneurons in and near the facial nuclei after presentations of stimuli leading to acquisition of a Pavlovian conditioned facial movement. Neurosci Res, 3:568–589.

McCormick DA, Guyer PE, Thompson RF (1982). Superior cerebellar peduncle lesions selectively abolish the ipsilateral classically conditioned nictitating membrane/eyelid response of the rabbit. Brain Res 244:347–350.

McCormick DA, Thompson RF (1984). Neuronal responses of the rabbit cerebellum during acquisition and performance of a classically conditioned nictitating membrane-eyelid response. J Neurosci 4:2811–2822.

Moyer JR, Deyo RA, Disterhoft JF (1990). Hippocampal lesions impair trace eye-blink conditioning in rabbits. Behav Neurosci 104:243–252.

Norman RJ, Villablanca JR, Brown KA, Schwafel JA, Buchwald JS (1974). Classical eyeblink conditioning in the bilateral hemispherectomized cat. Exp Neurol 44:363–380.

Rosenfield ME, Moore JW (1983). Red nucleus lesions disrupt the classically conditioned nictitating membrane response in rabbits. Behav Brain Res 10:393–398.

Rushworth G (1962). Observations on blink reflexes. J Neurol Neurosurg Psychiatry 25:93–108.

Sakai H, Woody CD (1980). Identification of auditory responsive cells in the coronal-pericruciate cortex of awake cats. J Neurophysiol 44:223–231.

Sanchez-Andres JV, Alkon DL (1991). Voltage-clamp analysis of effects of classical conditioning on the hippocampus. J Neurophysiol 65:796–807.

Steinmetz JE, Sears LL, Gabriel M, Kubota Y, Poremba A, Kang E (1991). Cerebellar interpositus lesions disrupt classical nictitating membrane conditioning but not discriminative avoidance learning in rabbits. Behav Brain Res 45:71–80.

Storozhuk VM, Ivanova SF, Sanzharovskii AV (1992a). Involvement of glutamatergic intracortical connections in conditioned reflex activity. Neirofiziologiya 24:701–712.

Storozhuk VM, Ivanova SPh, Stezhka VV (1992b). Analysis of extrathalamic synaptic influences on reactions of sensorimotor cortical neurons during conditioning. Neuroscience 46:605–615.

Thompson RF (1992). The cerebellum and memory. Behav Brain Sci 15:801–802.

Tremblay N, Warren RA, Dykes RW (1990). Electrophysiological studies of acetylcholine and the role of the basal forebrain in the somatosensory cortex of the cat: I. Cortical neurons excited by glutamate. J Neurophysiol 64:1199–1211.

Ukhtomsky AA (1926). Concerning the condition of excitation in dominance. Nov. Refl Fiziol Nerv Sist 2:3–15.

Voronin LL, Gerstein GL, Kudryashov IE, Ioffe SV (1975). Elaboration of a conditioned reflex in a single experiment with simultaneous recording of neural activity. Brain Res, 92:385–403.

Wang XF, Woody CD, Chizhevsky V, Gruen E, Landeira-Fernandez J (1991). The dentate nucleus is a short latency relay of a primary auditory transmission pathway. Neuroreport 2:361–364.

Welsh JP (1992). Changes in the motor pattern of learned and unlearned responses following cerebellar lesions: A kinematic analysis of the nictitating membrane reflex. Neuroscience 47:1–19.

Woody CD (1982). Memory, Learning, and Higher Function: A Cellular View. New York: Springer-Verlag, pp 1–483.

Woody CD (1984). The electrical excitability of nerve cells as an index of learned behavior. In D Alkon J Farley (eds), Princeton Symposium on Primary Neural Substrates of Learning and Behavioral Change. Cambridge: Cambridge University Press, pp 101–127.

Woody CD (1987). Reflex Learning. In G Adelman (ed), Encyclopedia of Neuroscience. Boston: Birkhauser, vol 2, pp 1032–1035.

Woody CD, Baranyi A, Szente MB, Gruen E, Holmes W, Nenov V, Strecker GJ (1989). An aminopyridine sensitive, early outward current recorded in vivo in neurons of the precruciate cortex of cats using single electrode voltage clamp techniques. Brain Res 480:72–81.

Woody CD, Black-Cleworth P (1973). Differences in excitability of cortical neurons as a function of motor projection in conditioned cats. J Neurophysiol 36:1104–1116.

Woody CD, Brozek G (1969a). Gross potential from facial nucleus of cat as an index of neural activity in response to glabella tap. J Neurophysiol 32:704–716.

Woody CD, Brozek G (1969b). Changes in evoked responses from facial nucleus of cat with conditioning and extinction of an eye blink. J Neurophysiol 32:717–726.

Woody CD, Engel J (1972). Changes in unit activity and thresholds to electrical microstimulation at coronal-pericruciate cortex of cat with classical conditioning of different facial movements. J Neurophysiol 35:230–241.

Woody CD, Gruen E (1987). Acetylcholine reduces net outward currents measured in vivo with single electrode voltage clamp techniques in neurons of the motor cortex of cats. Brain Res 424:193–198.

Woody CD, Gruen E (1988). Evidence that acetylcholine acts in vivo in layer V pyramidal cells of cats via cGMP and a cGMP-dependent protein kinase to produce a decrease in an outward current. In M Avoli (ed), Neurotransmitters and Cortical Function. New York: Plenum, pp 313–319.

Woody CD, Gruen E (1993). Cholinergic and glutamatergic effects on neocortical neurons may support rate as well as development of conditioning. Prog Brain Res 98:365–370.

Woody CD, Gruen E, Birt D (1991a). Changes in membrane currents during Pavlovian conditioning of single cortical neurons. Brain Res 539:76–84.

Woody CD, Gruen E, Melamed O, Chizhevsky V (1991b). Patterns of unit activity in rostral thalamus of cats related to short latency discrimination between different auditory stimuli. J Neurosci 11:48–58.

Woody CD, Kim E H-J, Berthier NE (1983). Effects of hypothalamic stimulation on unit responses recorded from neurons of sensorimotor cortex of awake cats during conditioning. J Neurophysiol 49:780–791.

Woody CD, Knispel JD, Crow TJ, Black-Cleworth P (1976). Activity and excitability to electrical current of cortical auditory receptive neurons of awake cats as affected by stimulus association. J Neurophysiol 39:1045–1061.

Woody CD, Swartz BE, Gruen E (1978). Effects of acetylcholine and cyclic GMP on input resistance of cortical neurons in awake cats. Brain Res 158:373–395.

Woody CD, Vassilevsky NN, Engel J (1970). Conditioned eye blink: Unit activity at coronal-precruciate cortex of the cat. J Neurophysiol 33:851–864.

Woody CD, Wang X-F, Gruen E (1994). Activity to acoustic stimuli increases in ventral cochlear nucleus after stimulus pairing. Neuroreport 5:513–515.

Woody CD, Wang XF, Gruen E, Landeira-Fernandez J (1992). Unit activity to click CS changes in dorsal cochlear nucleus after conditioning. Neuroreport 3:385–388.

Woody CD, Yarowsky PJ (1972). Conditioned eye blink using electrical stimulation of coronal-precruciate cortex as conditional stimulus. J Neurophysiol 35:242–252.

Woody C, Yarowsky P, Owens J, Black-Cleworth P, Crow T (1974). Effect of lesions of cortical motor areas on acquisition of conditioned eyeblink in the cat. J Neurophysiol 37:385–394.

Yeo CH, Hardiman MJ, Glickstein M (1984). Discrete lesions of the cerebellar cortex abolish the classically conditioned nictitating membrane response of the rabbit. Behav Brain Res 13: 216–266.

III Visually Guided Movement

10 A Cerebellar Role in Acquisition of Novel Static and Dynamic Muscle Activities in Holding, Pointing, Throwing, and Reaching

W. Thomas Thach

Based on intuitions about both certain features of motor learning and cerebellar circuit structure and function, Brindley (1964), Marr (1969), and Albus (1971) proposed that the adaptation of previous patterns of movement and the acquisition of new ones was a cardinal function of the cerebellum. This "theory" has since resulted in a number of experimental tests that have been interpreted variously to support opposing opinions identified with the members of two groups. One group holds that much evidence supports the theory and is optimistic about its future acceptance. The other group holds that the evidence is flimsy, in the aggregate constituting only a "house of cards", and that the theory is wholly or substantially incorrect. Meanwhile, onlookers sit on the sidelines, waiting for some definitive statement that may help to decide the issue.

Among the first group are those who believe (1) that cerebellar single-unit recording data show specific correlations with performance errors (Simpson and Alley, 1974; Stone and Lisberger, 1990) and learning (Gilbert and Thach, 1977; Ojakangas and Ebner, 1992); (2) that ablation prevents learning (Ito, Shiida, Yagi, and Yamamoto, 1974; Robinson, 1976; McCormick et al., 1981; Leaton and Supple, 1986); (3) that conjoint stimulation of climbing and mossy fiber reproduces learning (Ito, Sakurai, and Tongroach, 1982; Rawson and Tilokskulchai, 1982; Ekerot and Kano, 1985; Kano and Kato, 1987); and (4) that successful network simulation of learning (Tyrell and Willshaw, 1992) is consistent with the original theory. A splinter of the first group proposed a different model in which the cerebellum assists in motor learning by detecting and signaling errors in performance. The proposed model also would cause corrective changes to occur in synapses located on target neurons downstream from the cerebellar cortical output and in structures more directly involved in controlling the behavior in the brainstem (Lisberger, 1988a,b).

In the second group are those who believe that (1) motor learning is a distributed function that cannot be localized to the cerebellum (Llinas, 1981); (2) some types of motor learning attributed to the cerebellum can be conditioned at a brainstem level after the cerebellum is removed (chapter 8); (3) the single-unit recording data neither localize storage site nor show cause and effect; (4) ablation so affects performance as to confound imputation of learning (Welsh and Harvey, 1989; chapter 6); and (5) conjoint stimulation experiments are neither reproducible nor robust under natural conditions. A splinter of this second group proposed that the olivocerebellar system is more properly concerned with the "clocking" of movements than with their learning (Llinas and Welsh, 1993; cf. Keating and Thach, 1995).

Our opinion is that much evidence does favor the Marr-Albus theory for trial-and-error modification of certain kinds of behavior within the province of cerebellar control. Those behaviors that we have studied include the "functional" stretch reflex, feed-forward compensation for interactive torques in reaching, and eye-hand coordination in pointing and throwing.

FUNCTIONAL STRETCH REFLEXES: DISCHARGE OF PURKINJE CELLS DURING ADAPTATION

In trying to find a very simple movement to avoid various possible confounds, we first trained monkeys to hold a manipulandum against constant torque loads by flexing or extending the wrist tonically so as to maintain a fixed position (Gilbert and Thach, 1977). The position window was 10 degrees wide and was displayed as a vertical band on an oscilloscope screen. The wrist position was measured by a potentiometer coupled to the manipulandum and was displayed as a vertical-line cursor on the oscilloscope screen. The task required a monkey to hold the cursor within the window for randomly varied intervals of several seconds, at the end of which time the load switched to an equal and opposite value, displacing the wrist from the held position. The monkey then had to return the manipulandum quickly to within the position window within a few hundred ms to obtain a fruit juice reward. After the monkey had performed this task at an 80 to 90 percent success rate, the activity of single Purkinje cells was recorded during task performance. Novelty was introduced unexpectedly by changing the magnitude of one of the torque loads. An increase in load displaced the wrist by an amount greater than customary and led to an undershoot of the target window on the return movement. A decrease in load displaced the wrist by a lesser amount and led to an overshoot of the target window on the return. Having under- or overshot the target window, the monkey's movements were unsuccessful and were not rewarded. Nevertheless, within 12 to 100 trials, the animal adapted to the novel torque load, and after displacement it returned to the position window within the prior reaction time limits. The behavioral adaptation was within the time period and had the characteristics that others have attributed to the long-loop functional stretch (Evarts, 1973; Meyer-Lohmann, Conrad, Matsunami, and Brooks, 1975; Evarts and Tanji, 1976).

Purkinje cells were identified as generating action potentials of two different waveforms, called *simple spikes* and *complex spikes*, as previously described (Thach, 1967, 1968, 1970). Ninety cells had simple spikes changing frequency in relation to the wrist displacement and return. Of these transient-related cells, 28 were isolated sufficiently well to permit analysis in relation to changes in loads. Eight Purkinje cells had maintained simple spike discharge related also to the maintained load. Fourteen of the transient-related simple-spike cells and five of the load-related Purkinje cells also showed complex spikes occurring in relation to the introduction of the novel load. The remainder exhibited alterations in the simple-spike frequency only. Both the transient-related simple-spike plus complex-spike cells and the load-related simple-spike plus complex-spike types of Purkinje cell showed similar alterations in transient-related activity with load changes, and the results were combined. In both groups, there was a progressive trial-by-trial change in the simple-spike discharge rate that correlated with the occurrence of the complex spike. This change was in the direction of a decrease. SS firing continued to decrease as long as the complex spike was present. Once it had returned to its baseline firing rate of around once per second, no longer in relation to the behavior, the simple-spike frequency stabilized at a new level. These Purkinje cells whose simple and complex spikes were both related to the introduction of the novel load were located preferentially in lobules III, IV, and V of an intermediate portion of the anterior lobe. Those that were transient-related only were more widespread than those that were also load-related. These results were interpreted as being consistent with the Marr-Albus prediction that climbing fiber action potentials occur preferentially during adaptation and serve to change the input-output function of the parallel fiber–Purkinje cell synapse. More specifically, the results suggested that the direction of change was that predicted by Albus: a decrease in parallel fiber–Purkinje cell synaptic efficacy. The authors pointed out that the results did not prove that the occurrence of complex spikes altered the parallel fiber–Purkinje cell synapse; the decrease in simple-spike frequency could have been due to dropoff in the firing frequency of mossy fiber spinocerebellar feedback. However, the cause-effect relationship was demonstrated subsequently in the reduced preparation by conjoint stimulation of the climbing fiber and mossy fiber pathways (Ito et al., 1982). Both these results are necessary to the acceptance of the theories that (1) complex spikes can change the parallel fiber–Purkinje cell synapse and (2) complex spikes do occur preferentially during the behavior modification.

VISUALLY GUIDED WRIST MOVEMENT: DISSOCIATION OF MOVEMENT ADAPTATION AND PERFORMANCE

It has long been believed that the cerebellum participates in proprioceptively controlled tasks, such as the one described earlier. Thus it is not surprising that the cerebellum should be able to tune its reflex components so as to adapt them to changes in the task. However, does the cerebellum participate in the adaptation of other, or indeed all, motor tasks? What is the range and limit of its adaptive control? Does it participate in adapting those motor tasks that are more under teleceptive and voluntary control? To address this question of generality, rhesus monkeys and humans were trained to place a hand in a manipulandum that controlled the position of a cursor on a screen in front of them (Keating and Thach, 1990; Keating, Martin, Mink, and Thach, 1995). The subject held the cursor in a target zone; the target zone then stepped instantaneously to a new position (a *JUMP* in our terminology), and the subject had to replace the cursor within the target zone in one quick movement by flexing or extending the wrist. After a series of control trials, the gain was altered so that the hand-cursor relationship changed during the quick movement to a novel value (see chapter 11). The previously performed movement was thus no longer of the correct magnitude to place the cursor in the target zone; the correct magnitude could not be inferred by lesser movements in the hold position and had to be acquired by trial-and-error-practice. Over several trials, the movement magnitude did change to produce the proper range. The endpoints of the initial ballistic movement from a series of trials were fit by regression to an equation of the form $f(x) = a + be^{-x/c}$. This is the general formula for an exponential decay curve; in this case, it becomes a "learning" curve, in which the rate of adaptation (time-constant) is expressed as the number of trials needed for 70 percent completion of the adaptation. Residuals were trial-invariant and had normal distributions; c, analogous to a time-constant, was used as a measure of the rate of adaptation. Performance was measured in terms of trial-to-trial variability, specifically the standard deviation of regression of the curve fit, and was independent of adaptation. Under normal circumstances, adaptation is enduring. Twenty-four hours after subjects were adapted to a novel JUMP condition, the first-trial movements ended in the adapted target zone, not the overtrained control zone (Keating and Thach, 1992).

In the monkeys (Keating and Thach, 1991), inactivation of cerebellar cortex by small injections of the gamma aminobutyric acid (GABA) agonist, muscimol, impaired adaptation of the JUMP task. The critical area was within the somatosensory "arm" receiving area of lobules III, IV, and V, and lateral within Crus I. An "inactivation map" of cerebellar cortex was made by systematic injection at 24 sites of 2 μl of 1-μg/μl muscimol and an attempt to induce adaptation. Inactivation of a small area (2 mm $\times$ 2 mm) of cortex in the extreme lateral hemisphere resulted in a marked slowing of adaptation, with no significant change in the performance of the task.

A 61-year-old right-handed patient suffered an infarct of the right superior cerebellar artery (SCA). His right hand (previously dominant) showed normal reaction time and endpoint control on the JUMP task but showed impairment of combined finger movements and hypermetric and decomposed reaching. Yet on the JUMP task, his right wrist adapted more slowly, one third as fast as the left (Keating and Thach, 1990). Taken together, these data show that the cerebellar cortex can play an essential role in producing changes of at least 24 hours duration in the JUMP type of movement adaptation.

THROWING REQUIRES ADAPTATION EYE-HAND COORDINATION

In throwing, the eyes (and head) fixate the target and serve as reference aim for the arm. Coordination between gaze direction and arm throw is a skill; it is developed and maintained by practice. When wedge-prism spectacles are placed over the eyes with the base to the right, the optic path is bent to the right, and the eyes (and head) move to the left to fixate the target. The arm, calibrated to the line of sight, throws to the left of the target (see chapter 13). With practice the calibration changes, the gaze-throw angle widens, and the arm throws closer to (and finally on) the target. Proof that the gaze position is the reference aim for the arm throw trajectory occurs when the prisms are removed and the arm throws. The calibration of a widened gaze-throw angle, compensating for the previously left-bent gaze, persists; the eyes are now on-target, and the arm throws to the right of the target an amount of times almost equal to the original leftward error. With practice, the angle between gaze direction and throw direction is again recalibrated; each throw moves closer to (and finally on) the target (Kane and Thach, 1989; Thach et al., 1992a).

How specific is this adaptation to the task and to the body parts? Our data show that prism adaptation in throwing is specific for arm and type of throw (Thach, Goodkin, Keating, and Martin, 1992c). In one experiment varying the throwing arm, subjects threw with (1) one arm, (2) the other arm, (3) the first arm with prisms, (4) the other arm, and (5) the first arm. Prism adaptation occurred in all subjects in the throwing arm (3), did not affect or abate with throws by the other arm (4), and readapted during throws by the first arm (5). In a second experiment varying the type of throw, subjects threw (1) underhand, (2) overhand (same arm), (3) overhand with prisms, (4) underhand, and (5) overhand. While wearing prisms, all subjects adapted the overhand throw (3). In most (6 of 8 subjects), subsequent underhand throws showed no effect of prior overhand adaptation (4). In these subjects, prior overhand adaptation persisted in subsequent overhand throws despite intervening underhand throws, and readapted only with repeated overhand throws (5). Two subjects showed carryover from prior overhand adaptation (3) to underhand throws, which disappeared with underhand throwing (4), and the amount of residual overhand adaptation (5) was less. Thus, in most subjects adaptation involved one task and not another task, although many (or the same) body parts participated in both tasks. This implies separate central channels for adaptation of muscle actions for each task.

How many gaze-throw calibrations can be stored? Following extended training with a specific diopter strength of wedge-prism spectacles (12,000 throws, 6 weeks of alternate prism versus no-prism throws), subjects stored two eye-hand calibrations (the no-prism calibration and the trained-prism calibration; see Martin, Keating, Goodkin, Bastian, and Thach, 1993). Trained subjects

Acquisition of Static and Dynamic Muscle Activities

threw successfully on-target immediately on donning the trained prisms (even though the prisms bent the light path and the gaze was directed away from the actual target) and immediately on removing them (the gaze-throw angle now normal). When donning a novel pair of prisms, subjects adapted as in the preceding naive state; they threw off-target in the same direction as the prism-bent gaze, gradually adapted throws onto target, and then threw off-target in the opposite direction when the novel prisms were removed. This adaptation affected both the no-prism and trained-prism calibrations; each calibration had to be independently readapted. This showed that two (or more) gaze-hand calibrations can be stored simultaneously.

Is the cerebellum necessary for prism adaptation of throwing? To test prior assertions that the cerebellum is involved in wedge-prism adaptation of limb movements directed to visual targets (chapter 13), we studied patients with cerebellar damage. Our preliminary results (Thach, Goodkin, and Keating, 1991) supported the hypothesis that the olivocerebellar system plays an important role in this visuomotor adaptation. Investigators have further studied patients with specific lesions of the cerebellum or its inputs or outputs to localize the regions of the olivocerebellar system that are necessary for normal prism adaptation (Martin, Keating, Goodkin, Bastian, and Thach, 1996a,b). Patients with generalized cerebellar atrophy, lesions of the superior vermis, damage of the inferior olive, infarcts in the distribution of the posterior inferior cerebellar artery (PICA; possibly with inferior cerebellar peduncle involvement), and focal infarcts in the contralateral basal pons or ipsilateral middle cerebellar peduncle had absent or impaired ability for prism adaptation. This group often showed mild or no limb ataxia. By contrast, subjects usually adapted normally despite infarcts in the distribution of the SCA (involving the anterior superior surface of the cortex and the dentate nucleus) or in the cerebellar receiving zones of the thalamus. This group often had marked limb ataxia. These results implicate climbing fibers from the contralateral inferior olive via the ipsilateral inferior cerebellar peduncle, mossy fibers from the contralateral pontocerebellar nuclei via the ipsilateral middle cerebellar peduncle, and the superior vermal cerebellar cortex as being critical for this adaptation. Apparently not necessary are lateral hemisphere cortex and the dentatothalamic projection.

What is the specific adapted variable in throwing? We tested the hypothesis that it was the body-part components contributing to the gaze-throw angle (Martin et al., 1993, and 1996b). To determine the body parts involved in the gaze-throw recalibration, in the two long-term prism versus no-prism trained subjects (Martin et al., 1993), we videorecorded positions of head-in-space and shoulders-in-space while subjects were throwing with and without prisms. Knowing that eyes foveated the target and that throws hit the target, we computed the angular positions of eyes-in-head, head-on-trunk, and trunk-on-arm. We found that for both subjects, the gaze adjustment was not confined to any one set of two members (e.g., eyes-in-head), but instead was distributed across all three sets of coupled body parts. Moreover, each subject had a different distribution of coupling changes across the three sets of coupled body parts.

These results are in accord with classic views of the nature of cerebellar control. Coordination of the many body parts to achieve smooth movements is generally agreed to be the specific role of cerebellar control. This is often thought of as being due to a "fine tuning" of the many movement pattern generators downstream from the cerebellum in the spinal cord, brainstem, and motor cortex (Holmes, 1939). We have argued elsewhere in support of an additional mechanism for coordination of body parts in posture and movement (Thach, Goodkin, and Keating, 1992a). Flourens (1984) and Babinski (1899 and 1906) suggested that cerebellar damage interrupts a specific control of coordination of compound movements, sparing simple movements. Elsewhere we have presented evidence supporting a dissociation in the control of compound movements and simple movements. Monkeys (Goodkin and Thach, 1991, 1992; Thach, Kane, Mink, and Goodkin, 1992b; Thach, Perry, Kane, and Goodkin, 1993) and humans (Goodkin, Keating, Martin, and Thach, 1993) with lateral cerebellar lesions show impairment of compound movements (across several joints) with relative or absolute sparing of simple movements (made at a single joint by loaded-agonist muscles only). By contrast, inactivation of the motor cortex is known to impair both compound and simple movements (Schieber, Kim, and Thach, 1991). Single-unit recording in lateral cerebellar nuclei and in the motor cortex of monkeys has also suggested a direct and preferential control of such simple movements by the motor cortex and not by the cerebellum (Schieber and Thach, 1985a,b; Thach et al., 1993). We have elsewhere extended the Marr-Albus model to propose that the parallel fiber contact on the beam of many somatomotor-coded Purkinje cells could be the mechanism that combines downstream elements (Thach et al., 1992a,b, 1993; Thach, Martin, Keating, Goodkin, and Bastian, 1995; Martin et al., 1996a). The resulting combinations of linked downstream components would be larger, more varied, and more specific to the triggering motor contexts than is provided for in the wiring of the motor pattern generators themselves.

In the prism experiments, we have studied a behavior that requires the static coordination across a number of joint positions before the throw is launched. The behavior is easily and quickly modifiable over a wide range of joint angles, shows specificity as to involved body part and to task, is capable of storing multiple calibrations across body parts, and is dependent on the cerebellar cortex. Whereas the behavior does indeed exhibit "fine control," the great range of variation over which it is normally capable, plus the results of the simple movement–compound movement studies, suggest to us that the mechanism of control is at the level of coordination itself, and not simply and solely fine tuning of downstream elements. In the next experiments to be described, we explore dynamic aspects of compound movements that also may require and use the mechanism of adaptive coordination that we have proposed.

CONTROL OF INTERACTION TORQUES DURING REACHING IN NORMAL AND CEREBELLAR PATIENTS

From a mechanical standpoint, a multijointed movement is more complex than a summed combination of single-jointed movements. This is due to the interaction torques (e.g., inertial, centripetal, and Coriolis) generated by one linkage moving on another. We have studied normal and cerebellar subjects performing two-jointed reaching movements under two conditions. For the "accurate" condition, seated subjects were asked to make a self-paced reach to touch a 1-cm target on a 4-cm ball hanging in front of them. For the "fast" condition, seated subjects were instructed to move as fast as possible and touch any part of the 4-cm ball. Subjects were videotaped with markers at the index finger, shoulder, elbow, and wrist joints. Marker positions were digitized (at 60 Hz) and joint angles and trajectories were calculated. Inverse dynamic equations (Soechting and Lacquaniti, 1981) were used to estimate net torques and interaction torques at the elbow and shoulder joints. Preliminary data (Bastian, Mueller, Martin, Keating and Thach, 1994; Bastian and Thach, 1995a; Bastian, Martin, Keating, and Thach, 1996) indicate that, under the "accurate" condition, cerebellar subjects moved in a manner that reduced the complexity of torques by decomposing the reach or slowing it down. Slowing the reach also permitted use of peripheral feedback to help shape the ongoing movement. Under the "fast" condition, cerebellar subjects produced abnormal torque profiles and often overshot the target (see also chapter 13). Fast reaching movements increase the magnitude of interaction torques (Soechting and Lacquaniti, 1981) and normally require subjects to account for them in a predictive manner.

We do not know yet whether abnormalities in the "fast" movements made by cerebellar patients reflect the inability to account for only interaction torques or increasing magnitudes of all torques. However, preliminary data show that cerebellar patients made increased errors in the initial direction of movement compared with control subjects, a finding that suggests a principal problem in accounting for interaction torques. As the reach velocity increased, these errors increased in a direction that is consistent with an inability to adjust for the interaction torques generated at the elbow. An electromyographic (EMG) analysis showed that the onset of the entire pattern of muscle activity was delayed, but the relative timing of the two muscles active during early phases of movement was normal. These findings support the idea that the cerebellum helps to initiate movement and learns to send predictive signals that correct for errors caused by interaction torques. We speculate that the cerebellum compensates for interaction torques in the early phases of the movement by scaling of amplitude or duration of muscle activity (see also chapter 4).

CONCLUSIONS

These studies have examined a number of different paradigms of adaptation and of *acquisition of skill*—defined as a movement specialized to meet a certain goal and gained through practice. In each of several paradigms, change has been shown to be achieved through trial-and-error performance (functional stretch reflex, visually initiated JUMP movements, and prism-adapted throwing). In some of the tasks, damage of the cerebellar cortex has been shown to impair adaptation independently of (or at least disproportionately to) performance (visually initiated JUMP movements and prism-adapted throwing). Therefore, deficits in performance cannot have explained the deficits in adaptation (cf. chapter 6). In some of the tasks, the discharge of Purkinje cells and (by inference) the discharge of inferior olive cells and mossy fibers has behaved in a manner consistent with the Marr-Albus theory of motor learning (functional stretch reflex, JUMP movements). The theory has been extended (Thach et al., 1992; Martin et al., 1996a,b) to show how parallel fibers could implement roles both in the coordination of all complex movements and in the learning of new movements. The cardinal logical functions of the cerebellum, in contrast to other elements within the motor circuitry, would be that of context-response linkage and combination of downstream elements. The context-response linking element would be the parallel fiber. The linkage would be formed through trial-and-error practice, through the action of the inferior olive climbing fiber. The memory capacity for storage of different context-response linkages would be proportionate to the number of granule cells. The size of the response combinations would be proportionate to the length of parallel fibers. We do not mean to imply that motor adaptation is restricted to the cerebellum. Compensations for muscle weakness or vestibular hair cell damage, for example, should more properly extend equally across all behaviors in which those elements are employed. Their underlying synaptic adjustments properly would be made at a more peripheral level, (e.g., on the input to the motor neuron, or in the primary afferent terminal, respectively). It is probable that adjustments occur at every point where there are synapses. By contrast, the mechanism proposed here would permit optimized complex movement behaviors to respond to specific behavioral contexts rapidly, stereotypically, and automatically. The mechanism would permit storage of many context-response couplings, and many complex responses. The mechanism would permit complex linkages across many muscle groups both statically (as in prism-adapted throwing) and dynamically (as in compensation for interactive torques). The mechanism would permit privacy, individuality, and a large number of behavioral responses. These features would constitute the essence of cerebellar operation in motor learning.

ACKNOWLEDGMENTS

This work was supported by grants to WT Thach from the National Institutes of Health (NS12777) and the Office of Naval Research (N00014-92-J-1827). Additional support was provided by an NIH training grant (NRSA 5 T32 GM0700) for T Martin, H Goodkin, S Kane, and M Schieber, and by a grant from the Foundation for Physical Therapy Research (94D-18-BAS-01) to A Bastian.

REFERENCES

Albus JS (1971). A theory of cerebellar function. Math Biosci 10:25–61.

Babinski J (1899). De l'asynergie cerebelleuse. Rev Neurol 7:806–816.

Babinski J (1906). Asynergie et inertie cerebelleuses. Rev Neurol 14:685–686.

Bastian AJ, Martin TA, Keating JG, Thach WT (1996). Cerebellar ataxia: Abnormal control of interaction torques across multiple joints. J Neurophysiol (in press).

Bastian AJ, Mueller MJ, Martin TA, Keating JG, Thach WT (1994). Control of interaction torques during reaching in normal and cerebellar patients. Soc Neurosci Abstr 20:993.

Bastian AJ, Thach WT (1995). Cerebellar patients make initial directional errors consistent with impaired control of limb dynamics. Soc Neurosci Abstr 21:1921.

Brindley GS (1964). The use made by the cerebellum of the information that it receives from the sense organs. Int Brain Res Org Bull 3:80.

Ekerot C-F, Kano M (1985). Long-term depression of parallel fibre synapses following stimulation of climbing fibres. Brain Res 342:357–360.

Evarts EV (1973). Motor cortex reflexes associated with learned movement. Science 179:501–503.

Evarts EV, Tanji J (1976). Reflexes and intended responses in motor cortex pyramidal tract neurons of monkey. J Neurophysiol 39:1069–1080.

Flourens P (1824). Recherches experimentales sur les proprietes et les fonctions du systeme nerveux, dans les animaux vertebres. Paris: Cervot.

Gilbert PFC, Thach WT (1977). Purkinje cell activity during motor learning. Brain Res 128:309–328.

Goodkin HP, Keating JG, Martin T, Thach WT (1993). Preserved simple and impaired compound movement after infarction in the territory of the superior cerebellar artery. Can J Neurol Sci 20 (suppl. 3):S93–S104.

Goodkin HP, Thach WT (1991). Does the cerebellum preferentially control multijoint movements? Soc Neurosci Abstr 17:1380.

Goodkin HP, Thach WT (1992). How does the cerebellum control compound movements? Soc Neurosci Abstr 18:516.

Holmes G (1939). The cerebellum of man. The Hughlings Jackson memorial lecture. Brain 62:1–30.

Ito M, Sakurai M, Tongroach P (1982). Climbing induced depression of both mossy fiber responsiveness and glutamate sensitivity of cerebellar Purkinje cells. J Physiol (Lond) 324:113–134.

Ito M, Shiida T, Yagi N, Yamamoto M (1974). The cerebellar modification of rabbit's horizontal vestibulo-ocular reflex induced by sustained head rotation combined with visual stimulation. Proc Jpn Acad. 50:85–89.

Kane SA, Thach WT (1989). Palatal myoclonus and function of the inferior olive: Are they related? Exp Brain Res 17:427–460.

Kano M, Kato M (1987). Quisqualate receptors are specifically involved in cerebellar synaptic plasticity. Nature 325:276–279.

Keating JG, Martin TA, Mink JW, Thach WT (1995). Gaze direction plays a role in guiding a natural but not an instrumented wrist movement. Soc Neurosci Abstr 21:422.

Keating JG, Thach WT (1990). Cerebellar motor learning: Quantitation of movement adaptation and performance in rhesus monkeys and humans implicates cortex as the site of adaptation. Soc Neurosci Abstr 16:762.

Keating JG, Thach WT (1991). The cerebellar cortical area required for adaptation of monkey's "Jump" task is lateral, localized, and small. Soc Neurosci Abstr 17:1381.

Keating JG, Thach WT (1992). Adaptation of a ballistic movement to a novel endpoint is enduring. Soc Neurosci Abstr 18:516.

Keating JG, Thach WT (1995). Nonclock behavior of inferior olive neurons: Interspike interval of Purkinje cell complex spike discharge in the awake behaving monkey is random. J Neurophysiol 73:1329–1340.

Leaton RN, Supple WF (1986). Cerebellar vermis: Essential for long-term habituation of the acoustic startle response. Science 232:513–515.

Lisberger SG (1988a). The neural basis for motor learning in the vestibulo-ocular reflex in monkeys. Trends Neurosci 11:147–152.

Lisberger SG (1988b). The neural basis for learning of simple motor skills. Science 242:728–735.

Llinas R (1981). Electrophysiology of cerebellar networks. In VB Brooks (ed), Handbook of Physiology, section 1, volume II, part 2. Bethesda: American Physiological Society, pp 831–876.

Llinas R, Welsh JP (1993). On the cerebellum and motor learning. Curr Opin Neurobiol 3:958–965.

Marr DA (1969). A theory of cerebellar cortex. J Physiol (Lond) 202:437–470.

Martin TA, Keating JG, Goodkin HP, Bastian AJ, Thach WT (1993). Storage of multiple gaze-hand calibrations. Soc Neurosci Abstr 19:980.

Martin TA, Keating JG, Goodkin HP, Bastian AJ, Thach WT (1996a). Throwing while looking through prisms: I. Focal olivocerebellar tesions impair adaptation. Brain (in press).

Martin TA, Keating JG, Goodkin HP, Bastian AJ, Thach WT (1996b). Throwing while looking through prisms. II. Specificity and storage of multiple gaze-throw calibrations. Brain (in press).

McCormick DA, Lavond DG, Clark GA, Kettner RE, Rising CE, Thompson RF (1981). The engram found? Role of the cerebellum in classical conditioning of nictitating membrane and eyelid responses. Bull Psychon Soc 18:103–105.

Meyer-Lohmann J, Conrad B, Matsunami K, Brooks VB (1975). Effects of dentate cooling on precentral unit activity following torque pulse injections into elbow movements. Brain Res 94:237–251.

Ojakangas CL, Ebner TJ (1992). Purkinje cell complex and simple spike changes during a voluntary arm movement learning task in the monkey. J Neurophysiol 68:2222–2236.

Rawson JA, Tilokskulchai K (1982). Climbing modification of cerebellar Purkinje cell responses to parallel fiber inputs. Brain Res 237:492–497.

Robinson DA (1976). Adaptive gain control of the vestibuloocular reflex by the cerebellum. J Neurophysiol 39:954–969.

Schieber MH, Kim L, Thach WT (1991). Muscimol in monkey area 4 impairs individuated finger movements, in area 6 produces contralateral neglect. Soc Neurosci Abstr 17:1021.

Schieber MH, Thach WT (1985a). Trained slow tracking: I. Muscular production of wrist movement. J Neurophysiol 55:1213–1227.

Schieber MH, Thach WT (1985b). Trained slow tracking: II. Bidirectional discharge patterns of cerebellar nuclear, motor cortex, and spindle afferent neurons. J Neurophysiol 55:1228–1270.

Simpson JI, Alley KE (1974). Visual climbing fiber input to rabbit vestibulocerebellum: a source of direction-specific information. Brain Res 82:302–308.

Soechting JF, Lacquaniti F (1981). Invariant characteristics of a pointing movement in man. J Neurosci 7:710–720.

Stone LS, Lisberger SG (1990). Visual responses of Purkinje cells in the cerebellar flocculus during smooth-pursuit eye movements in monkeys: II. Complex spikes. J Neurophysiol 63: 1262–75.

Thach WT (1967). Somatosensory receptive fields of single units in cat cerebellar cortex. J Neurophysiol 30:675–696.

Thach WT (1968). Discharge of Purkinje and cerebellar nuclear neurons during rapidly alternating arm movements in the monkey. J Neurophysiol 31:785–797.

Thach WT (1970). Discharge of cerebellar neurons related to two maintained postures and two prompt movements: II. Purkinje cell output and input. J Neurophysiol 33:537–547.

Thach WT (1996). On the specific role of the cerebellum in motor learning and cognition: clues from PET activation and lesion studies in man. Behav Brain Sci (in press).

Thach WT, Goodkin HP, Keating JG (1991). Inferior olive disease in man prevents learning novel synergies. Soc Neurosci Abstr 17:1380.

Thach WT, Goodkin HP, Keating JG (1992a). Cerebellum and the adaptive coordination of movement. Annu Rev Neurosci 15:403–442.

Thach WT, Goodkin HP, Keating JG, Martin TA (1992c). Prism adaptation in throwing is specific for arm and type of throw. Soc Neurosci Abstr 18:516.

Thach WT, Kane SA, Mink JW, Goodkin HP (1992b). Cerebellar output: Multiple maps and modes of control in movement coordination. In R Llinas, C Sotelo (eds), The Cerebellum Revisited. New York: Springer-Verlag.

Thach WT, Martin TA, Keating JG, Goodkin HP, Bastian AJ (1995). Schematic model of short- and long-term adjustments of eye-hand coordination in throwing. Soc Neurosci Abstr 21:917.

Thach WT, Perry JG, Kane SA, Goodkin HP (1993). Cerebellar nuclei: rapid alternating movement, motor somatotopy, and a mechanism for the control of muscle synergy. Rev Neurol 149:607–628.

Tyrell T, Willshaw D (1992). Cerebellar cortex: Its simulation and the relevance of Marr's Theory. Philos Trans R Soc Lond B 336:239–257.

Welsh JP, Harvey JA (1989). Cerebellar lesions and the nictitating membrane reflex: Performance deficits of the conditioned and the unconditioned response. J Neurosci 9:299–311.

11 The Cerebellum's Role in Voluntary Motor Learning: Clinical, Electrophysiological, and Imaging Studies

Timothy J. Ebner, Didier Flament, and
Sharad J. Shanbhag

The cerebellum's role in motor learning has been the subject of considerable and intense debate (Miles and Lisberger, 1981; Ito, 1982, 1989; Lisberger, 1988; Llinas and Welsh, 1993). Marr (1969), then Albus (1971) proposed the initial theories, both speculating on the function of the unique physiological and anatomical properties of the cerebellar cortex and its two afferent systems, the mossy and climbing fibers. The powerful, all-or-none, climbing fiber action on a Purkinje cell was hypothesized to alter the strength of the excitatory, parallel fiber synapses on the same cell, a form of heterosynaptic modification. Marr (1969) hypothesized an augmentation of the parallel fiber synaptic strength, but Albus (1971) proposed a decrease. Subsequently, a prolonged reduction in parallel fiber synaptic strength resulting from the conjunction of climbing fiber and parallel fiber inputs was described (Ito, Sakurai, and Tongroach, 1982; Ekerot and Kano, 1985; Sakurai, 1987). This so-called long-term depression (LTD) was hypothesized to provide the neural substrate underlying cerebellar motor learning (Ito, 1982, 1989). A form of long-term potentiation in the cerebellar cortex also has been described (Kano, Rexhausen, Dreesen, and Konnerth, 1992).

Most behavioral investigations into the cerebellum's role in motor learning have emphasized and used models of reflex adaptation. Emphasis was first placed on the plasticity of the vestibuloocular reflex (Robinson, 1976; Ito, 1982; see also chapter 2). Others have championed a role for the cerebellum as the site of storage for classical conditioning (Thompson, 1988; see also chapter 5), a hypothesis challenged by several studies and investigators (Welsh and Harvey, 1989; Kelly, Zou, and Bloedel, 1990; see also chapters 6 and 8). However, the cerebellum's role in motor learning is theorized to extend beyond reflex adaptation and classical conditioning, encompassing voluntary motor learning (Eccles, 1977; Gomi and Kawato, 1992; Kawato and Gomi, 1992; see also chapters 10 and 13).

The cerebellum's role in voluntary motor learning has been evaluated from several perspectives, including studies in patients with cerebellar disease, electrophysiologic studies in behaving nonhuman primates, and human functional imaging studies using positron emission tomography (PET) and, more recently, magnetic resonance imaging (MRI). The findings have been divergent and have prompted different interpretations. In this chapter, we will examine the existing evidence for the cerebellum's role in voluntary movement learning.

DEFINITIONS, INTERNAL MODELS, AND THEIR NEURAL REPRESENTATIONS

Any attempts to elucidate the neural substrates for voluntary motor learning are prone to confusion unless a clear conception of motor learning is present. In the realm of psychological approaches to motor learning, Schmidt (1982) has presented a cogent definition: "Motor learning is a set of processes associated with practice or experience leading to relatively permanent changes in skilled behavior." Motor learning thus is defined as the process of acquiring the capability for producing skilled actions; the underlying events and changes that occur during practice or experience are the constituents of motor learning. The result of learning is a long-lasting capacity for skilled performance. We will adopt Schmidt's concept as a working definition.

The goal of a physiological understanding of motor learning is the elucidation of the processes in Schmidt's definition. From a control systems standpoint, Atkeson (1989) specifies two general processes required in motor learning. One objective is the specification of internal models of the motor apparatus (the limb and its musculotendinoskeletal structure) and the environment in which the motor system operates. These models then are used to generate motor output commands and to process and interpret feedback regarding the motor output and the environment. Second, any mismatch between the specific output and the feedback of the motor output then must be transformed into an appropriate form so that the internal model may be corrected to improve performance.

The use of internal models stems from the conceptualization of motor control as resulting from a series of transformations (Atkeson, 1989; Zajac and Gordon, 1989; Soechting and Flanders, 1992; see also chapter 20). For example, in reaching movements, a kinematic plan of hand motion may be converted to a motor command in terms of muscle activations by an inverse transformation. The motor command then could be transformed into movement of the limb, thus expressing the forward model. To obtain a measure of the command error, the movement may be converted back to a motor command form through a second inverse transformation. Thus, the inverse model may be used both for specifying and evaluating the motor command. This schema for reaching may be expressed as follows: The kinematic plan must include the final, or intended, position of the hand in space and also may incorporate information about the trajectory and movement kinematics (which requires knowledge of the starting limb position). To reach the final position, muscle activity must produce sufficient force to overcome the limb's own inertia, plus any other loads that may be encountered. Therefore, the motor command must be generated in terms of movement dynamics rather than kinematics (i.e., the first inverse transformation). This command produces a movement of the limb, with all its kinematic properties (displacement, velocity, etc.). This is the expression of the original goal, or forward model. To measure errors in the motor command, the limb kinematics may be converted back to the forces that produced them (second inverse transformation). These actual forces can be compared with the desired forces to make modifications to the motor command.

Given the concept of an internal model, a second issue concerns its form. Two basic classes of representations have been developed for use in the control of robotic manipulators, systems which are forced to contend with the same control problems as biologic limbs (Atkeson, 1989). One form is a structured representation that explicitly defines the physical structure of the motor output system and uses this information to perform a transformation from a behavioral goal to a movement plan specifying the motor output. The other form is a tabular representation, with particular locations in a table or map corresponding to a particular transformation.

These two representations predict different types of capabilities with regard to motor learning (Atkeson, 1989). Because a structured representation requires the specification of relatively few parameters for a given transformation, a fast rate of learning may be achieved. Furthermore, once a few combinations of inputs and outputs are learned for a given transformation, the model may be generalized to other inputs and outputs. However, if poor information exists about the parameters describing the output structure, the structured representation becomes less accurate and less effective. A tabular model allows for flexibility of coordinate systems and rapid learning of similar input-output transformations. Drawbacks of a tabular representation include difficulties in generalization and the fundamental requirement for the storage of a large number of parameters.

Psychophysical and electrophysiological investigations support the concept that internal models of kinematics exist (Georgopoulos, 1990; Soechting and Flanders, 1991). Studies evaluating adaptation to visuomotor transformations suggest that these kinematic representations are readily modifiable (Cunningham, 1989; Ojakangas and Ebner, 1991; Shanbhag and Ebner, 1994). Recently, two studies have shown that some internal representation of limb dynamics also must exist. In one of these studies, Coriolis-force perturbations were applied to human subjects performing pointing movements in the dark (Lackner and Dizio, 1994). Subjects were able to compensate for the velocity-dependent perturbations, a correction requiring a specific representation of limb dynamics. In the second study, subjects performing a center-out reaching task regained straight trajectories while a novel viscous field perturbation was applied with a robotic arm (Shadmehr and Mussa-Ivaldi, 1994). The finding that the adaptation to the perturbation field could be generalized to positions outside the training workspace supports the presence of a structured internal representation of limb dynamics.

The early major theoretical formulations of motor learning in the cerebellum have been framed in terms of a tabular organization. This may not be an unreasonable assumption, given the highly regular and uniform cellular organization and circuitry of the cerebellar cortex. In the Marr-Albus theory (Marr, 1969; Albus, 1971), the cerebellum can be said to learn by storing a sequence of movement primitives (specified by climbing fiber input from the inferior olive) needing to be assembled to create a complex movement. Thus, a tabular representation of movement elements is created (Thach, Goodkin, and Keating, 1992).

Building on the Marr-Albus model, Ito has proposed a model in which the cerebellum is an adaptive feedforward controller (Ito, 1984). The cerebellum's role in learning is to modify output based on feedback. However, this feedback is not an on-line process; rather, the cerebellum works as an intermediate locus of adaptation to separate the feedback from the feed-forward control mechanism. In a variant of this concept, Kawato and Gomi (Gomi and Kawato, 1992; see also chapter 20) proposed that the cerebellum develops, stores, and updates an inverse model of the effector system. This model is then used as a modifiable controller for dynamics during movement. The Ito and Kawato models suggest a "mixed" representation having tabular and structured elements. In both models, cerebellar microzones form a tabular representation of movement elements defined by premotor networks in the brainstem, spinal cord, and cerebral cortex. Each microzone receives error signals in the coordinate space of the motor command via the climbing fiber input, and parallel fibers carry sensory input and motor command signals. As learning proceeds, the cerebellar microzones acquire an inverse model of the controlled object. Therefore, each microzone represents a structured inverse model of the controlled object and the "network" of cerebellar microzones constitutes a tabular representation of controlled objects.

In general, few experiments have tested directly the types of motor learning that are described in the formal models. According to Kawato's model, the cerebellum is involved in the generation, maintenance, and storage of an internal model of the inverse dynamics of the controlled object (Kawato and Gomi, 1992). Additionally, Atkeson's definition states that the internal model is used both in the generation of movements and in the interpretation of movement errors (Atkeson, 1989). These control-system models do not predict explicit cerebellar involvement in associative learning, classical conditioning, or cognitive function. Instead, one would expect involvement with the execution and "adaptive control of movement" (Thach et al., 1992).

This prediction raises an important caveat in the interpretation of experimental data regarding motor learning in general. If a structure is involved in both the generation and execution of movement in a behavioral task, one must ascertain whether the activity that one monitors using electrophysiological or imaging techniques is associated with learning parameters or with movement parameters such as limb kinematics or dynamics. In behavioral psychophysics using normal and patient subject populations, the issue becomes still more critical and troublesome, as we shall discuss in the next section.

VOLUNTARY MOTOR LEARNING IN CEREBELLAR PATIENTS

One approach to elucidate the processes subserved by the cerebellum in voluntary motor learning in humans is the examination of the effects of cerebellar lesions (see chapters 4 and 10). Investigations using this strategy rely on behavioral measures to access the processes underlying learning. Behavior is almost invariably the sole window into learning, and this involves movement. However, the classic clinical manifestations of cerebellar lesions are deficits in movement, such as ataxia and dysmetria (Holmes, 1939). According to the models for cerebellar function in motor learning discussed in the previous section, lesions to the cerebellum should create deficits in movement execution along with motor learning. Therefore, interpretation of experimental results becomes contingent on an experimental design that discriminates between performance deficits due to motor output disruption and deficits due to lack of motor learning. Achieving this goal in human behavioral studies poses a significant but necessary challenge to experimenters.

These difficulties in interpretation are illustrated in the results of a visuo-motor adaptation task analogous to that used in our single-cell recording and functional imaging studies (Ojakangas and Ebner, 1991, 1992, 1994; Flament, Ellermann, Ugurbil, and Ebner, 1994; Flament, Lee, Ugurbil, and Ebner, 1995). Subjects were seated in front of a video display where they controlled the movement of a cursor on the display using a planar two-joint manipulandum. The task consisted of maintaining the cursor in a central "start box" until one of eight equidistant "target" boxes appeared; the cursor then had to be moved to, and held in, the target box. After practicing on a normal hand-to-cursor movement relationship, a reversed cursor-to-hand relationship for both x- and y-directions was introduced, forcing the subjects to learn a new relationship between hand and cursor movement. Once the subjects' performance had returned to an acceptable level, the gain was restored to the initial conditions. The task does not require the subject to learn a new movement. For example, a cursor movement to a target at 15 degrees under the normal condition requires a hand movement identical to a cursor movement to a 195-degree target under the learning condition. What is changed is the visual feedback that requires the subject to learn a new transformation from visual feedback to motor output. Normal subjects rapidly reconfigure the initial, feed-forward portion of the movement and slowly minimize the number of feedback-related corrective movements (Shanbhag and Ebner, 1994).

The performance in this task of one male subject with an isolated, left-hemisphere cerebellar stroke due to an arteriovenous malformation is illustrated in figure 11.1. The cerebellar patient's performance using the left hand (lesioned side) under the practiced normal cursor gain condition is slightly less accurate than the performance of a control subject. The patient did not

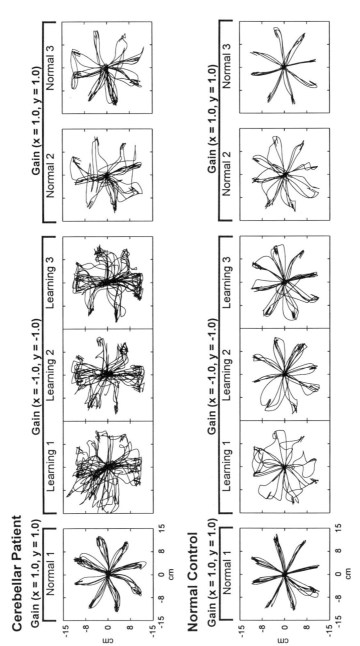

Figure 11.1 Comparisons of the handpaths from a normal subject (bottom) and a patient with a left cerebellar lesion (top) in the visuomotor adaptation task. The feedback gains used are shown above the plots of the handpaths. Both complete and incomplete movements are included, accounting for the large number of handpaths plotted in the learning sets for the cerebellar patient. Both subjects used the left hand.

adapt as rapidly as the control subject during the reverse gain period. Additionally, the patient did not regain the initial performance level on restoration of the normal gain condition. Did the cerebellar patient learn?

There was some degree of adaptation to the change in gain in the hand trajectories. Furthermore, the poor performance after the change from reversed to normal gain indicates an aftereffect. Pascual-Leone et al. (1993) have reported that patients with cerebellar cortical atrophy are unable to transfer procedural knowledge to declarative knowledge in a serial-reaction time task. In contrast to those results, this patient had no difficulty in transferring procedural- to declarative knowledge, as the subject was able accurately to describe the reverse condition when asked at the end of the experiment. Nevertheless, the patient is impaired when compared to the control subject. We are faced with the question of how to separate a motor performance deficit from a motor learning deficit.

In the study by Sanes, Dimitrov, and Hallett (1990; see also chapter 13), patients were placed into two groups: one with primarily cerebellar cortical atrophy, the other with olivopontocerebellar atrophy (OPCA). Subjects were asked to trace polygonal templates mounted on a graphics tablet, with a stylus, under conditions of full view of the arm and with mirror-reversed vision of the arm. During the full-vision condition, both groups of patients showed prolonged movement times (MT) relative to normal subjects. Only the OPCA patients demonstrated significant differences in MT in comparison to normal subjects. However, other quantitative measures of movement error (average error, end-point error, and constant-peak error) increased with practice for all subjects, suggesting a failure to learn on the part of all subjects (including normal controls). In the mirror-reversed condition, MT decreased significantly for cerebellar hemisphere and normal groups, whereas the OPCA group MT remained constant. Average error remained constant for all groups in comparison with the normal vision task. Because MT and accuracy decreased with practice, the authors argued that learning is not occurring in the OPCA group, instead calling the observed performance changes an alteration in performance strategy. However, even if the results had shown that normal subjects' performance improved in comparison to that of cerebellar patients, the problem remains of distinguishing between deficits in motor learning and deficits in movement execution.

Other studies of motor learning in humans with cerebellar lesions have focused on the visuomotor adaptation to displacement of the visual field from the use of prism glasses or to visual field distortions caused by magnifying lenses. The results have been inconsistent. Gauthier, Hofferer, Hoyt, and Stark (1979) showed that one patient with persistent cerebellar signs was unable to adapt to a magnifying visual-field perturbation in a drawing task. The patient had a clinical course and findings consistent with involvement beyond the cerebellum. However, four other patients with less dramatic long-term cerebellar signs showed no deficits, even though some had extensive but relatively localized cerebellar lesions. In another study, subjects threw darts at a target while wearing prism glasses (Thach et al., 1992). Two subjects with inferior olive hypertrophy showed an inability to recalibrate their throws under the shifted visual field caused by the glasses, with little or no after-effect. No data are presented with respect to the variability of the throws. Many factors can influence the trajectory of a thrown object, such as the path taken by the hand during the throw, the time of release of the thrown object, and the type of grip used. Therefore, additional information on performance would be useful to interpret these latter findings.

Weiner, Hallett, and Funkenstein (1983; see also chapter 13) used a task in which subjects were asked to make horizontal pointing movements with the hand to a visual target without vision of the hand under both normal and prism-shifted visual conditions. Cerebellar patients (five with degenerative disease, one with infarct damage, one with drug-induced cerebellar signs) did not adapt as completely nor as quickly as did normal subjects. Furthermore, the trial-to-trial variability of the cerebellar patients was much larger than that of normal subjects, suggesting that the patients were not able to make a coordinated accurate pointing movement. On removal of the prism glasses, normal subjects showed an aftereffect of adaptation manifested as a pointing error to the side opposite that of the displacement induced by the glasses. This aftereffect was reduced in the cerebellar patients, suggesting that the internal model for visuomotor transformations was not changed during the adaptation period. However, the subjects performed only 20 trials under the prism-shifted conditions. It would have been interesting to see whether the cerebellar patients could demonstrate aftereffects with longer adaptation periods, because even normal subjects did not reduce their pointing errors fully in the short adaptation time used.

A recent study by Timmann et al. (1994; see also chapter 13) has demonstrated that cerebellar patients are able to improve their performance in a visuomotor task. Patients with isolated cerebellar lesions were asked to trace and then draw from memory an irregular template. In another memory condition, subjects were asked to draw the template rotated 90 degrees to the left. Feedback of their performance was given by showing the template between trials. Under these tasks, cerebellar patients were able to improve their performance significantly after 20 trials. It is interesting to note that performance improvements on the rotation memory task were greater than on the nonrotation memory task. Additionally, the baseline performance of the cerebellar patients was poorer than that of the age-matched control subjects. These results challenge the hypothesis that the cerebellum is the locus of storage for motor memory. Because the patients did show deficits in performance and a deterioration in the total capacity for improvements in performance, the role of the cerebellum in acquisition of the task remains unclear.

Clearly, patients with cerebellar disease have difficulty adapting their movements under visuomotor transformations. We have emphasized the problem of deconvolving performance and learning deficits. One additional caveat to the interpretation should be stressed: Those patients with the most difficulty in learning have had primarily degenerative disease processes such as OPCA (Weiner et al., 1983; Sanes et al., 1990; Thach et al., 1992), in which the pathology is not restricted to the cerebellum (cortex or nuclei) proper. Comparable studies are needed of patients with well-defined, isolated cerebellar lesions.

ELECTROPHYSIOLOGICAL STUDIES

Adaptation to a mechanical perturbation delivered during a wrist movement was evaluated in the first study to examine Purkinje cell discharge during a form of voluntary motor learning (Gilbert and Thach, 1977). There were two key findings: First, the perturbation evoked transient increases and some decreases in complex-spike activity, and these complex-spike responses were likened to an error signal. The second crucial finding was the documentation of changes in simple-spike activity (particularly decreases) that persisted even though the animal had adapted to the perturbation. The authors interpreted these findings as consistent with the Marr-Albus hypothesis (i.e., climbing fiber activation modified the strength of the parallel fibers' synapses on the Purkinje cell). The importance of this seminal study led us to reevaluate Purkinje cell simple- and complex-spike activity during voluntary motor learning in primates.

Our study attempted to address several issues raised in our discussion of the internal models and clinical learning studies. First, electrophysiological studies have the same difficulty in dissociating motor performance from learning. Therefore, efforts were made to control for performance-related firing changes versus learning-related changes. Second, the learning paradigm was based on adapting to a visuomotor transformation, bearing in mind that cerebellar patients are known to have difficulties in similar tasks (Weiner et al., 1983; Sanes et al., 1990; see figure 11.1). Third, the goal was to evaluate voluntary movement in a paradigm in which the task requirements are explicitly controlled and in which the learning process and improvement in motor performance are well-defined. The task consisted of a two-dimensional arm reaching movement in rhesus monkeys (*Macaca mulatta*) as described earlier for the human subject studies. Purkinje cell activity was evaluated during a visuomotor transformation consisting of a change in the displacement gain between hand and cursor movement (Ojakangas and Ebner, 1991, 1992, 1994). For example, with a gain of 2.0, the cursor moved twice as far as the hand (i.e., the manipulandum) moved, and for a gain of 0.5, the cursor moved one-half the distance that the hand moved. Completion of the task required compensating for this "error," matching the hand movement to the visuomotor transformation.

Primates adapt to the visuomotor transformation by scaling movement kinematics. An example of the scaling of tangential velocity as an animal learned a gain of 2.0 is depicted in figure 11.2. The experiments consisted of three phases. During the first (control) phase (gain = 1.0), the tangential

TANGENTIAL VELOCITY PROFILES DURING LEARNING PARADIGM
(averaged over trials specified)

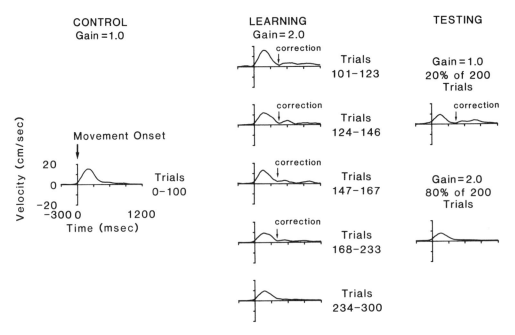

Figure 11.2 Averaged tangential velocity profiles using a gain of 2.0 during the learning phase. The profiles are averaged over the trials indicated, and the learning phase is partitioned. The peak velocity for the control phase (far left) profile is 15 cm/s, and the profile is asymmetrical but relatively smooth with one peak. During learning (middle column), as the novel gain is introduced, corrections are seen as indicated by secondary peaks in the averaged profiles. By trials 168 to 223, the secondary correction peak is decreasing, and by trials 234 to 300, the corrections have disappeared. Note that the peak velocity has decreased to 8 cm/s and the profile is smooth. During the testing phase (far right), the trials with the randomly interspersed gain of 1.0 show secondary velocity peaks, indicating corrections, whereas the average tangential velocity profile for the majority of the trials (gain of 2.0) is single-peaked and smooth. (Reprinted with permission from Ojakangas and Ebner, 1991.)

velocity profile was single-peaked, smooth, and slightly asymmetric, as is typical of reaching movements (Georgopoulos, 1986). The second (learning) phase consisted of 100 to 200 movements to a new visuomotor gain. At the onset of the learning phase, the first peak of the velocity profile was similar in amplitude and timing but was followed by several corrective movements. The amplitude of the corrections decreased as the animal adapted, with a gradual reduction in the peak of the bell-shaped velocity profile. On average, the peak amplitude was reduced by 49 percent for a gain of 2.0 (i.e., the velocity scaled to match precisely the new movement amplitude needed). In the third (testing) phase, random presentations of the control gain occurred for 20 percent of the trials and were used to demonstrate that learning occurred. When the gain was 1.0, the initial velocity component remained scaled back, and secondary velocity corrective components reappeared (i.e., an aftereffect was evident).

Analysis of the kinematics revealed that in adapting to a novel gain, primates adopt a consistent strategy of scaling movement amplitude, velocity, and duration in proportion to the distance the hand needs to travel for a new visuomotor gain (Ojakangas and Ebner, 1991). Two distinct movement phases were evident. The first was an initial, stereotypical, open-loop phase beginning at movement onset and lasting to peak velocity. The second, later phase involved the movement corrections needed to adjust for the visuomotor transformation. Learning involved utilizing the errors from previous trials to scale the initial phase of the movement. Having a consistent learning strategy with objective improvement in performance, we could evaluate Purkinje cell complex-spike and simple-spike activity before, during, and after the adaptation to the visuomotor transformation. The goal was to test two predictions of the Marr-Albus hypothesis: (1) that climbing fiber activity increases during motor learning and (2) that "persistent" alterations in the simple-spike discharge of Purkinje cells occur as a consequence of the complex-spike activation.

Of the 170 Purkinje cells recorded throughout the learning process, over 70 percent had statistically significant increases in complex-spike discharge (Ojakangas and Ebner, 1992, 1994). The cells were located primarily in the intermediate zone and adjacent hemispheres of lobules V and VI. Furthermore, the majority of the complex-spike responses were transient, the increased discharge occurring during the learning phases of the task but then returning to the control levels. An example is shown in figure 11.3 in which, for purposes of the analysis, the learning trials were subdivided into three periods. For this Purkinje cell, significant increases in complex-spike discharge occurred during the response window in the first, second, and third learning periods. The transient nature of the increased climbing fiber afferent discharge is evident, beginning in the first learning period, becoming maximal by the second learning period, and decreasing again in the third period. In the testing phase, the complex-spike activity in the window was no longer significantly different from the control gain. In support of the first prediction of the Marr-Albus hypothesis, complex-spike discharge changed transiently during the process of motor learning.

The next question addressed was whether the increased, transient complex-spike discharge was associated with long-term changes in the simple-spike discharge. For the Purkinje cell shown in figure 11.3, the simple-spike response modulated with learning. In both the third phase of learning and the testing phase, the simple-spike response increased significantly over the control phase. However, this observation alone cannot be taken as evidence for a learning-related, persistent change in simple-spike activity because the movement amplitude and kinematics after adaptation differ from the control movements. The assessment of any persistent alteration in simple-spike modulation must account for this change in performance. Consequently, we introduced an

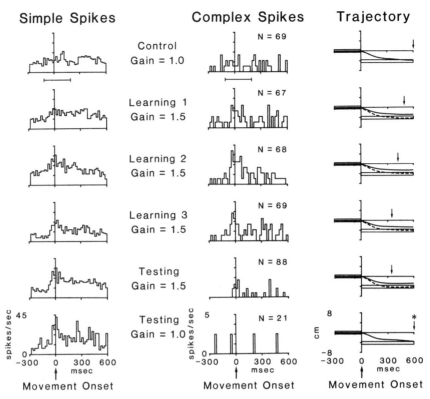

Figure 11.3 Simple and complex spike activity from a Purkinje cell showing a transient increase in complex spike activity during learning using a gain of 1.5. Simple-spike histograms are on the left, complex spike histograms in the middle, and hand-cursor trajectories on the right. Arrows on the trajectories denote the end of movement. Asterisk in the last test phase denotes that movement end had not occurred in the 600 ms shown. The learning phase is divided into thirds. Each histogram is the accumulated activity for the number of trials indicated and is aligned on movement onset. Spike activity was analyzed for the response window of 120 ms before to 190 ms after movement onset (bar under the two histograms in control phase). Complex spike firing rates in spikes per second during window for the six phases, in order from top to bottom, were 0.86, 1.33, 2.11, 1.53, 0.56, and 0.16. The ratio of simple-spike firing rate during window compared with background for each phase was, from top to bottom, 142, 159, 153, 280, 248, and 294%. Simple- and complex-spike responses are plotted in 20-ms binwidths. (Reprinted with permission from Ojakangas and Ebner, 1992.)

additional control, the distance control. Prior to the visuomotor adaptation, the monkeys were required to move with a gain of 1.0 to the target box placed at the distance and in the direction the hand would have to move in the adapted state. This distance control provided an exact match for the distance of the learned movement and allowed a close approximation of the learned velocity (Ojakangas and Ebner, 1992). Using this distance control, we determined whether the simple-spike changes with learning could be accounted for by the kinematics. Next, we determined whether the transient increases in complex spikes were correlated with the changes in simple-spike modulation by dividing the Purkinje cells into two groups, those with learning-related complex-spike responses and those without. Two findings led to the conclusion that the changes in simple-spike modulation were not correlated with the transient climbing fiber activation occurring during the learning. First, a similar number of Purkinje cells with and without complex-spike learning responses demonstrated persistent changes in simple-spike modulation (i.e., the increased complex-spike discharge was not preferentially associated with persistent changes in the simple-spike activity). Furthermore, the onset time, location, receptive field, and magnitude of the simple-spike modulation were comparable for both groups of Purkinje cells. Second, the amplitude of the simple-spike changes was equally likely to increase or decrease, although a decrease in simple-spike activity has been predicted (Albus, 1971; Ito et al., 1982; Ito, 1989). These findings lead to the conclusion that the transient changes in complex-spike activity and the nonkinematic-related changes in the simple-spike responses are independent processes.

The question remains, "What is driving the transient increases in complex-spike discharge?" It must be emphasized that the complex-spike discharge was not related directly to the visuomotor error imposed by the paradigm. The visuomotor disparity remained throughout the learning and test phases, yet the complex-spike responses were predominantly transient. The complex-spike responses were not associated with the corrective movements that occurred after the initial bell-shaped velocity profile. Instead, the complex-spike responses occurred around movement onset. The average complex-spike response started approximately 100 ms before movement onset, and the increased firing was maintained until 200 ms after movement onset, too early for feedback mechanisms to have detected the visuomotor error.

A detailed analysis of the complex-spike discharge in relation to the movement kinematics helped provide insights into this question (Ojakangas and Ebner, 1994). For 141 Purkinje cells, the movements during the visuomotor adaptation were sorted into two groups: those in which a complex spike occurred in a defined response window, and those in which no complex spikes occurred. The occurrence of complex spikes was associated with changes in movement velocity in the majority of instances (78 percent). Figure 11.4 shows an example of the results of this analysis for 15 Purkinje cells with strong complex-spike responses around movement onset during the learning of the visuomotor transformation. Sorting of the movements on the presence or absence of a complex spike in the response window reveals that hand velocity is significantly different on the trials in which a complex spike occurred. These complex spike—associated velocity changes were significant whether the data were aligned on movement onset or aligned on the complex-spike times.

The velocity changes associated with complex-spike discharge consisted of unimodal increases and decreases or bimodal changes (increases followed by decreases, etc.). A contingency analysis showed that the relationship between the visuomotor gain and the change in velocity is a dependent one (Ojakangas

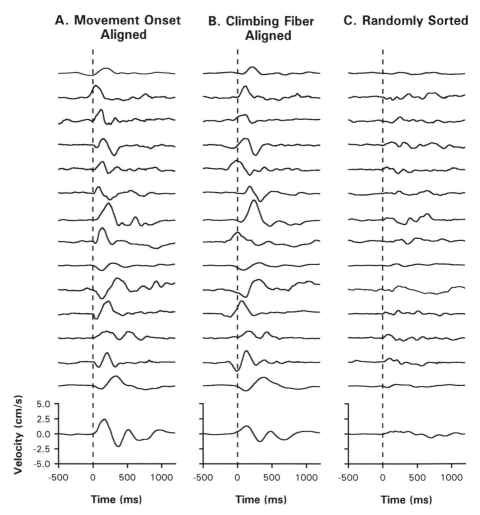

Figure 11.4 Velocity differences obtained from 15 Purkinje cells (A) aligned on movement onset, (B) aligned on CS, and (C) randomly sorted and aligned on movement onset. Velocity differences were determined by subtracting the velocity profiles from the movement trials in which complex spikes did *not* occur from those in the trials in which complex spikes *did* occur in a defined response window. Note increases and decreases and unimodal and bimodal differences. Scales for all cells shown at bottom of figure. The velocity difference for each cell was significant, based on a ±3.5-SD criterion from the randomly sorted trials. (Reprinted with permission from Ojakangas and Ebner, 1994.)

and Ebner, 1994). When adapting to high gains (i.e., movements requiring smaller adjustments), the complex spikes occur preferentially in movements with a larger velocity. Furthermore, when the feedback gain was less than one, the complex spike occurred preferentially during movements in which the velocity decreased. Simply stated, the complex spikes are more likely to occur in trials in which the velocity difference is inappropriate for the feedback gain. The absolute mean velocity change decreased monotonically as the gain increased, and the velocity changes were coupled to the time of complex-spike occurrence. In summary, the amplitude, size, and timing of the velocity changes are coupled to the visuomotor gain and the timing of the complex spike. The complex spikes act as a velocity-related error signal, in which the climbing fiber afferent discharge is evoked by the errors occurring in the previous movements. We postulated that the complex spikes contributed to the required adjustments in velocity. Although a velocity-related error signal could prove useful in the computations required to adapt to these visuomotor transformations, the electrophysiological evidence does not support the cerebellum as the site of the plasticity.

HUMAN NEUROIMAGING STUDIES

The ability to study in humans the changes in brain activity that occur in relation to motor learning first became possible with the advent of PET technology. The changes in regional cerebral blood flow (rCBF) or glucose metabolic rate (GMR) can be measured during the various stages of skill acquisition as subjects learn a new motor task. A recent development has been the use of MRI to map noninvasively human central nervous system (CNS) activity without the use of exogenous contrast agents (Bandettini, Wong, Hinks, Tikofsky, and Hyde, 1992; Kwong et al., 1992; Ogawa et al., 1992). The basis of this technique is that deoxyhemoglobin acts as an endogenous paramagnetic contrast agent, with neural activation leading to alterations in the local concentration of deoxyhemoglobin (Thulborn, Waterton, and Mathews, 1982; Ogawa, Lee, Kay, and Tank, 1990a; Ogawa, Lee, Nayak, and Glynn, 1990b). Functional fMRI now promises to reveal detailed spatial and temporal information about the changes in the CNS during learning. An advantage of PET and fMRI is that both techniques allow visualization of many different brain areas simultaneously. The use of these imaging methods in human subjects also means a considerable increase in the complexity and diversity of the motor learning paradigms that can be studied.

Given the power of neuroimaging techniques, the possibility exists to identify the CNS structures involved with motor learning and, specifically, the cerebellum's role in voluntary learning. Ideally, imaging techniques would make possible the identification of the site(s) of any internal model(s) and provide insights into the modifiable parameters represented. Specific tests of formal models should be possible. Judging from the literature (table 11.1), it is clear that the problem is far from simple. One of the first issues that needs clarification is the variety of paradigms deemed to be motor learning. Returning to Schmidt's definition (1982), motor learning is characterized by an enduring improvement in skilled behavior and falls under the broad category of procedural learning (Squire, 1986). In contradistinction, declarative learning is characterized by the ability to describe or explain what has been learned (Halsband and Freund, 1993). Although both elements may be involved in

Table 11.1   Activity Changes in Motor Areas Associated with "Motor Learning"

Task	Anatomic Structure							Technique	Performance Assay	Type	Reference
	Cblm	BG	M1	SC	SMA	PM	Cin				
Finger-thumb sequence	↑(↓?)	→	↑	—			→	1	Video, EMG	D	Seitz et al., 1990
Finger-thumb sequence	—	↑	↑	→	→	↑	↑	1	Video, EMG	D	Seitz & Roland, 1992
Finger-thumb sequence	—	—	↑[a]	↑[a]	—	↑	—	1	Veido, EMG	D	Schlaug et al., 1994
Finger-thumb opposition	→	—	—[a]	—	→	↑		2	Not measured	D	Friston et al., 1992
Keypresses	→	→	—[a]	↓[b]	↑	→	→	2	Count responses	D, P	Jenkins et al., 1994
Keypresses (Tetris)	→	→	→	→	↑	→	→	3	Game score	D, P	Haier et al., 1992
Point to screen	↓[c]	—	—		↑	—		2	Video	D	Decety et al., 1992
Point to screen	→	—	↑		↑	↑	→	2	Video	D	Kawashima et al., 1994
Pursuit rotor	—	—	↑		↑		→	2	Contact time[d]	P	Grafton et al., 1992
Pursuit rotor	→	↑	→		→	↑	→	2	Contact time[d]	P	Grafton et al., 1994
Virtual hand and motor imagery	?	?	?	?	?	?	?	2	No movement	D	Decety et al., 1994
Eyeblink conditioning	→	→					↑	2	Transducer[e]	P	Molchan et al., 1994
Tactile recognition	→	—	—	—	—	—		4	Video	D	Roland et al., 1989
Joystick tracking	→		↑		↑	↑	→	5	Trajectory A/D[f]	P	Flament et al., 1994, in press

Anatomic structures: Cblm = cerebellum; BG = basal ganglia; M1 = primary motor cortex; SC = somatosensory cortex; SMA = supplementary motor area; PM = premotor cortex; Cin = cingulate gyrus.

Technique: 1 = ¹¹O regional cerebral blood flow; 2 = ¹⁵O regional cerebral blood flow; 3 = 18-fluoro-2-deoxyglucose, glucose metabolic rate; 4 = regional cerebral oxidative metabolism; 5 = functional magnetic resonance imaging.

Type of learning: D = declarative learning; P = procedural learning.

[a] Primary motor and sensory cortices were grouped together.

[b] Refers to Brodman's area 7.

[c] The authors conclude no change, but data indicate a decrease.

[d] A digital clock was used to measure contact time of stylus to rotor plate.

[e] Output of a mechanical transducer measuring eyeblink was displayed on a chart recorder.

[f] Joystick output in x in y directions was digitized to measure movement trajectories.

the acquisition of motor skills, procedural learning should be a significant component of any motor learning paradigm.

The majority of the motor learning functional imaging studies to date have relied on tasks dominated by declarative learning (see table 11.1). For example, in the two PET studies evaluating the learning associated with preparation for reaching (Decety et al., 1994; Kawashima, Roland, and O'Sullivan, 1994), the subjects were briefly shown dots of different sizes projected onto a screen. The task consisted of learning the positions of the dots based on size; the subjects were then required to point to the dots in the correct order. When interpreting these studies in the context of voluntary motor learning, the declarative nature of the task must be emphasized. Several PET "motor" learning studies were based on remembering a finger-thumb sequence, again a primarily declarative form of learning (Seitz, Roland, Bohm, 1990; Friston, Frith, Passingham, Liddle, and Frackowiak, 1992; Seitz and Roland, 1992; Schlaug, Knorr, and Seitz, 1994). Tactile-recognition learning of novel objects is another example of a predominantly declarative form of learning (Roland, Eriksson, Widen, and Stone-Elander, 1989). An even more striking example is a recent PET study in which the subjects were imaged while watching a virtual hand grasp an object or while they imagined grasping the object (Decety et al., 1994). Because there was no limb movement or demonstrated improvement in a motor skill, the label of *motor learning* probably should not be applied to this interesting paradigm.

A second confounding problem is the needs to assay performance and to dissociate between performance-related changes in activity and learning-related activity. For example, the first PET motor learning study was based on acquisition of a finger-thumb sequence (Seitz et al., 1990). rCBF increased in the anterior lobe of the cerebellum with learning; however, because the frequency of finger movements nearly doubled from the start of the task to acquisition of the correct sequence, the blood flow in the cerebellum relative to the motor output may have remained constant or even decreased. In a simpler version of this task, opposition of the thumb to each digit in turn was studied, but the movement rate was maintained constant (Friston et al., 1992). Cerebellar rCBF decreased over time. A similar decrease occurred during the learning of a sequence of key presses in which the rate and amplitude of the movement were both constrained (Jenkins, Brooks, Nixon, Frackowiak, and Passingham, 1994). However, as in the lesion or electrophysiological studies, other aspects of the motor behavior may need to be controlled precisely to ensure the dissociation between performance and learning. In one of the few imaging studies attempting to normalize the rCBF based on performance (Grafton et al., 1992), cerebellar blood flow remained constant during the learning of a motor pursuit task. However, when this study was repeated in more subjects and at a higher resolution, it was found that the cerebellum was active during the early stages of learning when skill acquisition improved quickly; after learning had occurred and performance had stabilized, the cerebellum was no longer active (Grafton, Woods, and Tyszka, 1994).

Three steps are needed to sort out performance and learning: (1) a quantitative description of the motor behavior, (2) documentation of the motor improvement, and (3) rigorous comparison of the activation with the motor performance. The performance assays used in functional imaging studies have varied considerably from no measurement of the movements, to qualitative evaluation of video or EMG activity, to quantitative measurement of performance (see table 11.1). One of the more thorough examinations of these issues was a study by Grafton et al. (1992). In a procedural form of learning, the time of contact of a stylus tracking a spot on a rotating disk was used as a measure of performance. During the task, rCBF in the midline and right parasagittal zones of the cerebellum increased but remained constant as the subject's performance improved (weighted to performance). With the learning, rCBF increased in the primary motor cortex and the supplementary motor area. These findings suggest that the cerebellar blood flow changes are more closely linked to performance and raise the possibility that the motor cortical areas are the sites of the modifiable internal model (Karni, Meyer, Jezzard, Adams, Turner, and Ungerleider, 1994; Pascual-Leone, Grafman, and Hallett, 1994).

We recently have begun to study the cerebellum's involvement in human voluntary motor learning using fMRI (Flament et al., 1994). At high-field (4T) imaging, using blood-oxygen-level-dependent contrast imaging, we were able to identify with high spatial and temporal resolution the changes in activity that take place in the cerebellum during the learning of a visuomotor transformation analogous to that used in the single-cell recording studies (Ojakangas and Ebner, 1992, 1994). Emphasis was placed on evaluating a procedural type of motor learning in which (1) the movements would be explicitly monitored, (2) performance and its improvement would be documented, and (3) the degree of correlation between motor performance and functional activation would be determined. The basic task is similar to the visuomotor transformation task presented with figure 11.1, except that subjects used a joystick to move the cursor. The paradigm was generated on a computer video monitor and projected onto a screen near the end of the magnet's bore. The joystick positions were digitized, and the kinematics were reconstructed. After the subjects had practiced and acquired proficiency at this task, images were obtained under three task conditions. In the first, the subjects performed the center-out task in which the cursor moved with the normal visuomotor relationship. In the second condition, the relationship between movement of the joystick and movement of the cursor was changed randomly between four conditions for each movement: (1) reversed relationship in x- but not y-direction, (2) reversed relationship in y- but not x-direction, (3) reversed relationship for both x- and y-directions, and (4) normal relationship. For this random period, a new and unpredictable visuomotor relationship was encountered for each movement. In the third or learning condition, the joystick-to-cursor relationship was reversed in both x- and y-directions but remained constant throughout several imaging periods,

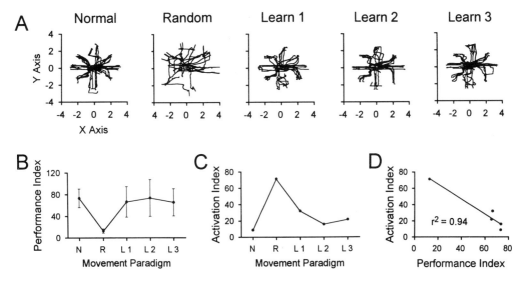

Figure 11.5 (A) Movement trajectories (x-y plots of displacement) made during each 3-min imaging period are shown. This subject rapidly learned the reversed gains. (B) The performance indices for each task period illustrate the rapidity of skill acquisition at the new task. (C) The activation index (product of area and intensity of activation) changed in a reciprocal fashion with the performance index, being highest for the random task period and lowest for the normal task. (D) A linear regression of the relationship between activation and performance in this subject produced a correlation coefficient (r^2) of 0.94.

allowing the subjects to learn the new visuomotor relationship. Learning this task consisted of reorganizing the initial feed-forward phase of the movement and minimizing feedback-related corrective movements occurring later (Shanbhag and Ebner, 1994), consistent with the modification of an internal model.

Figure 11.5 illustrates an example of the cursor trajectories made during the normal, random, and three consecutive learning task periods while imaging. During the normal task condition, the profiles of the trajectories were fairly accurate and stereotyped. In the 3-min normal task period the subject executed 45 movements. The random task was characterized by many inaccuracies, with corrections for movements whose initial direction was inappropriate. The number of movements completed during the random task period decreased to 20. Successive learning periods showed a progressive improvement in movement trajectories, as skill acquisition developed. Skill acquisition was relatively fast in this subject, and the number of completed movements was 42, 43, and 42, respectively, in the first, second, and third learning-task periods. A performance index based on the number of movements completed, movement path length, and movement duration was calculated for each task period and confirms the qualitative impression from the trajectories (figure 11.5B). A high performance index indicates proficiency at the task; a low index reflects poor performance. The worst performance occurred during the random task. The first learning period had a performance index lower than the normal task, but also striking was the increased variability in the trajectories (given by the larger standard deviation of the index, relative to that of the normal task). The performance index during the second and third learning periods was nearly equal to that of the normal task period.

The multislice activation maps of the subject's cerebellum were obtained using a 4T system with an actively shielded gradient and surface coil and a refocused FLASH imaging sequence. A detailed description of the imaging procedure is given in Ellermann et al. (1994). Relative to the normal task period, the highest amount of cerebellar activity occurred during the random task, when visuomotor errors were most frequent and the detection and correction for these errors was highest. The first learning period also exhibited a high level of cerebellar activity, decreasing in subsequent periods as learning of the new visuomotor relationship consolidated. We quantified the cerebellar activation using an activation index that is the product of the percent area with significant activation and the mean intensity of the significant activation for each task period (figure 11.5C). The highest level of cerebellar activity occurred during the random task and the second highest during the first learning period. The activation index during the second learning period approached that of the normal task period (where activation was lowest). During the third learning period, the activation index underwent a slight increase, paralleling the slight decrease in the performance index. In seven of eight subjects, cerebellar activation was greatest during the random period, remained elevated in the first learning period relative to the control task, and then decreased in the subsequent learning periods.

These findings suggest that motor performance and cerebellar activation change in a parallel but reciprocal manner. Additional regression analyses provided a statistical measure of the strength of this relationship. The tight coupling between movement performance and cerebellar activation is evident from the regression plot in figure 11.5D, in which the correlation coefficient r^2 was 0.94. This result typified the relationship between performance and correlation in seven of the eight subjects who mastered the visuomotor transformation (average $r^2 = 0.7$). In this regard, the eighth subject's failure to adapt is instructive. The area and intensity of activation in the cerebellum remained high throughout the learning periods, consistent with the subject's poor performance.

We considered the possibility that the progressive decrease in activation observed during sequential learning-task periods was due to factors other than changes in motor performance. For example, the progressive decrease in cerebellar functional activation could be due to nonspecific habituation of the hemodynamics underlying the MRI signal. To test this possibility, subjects were imaged during two additional experimental paradigms: (1) The normal task was repeated four times and (2) the random task was repeated four times after one period of the normal task. For the multiple normal task paradigm, we detected no differences between the means for the area of activation. Most importantly, there was no evidence for a decrease in activation for the

Ebner, Flament, and Shanbhag

repeated performance of the normal visuomotor relationship. There were no statistical differences between performance indices. For the multiple random task paradigm, the activity remained significantly above that for the normal task. The performance indices during the random tasks were all significantly lower than those calculated during the normal task. Therefore, the changes in cerebellar activation during the learning of the visuomotor transformation were not a consequence of such nonspecific effects as adaptation or familiarity with the paradigm. Cerebellar activation remained consistently high when subjects were continually challenged with visuomotor errors and continued to produce movement errors. Again, cerebellar activation and performance changed in parallel. Furthermore, preliminary results of an fMRI study of motor cortical areas and basal ganglia support the conclusion that the decreased activity observed in the cerebellum is not a consequence of a global decrease in activity with learning (Flament et al., 1995). Activity in cerebral cortical and subcortical motor structures does not necessarily follow the pattern described in the cerebellum. In a similar task, the area of activation in the primary motor cortex, premotor cortex, and supplementary motor cortex progressively increased while learning the visuomotor transformations.

We need to ask how the increases or decreases in activity, as assayed by the various functional imaging methodologies, should be interpreted in the context of voluntary motor learning. What constitutes evidence that a structure is involved in the storage of the motor engram or modification of an internal model? Consider first the problem of interpreting decreases in activity. From table 11.1, it is clear that decreases in cerebral blood flow, glucose metabolic rate, or cerebral oxidative metabolism or changes in the oxyhemoglobin-deoxyhemoglobin ratio have been reported in many regions. For most motor areas (e.g., the supplementary motor, premotor, or cingulate motor areas), the trend is not consistent. However, decreases in activity are prominent in two areas: the cerebellum and the somatosensory cortex. Our recent fMRI findings of a decrease in cerebellar activation agree with the results from most voluntary motor learning PET studies (table 11.1).

One explanation for the decrease in cerebellar activity is that it represents a decrease in synaptic strength (Friston et al., 1992) as theorized in the Albus (1971) and Ito (1982 and 1989) models. Specifically, the decrease in cerebellar activity has been related to LTD (Ito, 1989). Several additional points should be considered before embracing the concept that decreases in cerebellar activation reflect changes in synaptic strength. First, the cerebellar cortex is not the only CNS region in which decreases in activity occur (table 11.1). We have already pointed out the tendency for somatosensory cortex activity to decrease. Second, the decrease in cerebellar activation in the visuomotor adaptation task can be very dramatic (Flament et al., 1994). It is not obvious that large reductions in cerebellar activation would occur if LTD is localized to a few parallel fiber–Purkinje cell synapses specific to the task. Third, in the three studies attempting to relate motor performance quantitatively to the cerebral blood flow changes (Grafton et al., 1992; Grafton et al., 1994) or the fMRI changes (Flament et al., 1994), the activity measures are coupled to performance. In our study, an average 70 percent of the variance in cerebellar activation can be accounted for by motor performance. Last, the most common interpretation of functional images is that activated areas are involved in the task and that nonactivated areas are not. Interpretation of decreased activity as evidence for a site of learning counters the common view of functional activity maps.

The simplest interpretation is that the decreased cerebellar activation reflects the structure's diminishing role in the behavior. In this view, the cerebellum is playing a role in the feedback control of movement. A role for the cerebellum in error detection and correction is based on findings from a variety of behaviors (Kim, Wang, and Ebner, 1987; Wang, Kim, and Ebner, 1987; Stone and Lisberger, 1990; Lou and Bloedel, 1992; Ojakangas and Ebner, 1994). During the initial stages of learning a new task, performance is highly feedback-dependent (Atkeson and Hollerbach, 1985; Ojakangas and Ebner, 1991; Shadmehr and Mussa-Ivaldi, 1994; and Shanbhag and Ebner, 1994). Eventually, as the internal model is modified and as errors are minimized, a feedback controller's role in the behavior becomes progressively less important. A role in feedback control is completely consistent with the finding that the functional activation is inversely correlated with performance (figure 11.5D). A similar interpretation could be offered for the decreases in somatosensory cortex activity observed in several PET studies (Seitz and Roland, 1992; Jenkins et al., 1994). Last, this view provides for a reinterpretation of LTD's function in the cerebellar cortex. If the cerebellum acts as a feedback controller whose function is minimized as motor performance is optimized, LTD may act to remove the cerebellar cortex from the processing loop. In this interpretation, LTD does not serve as a storage mechanism but rather as a control function to reduce cerebellar participation in highly learned behaviors.

Persistent increases in activity in the CNS also occur during voluntary motor learning (see table 11.1). Many motor regions have been reported to have significant increases in activity with learning; however, the motor cortex has been identified consistently as a site of persistent increases. Our recent fMRI investigation into learning visuomotor transformations have observed similar increases in the motor cortical areas (Flament et al., 1995). Although it is tempting to speculate that this persistent activation reflects the modification of an internal model, additional studies are required to accept such an interpretation. In particular, the problem of dissociating performance- and learning-related activation will need to be addressed.

CONCLUSIONS

Several common themes emerge from the review of the clinical, electrophysiologic, and imaging studies of the cerebellum's role in voluntary motor learning. First, tasks based on procedural learning are needed. Although they are probably one of the more difficult types of motor learning to study, tasks in which motor performance is optimized based on practice provide the best opportunity for understanding motor learning. Second, the inevitable changes in motor performance that occur with voluntary motor learning must be subject to explicit control. One must evaluate whether the changes in single-cell activity or the activation seen in fMRI or PET studies are due to the modifications in motor behavior that occur as the result of learning. In both our electrophysiologic and fMRI studies, the changes in motor performance can account for much of the observed alterations in single-cell discharge and functional activation. Similarly, in clinical studies the analogous problem must be rigorously addressed. Performance deficits and motor learning deficits must be dissociated.

Our observation that the cerebellum is tightly linked to motor performance is certainly not surprising. The cerebellum is required for the production of smooth, coordinated movements. A role in the computations required to implement a novel visuomotor transformation is suggested by coupling these findings with the electrophysiologic and fMRI results showing that the cerebellum is preferentially activated during learning. The cerebellum's function in updating internal models may be to provide needed neural processing. The future goal is to define these computations precisely.

ACKNOWLEDGMENTS

We thank Linda King and Joan Bailey for typing the manuscript and Mike McPhee for preparing the illustrations. This work supported by National Institutes of Health grants NS18338, NS31530, and NS31318.

REFERENCES

Albus JS (1971). A theory of cerebellar function. Math Biosci 10:25–61.

Atkeson CG (1989). Learning arm kinematics and dynamics. Annu Rev Neurosci 12:157–183.

Atkeson CG, Hollerbach JM (1985). Kinematic features of unrestrained vertical arm movements. J Neurosci 5:2318–2330.

Bandettini PA, Wong EC, Hinks RS, Tikofsky RS, Hyde JS (1992). Time course EPI of human brain function during task activation. Magn Reson Med 25:390–398.

Cunningham HA (1989). Aiming error under transformed spatial mappings suggests a structure for visual-motor maps. J Exp Psychol 15:493–506.

Decety J, Perani D, Jeannerod M, Bettinardi V, Tadary B, Woods R, Mazziotta JC, Fazio F (1994). Mapping motor representations with positron emission tomography. Nature 371:600–602.

Eccles JC (1977). An instruction-selection theory of learning in the cerebellar cortex. Brain Res 127:327–352.

Ekerot C-F, Kano M (1985). Long-term depression of parallel fibre synapses following stimulation of climbing fibers. Brain Res 342:357–360.

Ellermann JM, Flament D, Kim S-G, Fu Q-G, Merkle H, Ebner TJ, Ugurbil K (1994). Spatial patterns of functional activation of the cerebellum investigated using high field (4T) MRI. NMR Biomed 7:63–68.

Flament D, Ellermann J, Ugurbil K, Ebner TJ (1994). Functional magnetic resonance imaging (fMRI) of cerebellar activation while learning to correct for visuomotor errors. Soc Neurosci Abstr 20:20.

Flament D, Lee JH, Ugurbil K, Ebner TJ (1995). Changes in motor cortical and subcortical activity, during the acquisition of motor skill, investigated using functional MRI (4T echo planar imaging). Soc Neurosci Abstr 21:1422.

Friston KJ, Frith CD, Passingham RE, Liddle PF, Frackowiak RS (1992). Motor practice and neurophysiological adaptation in the cerebellum: a positron tomography study. Proc R Soc Lond [B] Biol Sci 248:223–228.

Gauthier GM, Hofferer J, Hoyt WF, Stark L (1979). Visual-motor adaptation. Quantitative demonstration in patients with posterior fossa involvement. Arch Neurol 36:155–160.

Georgopoulos AP (1986). On reaching. Annu Rev Neurosci 9:147–170.

Georgopoulos AP (1990). Neurophysiology of reaching. In M Jeannerod (ed), Attention and Performance XIII: Motor Representation and Control. Hillsdale, NJ: Lawrence Erlbaum Associates, pp 227–263.

Gilbert PFC, Thach WT (1977). Purkinje cell activity during motor learning. Brain Res 128: 309–328.

Gomi H, Kawato M (1992). Adaptive feedback control models of the vestibulocerebellum and spinocerebellum. Biol Cybern 68:105–114.

Grafton ST, Mazziotta JC, Presty S, Friston KJ, Frackowiak RS, Phelps ME (1992). Functional anatomy of human procedural learning determined with regional cerebral blood flow and PET. J Neurosci 12:2542–2548.

Grafton ST, Woods RP, Tyszka M (1994). Functional imaging of procedural motor learning: Relating cerebral blood flow with individual subject performance. Hum Brain Map 1:221–234.

Halsband U, Freund H-J (1993). Motor learning. Curr Opin Neurobiol 3:940–949.

Holmes G (1939). The cerebellum of man. Brain 62:1–30.

Ito M (1982). Cerebellar control of the vestibulo-ocular reflex—Around the flocculus hypothesis. Annu Rev Neurosci 5:275–296.

Ito M (1984). The Cerebellum and Neural Control. New York: Raven Press.

Ito M (1989). Long-term depression. Annu Rev Neurosci 12:85–102.

Ito M, Sakurai M, Tongroach P (1982). Climbing fibre induced depression of both mossy fibre responsiveness and glutamate sensitivity of cerebellar Purkinje cells. J Physiol (Lond) 324:113–134.

Jenkins IH, Brooks DJ, Nixon PD, Frackowiak RSJ, Passingham RE (1994). Motor sequence learning: A study with positron emission tomography. J Neurosci 14:3775–3790.

Kano M, Rexhausen U, Dreessen J, Konnerth A (1992). Synaptic excitation produces a long-lasting rebound potentiation of inhibitory synaptic signals in cerebellar Purkinje cells. Nature 356:601–604.

Karni A, Meyer G, Jezzard P, Adams M, Turner R, Ungerleider LG (1994). Where practice makes perfect: A fMRI study of long-term motor cortex plasticity associated with the acquisition of a motor skill. Soc Neurosci Abstr 20:1291.

Kawashima R, Roland PE, O'Sullivan BT (1994). Fields in human motor areas involved in preparation for reaching, actual reaching, and visuomotor learning: A positron emission tomography study. J Neurosci 14:3462–3474.

Kawato M, Gomi H (1992). A computational model of four regions of the cerebellum based on feedback-error learning. Biol Cybern 68:95–103.

Kelly TM, Zou CC, Bloedel JR (1990). Classical conditioning of the eyeblink reflex in the decerebrate-decerebellate rabbit. Behav Brain Res 38:7–18.

Kim JH, Wang J-J, Ebner TJ (1987). Climbing fiber afferent modulation during treadmill locomotion in the cat. J Neurophysiol 57:787–802.

Kwong KK, Belliveau JW, Chesler DA, Goldberg IE, Weisskoff RM, Poncelet BP, Dennedy DN, Hoppel BE, Cohen MS, Tuner R, Cheng HM, Brady TJ, Rosen BR (1992). Dynamic magnetic resonance imaging of human brain activity during primary sensory stimulation. Proc Natl Acad Sci USA 89:5675–5679.

Lackner JR, Dizio P (1994). Rapid adaptation to Coriolis force perturbations of arm trajectory. J Neurophysiol 72:299–313.

Lisberger SG (1988). The neural basis for learning of simple motor skills. Science 242:728–735.

Llinas R, Welsh JP (1993). On the cerebellum and motor learning. Neurobiology 3:958–965.

Lou J-S, Bloedel JR (1992). Responses of sagittally aligned Purkinje cells during perturbed locomotion: Synchronous activation of climbing fiber inputs. J Neurophysiol 68:570–580.

Marr D (1969). A theory of cerebellar cortex. J Physiol (Lond) 202:437–470.

Miles FA, Lisberger SG (1981). Plasticity in the vestibulo-ocular reflex: A new hypothesis. Annu Rev Neurosci 4:273–299.

Ogawa S, Lee TM, Kay AR, Tank DW (1990a). Brain magnetic resonance imaging with contrast dependent on blood oxygenation. Proc Natl Acad Sci USA 87:9868–9870.

Ogawa S, Lee TM, Nayak AS, Glynn P (1990b). Oxygenation-sensitive contrast in magnetic resonance image of rodent brain at high magnetic fields. Magn Reson Med 14:68–78.

Ogawa S, Tank D, Menon R, Ellermann JM, Kim SG, Merkle H, Ugurbil K (1992). Intrinsic signal changes accompanying sensory stimulation: Functional brain mapping using MRI. Proc Natl Acad Sci USA 89:5951–5955.

Ojakangas CL, Ebner TJ (1991). Scaling of the metrics of visually-guided arm movements during motor learning in primates. Exp Brain Res 85:314–323.

Ojakangas CL, Ebner TJ (1992). Purkinje cell complex and simple spike changes during a voluntary arm movement learning task in the monkey. J Neurophysiol 68:2222–2236.

Ojakangas CL, Ebner TJ (1994). Purkinje cell complex spike activity during voluntary motor learning: Relationship to kinematics. J Neurophysiol 72:2617–2630.

Pascual-Leone A, Grafman J, Clark K, Stewart M, Massaquoi S, Lou J-S, et al. (1993). Procedural learning in Parkinson's disease and cerebellar degeneration. Ann Neurol 34:594–602.

Pascual-Leone A, Grafman J, Hallett M (1994). Modulation of cortical motor output maps during development of implicit and explicit knowledge. Science 263:1287–1289.

Robinson DA (1976). Adaptive gain control of vestibuloocular reflex by the cerebellum. J Neurophysiol 39:954–969.

Roland PE, Eriksson L, Widen L, Stone-Elander S (1989). Changes in regional cerebral oxidative metabolism induced by tactile learning and recognition in man. Eur J Neurosci 1:3–18.

Sakurai M (1987). Synaptic modification of parallel fibre-Purkinje cell transmission in *in vitro* guinea-pig cerebellar slices. J Physiol (Lond) 394:463–480.

Sanes JN, Dimitrov B, Hallet M (1990). Motor learning in patients with cerebellar dysfunction. Brain 113:103–120.

Schlaug G, Knorr U, Seitz RJ (1994). Inter-subject variability of cerebral activations in acquiring a motor skill: A study with positron emission tomography. Exp Brain Res 98:523–534.

Schmidt RA (1982). Motor Control and Learning. Champaign. Il: Human Kinetics.

Seitz RJ, Roland PE (1992). Learning of sequential finger movements in man: a combined kinematic and positron emission tomography (PET) study. Eur J Neurosci 4:154–165.

Seitz RJ, Roland PE, Bohm C, Greitz T, Stone-Elander S (1990). Motor learning in man: A positron emission tomographic study. Neuroreport 1:57–60.

Shadmehr R, Mussa-Ivaldi FA (1994). Adaptive representation of dynamics during learning of a motor task. J Neurosci 14:3208–3224.

Shanbhag SJ, Ebner TJ (1994). Analysis of kinematic and dynamic parameters of human motor learning. Soc Neurosci Abstr 20:1411.

Soechting JF, Flanders M (1991). Deducing central algorithms of arm movement control from kinematics. In DR Humphrey, HJ Freund (eds), Motor Control: Concepts and Issues, Chichester, Engl: Wiley, pp 293–306.

Soechting JF, Flanders M (1992). Moving in three-dimensional space: Frames of reference, vectors and coordinate systems. Annu Rev Neurosci 15:167–191.

Squire LR (1986). Mechanisms of memory. Science 232:1612–1619.

Stone LS, Lisberger SG (1990). Visual responses of Purkinje cells in the cerebellar flocculus during smooth-pursuit eye movements in monkeys: II. Complex spikes. J Neurosci 63:1262–1275.

Thach WT, Goodkin HP, Keating JG (1992). The cerebellum and the adaptive coordination of movement. Annu Rev Neurosci 150:403–442.

Thompson RF (1988). The neurobiology of learning and memory. Science 233:941–947.

Thulborn KR, Waterton JC, Mattews PM (1982). Dependence of the transverse relaxation time of water protons in whole blood at high field. Biochem Biophys Acta 714:265–272.

Timmann D, Shimansky Y, Larson PS, Wunderlich DA, Stelmach GE, Bloedel JR (1994). Visuomotor learning in cerebellar patients. Soc Neurosci Abstr 20:21.

Wang J-J, Kim JH, Ebner TJ (1987). Climbing fiber afferent modulation during a visually guided, multi-joint arm movement in the monkey. Brain Res 410:323–329.

Weiner MJ, Hallett M, Funkenstein HH (1983). Adaptation to lateral displacement of vision in patients with lesions of the central nervous system. Neurology 33:766–772.

Welsh JP, Harvey JA (1989). Cerebellar lesions and the nictitating membrane reflex: Performance deficits of the conditioned and unconditioned response. J Neurosci 9:299–311.

Zajac FE, Gordon ME (1989). Determining muscle's force and action in multi-articular movement. Exerci Sport Sci Rev 17:187–230.

12 Evolution of Neuronal Activity During Conditional Motor Learning

Steven P. Wise

Often we reach toward, look at, and move in relation to objects in space. However, we need not behave in such a habitual fashion. Through experience, we can learn to respond very differently and much more flexibly. Nonspatial cues can guide behavior as effectively as spatial aspects of stimuli. When used in this sense, the term *nonspatial* implies not that a cue lacks location but rather that the information relevant for guiding action is contained in its nonspatial aspects. For example, consider the color red. Regardless of its location, a red symbol or object relies for its import on the cue's hue, not its place. Red may indicate "stop" at a traffic light, "go" in a bull ring, "left" in political semiotics, or "right" in a laboratory. The ability to develop such multifarious and rapidly changeable stimulus-response relationships has been termed *conditional motor learning* or (more specifically) *conditional visuomotor learning* (Passingham, 1993). This chapter addresses some neuronal mechanisms that may underlie this sophisticated behavior.

Our focus will be on conditional motor learning in nonhuman primates. However, the neural mechanisms for conditional learning in those species almost certainly have homologues in our brains (see e.g., Halsband and Freund, 1990) and in those of other mammals (Passingham, Meyers, Rawlins, Lightfoot, and Fearn, 1988) as well. One might loosely characterize conditional motor learning as allowing the sensory-to-motor linkage of "anything" to "anything else." Conditional motor learning allows the performance of any learned motor action in any discriminable context. As such, it represents a highly intelligent problem-solving ability that undoubtedly confers significant adaptive advantages on the individual.

Conditional motor learning can be distinguished from such other kinds of motor learning as motor adaptation or skill learning, including the learning of movement sequences and either associative or nonassociative reflexes. These alternative forms of motor learning rarely exhibit the flexibility that characterizes conditional motor behavior. Motor learning as usually construed almost invariably entails a spatial context. As animals develop, they learn the relationships between their motor commands and such spatial consequences of those commands as movement of the limbs or body in space and the deviation of the fovea toward visual targets. Adaptation to prismatic distortion of visual input exemplifies this kind of motor learning (Thach et al., 1992, chapter 10). These motor mechanisms appear to adjust as necessary to bring the sensory world and motor commands into spatial compatibility, and subjects deprived of experience with the visual effect of their motor commands have profound abnormalities in visually guided movement (Held and Bauer, 1974; Hein, 1974). They can guide their movements with tactile information but, at least when first allowed vision of their hands, not through visual guidance. As Teuber (1972, p 648) put it: "[I]t is as if the animal's vision poisoned his motor system." As with the vestibuloocular reflex (see chapter 2), which adjusts eye position to eliminate "retinal slip" during head movements, these forms of motor learning are subject to severe spatial constraints. Associative conditioned reflexes (see chapters 5 and 15) show more flexibility in the spatial domain, but because they build on unconditioned reflexes in a rigidly time-dependent manner, they lack flexibility in the temporal domain. In conditional motor behavior, by contrast, a stimulus associated with an action can guide action through any combination of inherent spatial, nonspatial, or temporal (e.g., see Crowne, Dawson, and Richardson, 1988) information, and the action instructed seems to be limited only by the extent of the individual's motor repertoire.

NEUROPSYCHOLOGY OF CONDITIONAL MOTOR LEARNING

Petrides (1987) has dealt in detail with the neuropsychology of conditional motor learning, and Passingham has reviewed the subject specifically (Passingham, 1987), and in the context of the frontal lobe, generally (Passingham, 1993). This chapter will focus on those features of past discussions most relevant to the exploration of its neurophysiological mechanisms.

Conditional Motor Learning Defined

For the purpose of this chapter, *conditional motor learning* can be defined as the acquisition of a response, here termed *motor response 1*, to an arbitrarily linked stimulus, A. In general, subjects must learn simultaneously to emit response 2 to stimulus B. Thus, the subject's *problem* involves learning to select the "correct" response in the context of both stimuli A and B (denoted A1/B2). This kind of task can be termed a *two-problem set*, because the subject (e.g., or monkey) must learn which of two responses is associated with each of two stimuli. More complex stimulus-response mappings also have been studied. We will refer to the stimulus in its context as an *instruction stimulus*. In one special case of conditional motor learning, a response may involve "approaching" or "manipulating" the instruction stimulus (e.g., reaching toward or touching or tapping it), but more generally the required movement has no obligatory spatial relationship with the location of the instruction stimulus. Another special case of conditional motor learning involves go-no-go tasks, in which one instructed "response" is the withholding of any overt motor act. We will refer to these forms of conditional motor learning as *A1/B0 designs*.

The distinction between A1/B2 and A1/B0 designs has some theoretical significance. Most conditional motor learning involves so-called symmetric reward. Every correct response is reinforced, and this behavioral contingency may be denoted as *A1+/B2+* or *A1+/B0+*. In asymmetric reward, the "go" response and only that response is rewarded (A1+/B0−). As Petrides (1986) has demonstrated, these differing reward contingencies can determine whether a go-no-go task requires conditional motor learning or, alternatively, whether that subject can rely instead on simple sensory discrimination. To solve successfully the "problem" posed by the experimenter in an A1+/B0− task, the subject need only learn to discriminate the instruction stimuli from each other, associate the positive one with reward, and approach the reward-associated stimulus. Considerable research suggests that the brain structures and mechanisms differ for sensory discrimination versus conditional motor learning. For example, sensory discrimination learning, especially that which relies on stimulus-reward associations, often depend on the amygdala (Gaffan and Murray, 1990; Gaffan, 1994). By contrast, complete ablations of the amygdala have virtually no effect on the acquisition or retention of conditional motor associations (Murray and Wise, 1995). Conversely, ablations that include the dorsal premotor cortex (PMd) severely disrupt conditional motor learning (i.e., symmetrically rewarded [A1+/B0+] tasks) but cause no deficits in discrimination learning (i.e., asymmetrically rewarded [A1+/B0−] tasks) (Petrides, 1986).

Lesions Dramatically Affecting Conditional Motor Behavior

In its general sense, conditional motor learning (A1+/B2+ or A1+/B0+) appears to depend on the integrity of two brain structures. One of these structures, the PMd, is a part of Brodmann's area 6, lying dorsal and medial to the superior limb of the arcuate sulcus (figure 12.1) (Halsband and Passingham, 1982; Petrides, 1982, 1987; Passingham, 1985a, 1988, 1989, 1993; Kurata and Hoffman, 1994). Damage to this area severely impairs learning (Petrides, 1982) and relearning (Halsband and Passingham, 1982, 1985) conditional motor associations. Prior to the postoperative relearning experiments, subjects learn a simple pair of conditional motor problems (A1+/B2+) preoperatively. After undergoing experimental ablations, the subjects are retrained on the same two problems. The extent of deficit varies between individuals, but some animals with damage to PMd perform at nearly chance levels (50 percent) for more than 200 trials of postoperative training and testing. In different sets of experiments, Passingham showed that with or without a 3-s delay between the instruction and the response, two animals performed at chance (50 percent) levels for at least the first 500 trials after surgery and monkeys with premotor cortex lesions failed to relearn the task in 1000 trials. Subjects not operated on will, not surprisingly, perform better

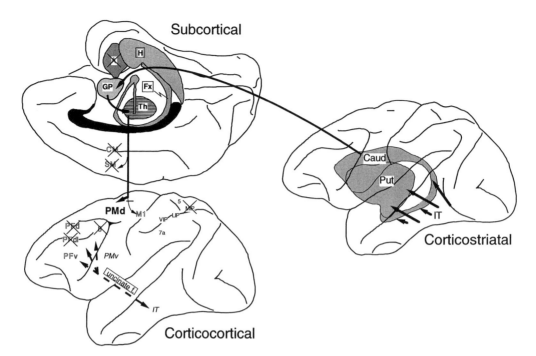

Figure 12.1 Surface views of a macaque monkey hemisphere. The results of damage to those areas or pathways on either new postoperative learning or relearning is noted by a code. An X over the area indicates that damage to that area does not affect conditional motor learning or relearning. Boldface type indicates the structures and pathways most needed for conditional motor learning. A box around the name suggests a less important involvement in conditional visuomotor learning. A, amygdala; H, hippocampus; GP, globus pollidus; Fx, fornix; Th, dorsal thalamus; CM, cingulate motor areas; SM, supplementary motor area; PMd, dorsal premotor cortex; PMv, ventral premotor cortex; M1, primary motor cortex; PFd, dorsal prefrontal cortex; PFdl, dorsolateral prefrontal cortex; PFv, ventral prefrontal cortex; IT, inferotemporal cortex; f, fascicle; VIP, ventral intraparietal area; LIP, lateral intraparietal area; MIP, medial intraparietal area; Caud, caudate nucleus; Put, putamen.

after the "surgery," i.e., a subsequent period that usually matches the duration of the surgery and postoperative recovery for a subject that has undergone surgery. These animals generally perform at 90 percent correct or better. Note than the subjects are not required to learn any new conditional motor associations in this testing phase but need only to relearn or retrieve two such associations acquired before ablations of PMd. Thus, the magnitude of the deficit after PMd damage is profound.

However, PMd is not the only brain region necessary for normal conditional motor learning. The largest deficits in such behavior follow damage to the thalamic relays of basal ganglionic output to the frontal cortex (Canavan, Nixon, and Passingham, 1989). In two cases involving the most extensive damage to the two main relay nuclei, the rostral part of the ventrolateral nucleus (VLo) and the ventroanterior nucleus (VA), animals failed to relearn (to a 90 percent correct criterion) a two-choice conditional task (A1 +/B2 +)

in 3,000 postoperative trials. A third subject needed 1,557 trials to relearn. Radiofrequency lesions centered on VA produced a much greater impairment than those centered on VLo. Unoperated controls tested in parallel made fewer than 50 errors, but two of the animals with lesions involving VA made more than 1,700 errors on this simple task. As discussed further, although damage to other pathways and structures causes modest impairments in conditional motor learning, PMd and the "basal ganglionic" thalamus appear to be the structures most important for this kind of associative learning and memory. It should be pointed out that the monkeys studied by Canavan et al. (1989) were impaired on tasks other than conditional motor associations, specifically delayed alternation and visual discrimination, and their lesions involved structures other than VA and VLo, including but not restricted to the mediodorsal nucleus (MD) and the mammilothalamic tract. Further, neurotoxin lesions of similar parts of the thalamus did not yield significant impairments in conditional motor relearning. Canavan et al. explain the delayed alternation deficits by invoking the incidental MD damage and the difference between neurotoxin and radiofrequency lesions in terms of greater damage done to lateral VA by the latter.

Ablations Not Affecting Conditional Motor Behavior

Based on the failure to demonstrate significant deficits after localized brain damage, neuropsychological studies indicate that conditional motor learning does not require the amygdala (Murray and Wise, 1995), the dorsal prefrontal cortex (Passingham, 1987), the periprincipal, dorsolateral prefrontal cortex (Petrides, 1982), "area 8," including the frontal eye field (Passingham, 1985b; Halsband and Passingham, 1982), supplementary or cingulate motor areas (Chen, Thaler, Nixon, Stern, and Passingham, 1995; Thaler, Chen, Nixon, Stern, and Passingham, 1995), the ventral premotor cortex (Kurata and Hoffman, 1994), or the posterior parietal cortex (Passingham, personal communication, 1994; cf., Halsband and Passingham, 1982). Figure 12.1 summarizes the brain regions and pathways that have been studied in conditional motor tasks.

The argument concerning the ventral premotor cortex needs some elaboration. Two rather different frontal lesions lead to deficits in conditional motor learning. One, involving ablations of the cortex dorsal to the arcuate spur (see figure 12.1), includes the cortex on both the rostral and caudal banks of the arcuate sulcus. This lesion combines parts of Brodmann's areas 8 and 6. Several studies, some dating back to the early 1970s, showed that behavioral deficits followed damage to this region of the frontal lobe but, because of the mongrel nature of the lesion (which includes both premotor and prefrontal areas), these studies were inconclusive. However, most (if not all) of the deficits observed after periarcuate lesions could be classed as conditional motor deficits, and the others can probably be construed as conditional learning impairments of a more general type (see discussion in Wise, 1984, pp 544–546, for citations and analysis of those early studies). Petrides (1987) showed that the caudal part of this periarcuate lesion, the region now known as PMd, is necessary for normal conditional motor learning. The rostral part of that lesion disrupts conditional visuovisual learning (Petrides, 1987) instead, which is not affected by the caudal aspect of the periarcuate (Halsband and Passingham, 1985; Petrides, 1987). The other experimental approach (Halsband and Passingham, 1982, 1985), by contrast, involves ablation area 6 exclusive of the supplementary motor area (SMA). This lesion includes both PMd and the ventral premotor cortex (PMv) but not area 8. Such lesions cause the severe deficits on relearning a simple, two-way conditional motor association, described earlier. Kurata and Hoffman (1994) separately inactivated parts of PMd and PMv with the GABAergic agonist, muscimol. Their task required monkeys to perform a well-learned, two-problem conditional motor task. They found that incorrect choices (i.e., errors in conditional motor behavior) followed PMd injections but not PMv inactivations. (After PMv injections, the amplitude of movement and other motor parameters were somewhat abnormal.) Thus, the area common to the periarcuate and the premotor lesion is PMd, and inactivation of parts of it causes mild impairments in retrieval of a well-learned conditional motor task. Taken together, the ablation and inactivation studies suggest that PMd, but neither area 8 rostral to it nor PMv, contain an essential part of the mechanism necessary for learning or retrieval of conditional motor associations.

Lesions Less Severely Affecting Conditional Motor Behavior

As previously mentioned, though both PMd and the thalamic relays from basal ganglia to frontal cortex are necessary for efficient conditional motor learning, damage to other brain structures can disrupt conditional motor learning to a lesser extent. Some of these deficits are bound to result from nonspecific factors. For example, inability to attend to instruction stimuli should cause deficits on conditional motor tasks. Similarly, problems with sensory information processing (especially for spatial information) or with motivation to learn and perform these tasks in an experimental setting may cause nonspecific deficits in conditional motor learning.

The most efficient and consistent learning of conditional motor relations requires an intact hippocampus (Murray and Wise, 1995), the output from the hippocampus through the fornix (Rupniak and Gaffan, 1987), and the pathway from the inferotemporal visual cortex (IT) to the ventral or ventromedial prefrontal cortex (PFv) (Eacott and Gaffan, 1992), known as the uncinate fascicle (see figure 12.1). Although damage to those structures and pathways causes significant slowing of conditional motor learning, subjects can sometimes learn individual conditional motor associations with minimal, if any, deficits. In these studies, subjects usually are presented with a set of two or more conditional motor problems to solve simultaneously. After disconnecting IT from PFv, a number of individual conditional motor problems were learned with as few as one error (see table 1 of Eacott and Gaffan, 1992), thus demonstrating an animal's ability to acquire conditional motor associations and behave in accordance with them. There was, however, a 2.3-fold increase in the number of postoperative errors made while learning 10 two-problem sets compared to preoperative learning of the same number of problems. With crossed disconnection of IT from PFv (Gaffan and Harrison, 1988), there was a slowing of the rate of learning from a mean of 147 trials to criterion (90 percent correct) to a mean of 360 trials. Whereas this might appear to be a serious deficit, it is noteworthy that these animals can learn (to a 90-percent-correct level) completely novel conditional visuomotor associations, and they can do so with only approximately 2.4 times as many presentations of the initially novel stimuli. Thus, whatever the role of IT input to PFv is in conditional visuomotor learning, it appears to be relatively dispensable.

Deficits that follow hippocampal ablations (Murray and Wise, 1995) or fornix transections (Rupniak and Gaffan, 1987) resemble those that follow uncinate disconnections. Rupniak and Gaffan found that the average number of errors to a criterion of 90 percent (for 100 trials) increased from 7.9 errors per problem in control monkeys to 21.2 errors in fornix-transected animals. This finding can be viewed as a significant 2.7-fold increase in the number of errors. Alternatively, the animals are able to achieve 90 percent of performance on a pair of conditional visuomotor problems and need only an additional 13 trials per problem. Murray and Wise (1995) found that after hippocampectomy, monkeys learned a three-choice conditional motor learning task moderately well, although clear deficits were observed. With chance levels of performance at 33 percent, the subjects learned within 50 trials to choose the correct response approximately 69 percent of the time. On certain three-problem sets, the subject's learning rates and performance were substantially better, although never as good as amygdalectomized monkeys or as the same monkeys preoperatively (96 percent correct). These deficits appear to be specific to spatially directed motor tasks, because similar lesions do not cause deficits in learning to tap versus continuously touch a visual instruction stimulus (Gaffan and Harrison, 1989).

Neuropsychology Summary

There appear to be two quantitatively distinguishable conditional motor syndromes. One, following damage to uncinate fascicle, hippocampus, or fornix, causes a modest and inconsistent deficit in the rate of learning new conditional visuomotor associations, especially when the response is spatial in nature. The other, following damage to PMd and the thalamic relays from basal ganglia to the frontal cortex, presents as a devastating inability to learn novel (or relearn previously learned) conditional visuomotor associations. Neither the modality or submodality of the instruction stimulus nor the exact effector system or response affects this syndrome dramatically.

One possibile explanation of the route of nonspatial visual information to the motor system may lie in the projection from IT to the PFv, and from there to the premotor areas. However, as noted above, that pathway does not appear to be essential in subserving conditional visuomotor learning. The mild deficits in conditional motor learning after disconnecting IT and PFv can be contrasted with the much more severe deficit in visuovisual learning. As described earlier, conditional motor learning consists of the association of the visual instruction stimulus with a motor response (A1+/B2+). An analogous visuovisual conditional association involves the association of one visual stimulus with another (Aa+/Bb+). Deficits on such conditional visuovisual learning after disconnection of the IT from PFv dramatically exceed those for visuomotor conditional learning. Eacott and Gaffan (1992) reported that animals with transections of the uncinate fascicle were unable to relearn a two-choice visuovisual task despite 4,000 test trials on a problem that had been learned to a 90-percent criterion preoperatively. Thus, the flow of information between IT and PFv appears to be necessary for visuovisual conditional associations, but this pathway appears to be less important for visuomotor conditional associations.

These findings argue against an obligatory role for PFv as a relay for nonspatial visual information to the motor system. Thus, it appears that the most likely possibilities for such information transfer involve either multiple, polysynaptic pathways from IT to PMd or pathways from IT to the basal ganglia (Passingham, 1993). A corticocortical route of nonspatial visual information to the premotor cortex would be simple and straightforward. However, the areas of parietal cortex that project to PMd appear to process visuospatial and proprioceptive information, rather than nonspatial aspects of visual stimuli. In the older neuroanatomical literature, there are some reports that suggest inputs from the superior temporal polysensory area (or "area 19") to the premotor cortex, but investigation with modern neuroanatomical methods has failed to confirm these reports (Boussaoud, di Pellegrino, and Wise, 1996; Wise, di Pellegrino, and Boussaoud, 1996). Thus, if nonspatial visual information arrives in PMd through corticocortical routes, it would appear to depend mainly on relays through the various prefrontal areas. However, as previously outlined, damage to the visual inputs from IT to prefrontal cortex (or of most other prefrontal areas that could relay such information to PMd) causes little, if any, impairment in conditional motor learning (figure 12.1). Thus, if a corticocortical route conveys nonspatial visual information to PMd, it must do so through a variety of pathways possibly including the "spatial" parietal areas but not depending on any particular one. The situation for oculomotor behavior is clearer. There is evidence that IT projects directly to the ventral (or small-saccade) aspect of the frontal eye field (FEF) (Webster, Bachevalier, and Ungerleider, 1994). IT also projects to other parts of PFv that, along with FEF, reciprocally interconnect with the supplementary eye field (SEF) (Schall, Morel, and Kaas, 1993).

Alternatively, nonspatial visual and motor information could converge at subcortical levels. On the basis of the results cited previously and some results from noninvasive imaging of regional cerebral blood flow (Jenkins, Brooks, Nixon, Frackowiak, and Passingham, 1994; Passingham, 1993), Passingham (1987, 1993) has argued that visual information converges with motor information at the level of the striatum or perhaps the striatopallidal projection. The convergence of visual signals onto the motor and premotor parts of the striatum presents attractive possibilities for confirming the neural basis of conditional motor learning (Deiber et al., 1991; Marsden and Obeso, 1994; Dominey, Arbib, and Joseph, 1995). However, on the basis of currently available neuroanatomical data, it is difficult to make a strong case for such convergence, especially for the skeletomotor areas of the cortex and the analogous parts of the striatum. For the oculomotor system, there is somewhat more evidence of convergence of nonspatial visual information and premotor cortical output, taking SEF and FEF as the ocular premotor areas in question. This evidence will be discussed in some detail later. However, in considering corticostriatal convergence, one must be aware that apparent convergence may represent overlapping interdigitation (regional convergence) rather than frank convergence (Selemon and Goldman-Rakic, 1985) and that there remains no direct evidence for convergence at the cellular level. It has been suggested that reciprocally connected cortical areas send convergent corticostriatal projections (Yeterian and Hoesen, 1978), but it appears unlikely that this general principle holds for all cortical areas. Accordingly, it must be stressed that this analysis of data published to date can reveal only the possibility of convergence at the cellular level.

Comparison of the distribution of corticostriatal projections from the IT (Saint-Cyr, Ungerleider, and Desimone, 1990; Webster, Bachevalier, and Ungerleider, 1993) with those from SEF (Parthasarathy, Schall, and Graybiel, 1992) and FEF (Stanton, Geldberg, and Bruce, 1988; Parthasarathy et al., 1992) indicates some possible areas of overlap. The most significant areas of common projection to the striatum involve the ventromedial aspect of the body of the caudate nucleus and the posterior limit of the putamen (see figure 7 of Webster et al., 1993, and figure 8 of Stanton et al., 1988, for examples). The case for corticostriatal overlap from IT and PMd is even more tenuous but the available evidence precludes ruling it out definitively. Again, the posterior limit of the putamen appears to be the area most likely to receive both PMd (Stanton et al., 1988) and IT (Saint-Cyr et al., 1990; Webster et al., 1993) inputs. Clearly, there is a need for multiple-label neuroanatomical experiments and transynaptic transport methods (Hoover and Strick, 1993; Lynch, Hoover, and Strick, 1994). Passingham (1987, 1993) has stressed the possibility that convergence at the striatopallidal (if not the corticostriatal) level could underlie conditional motor learning. This idea, too, requires further neuroanatomical support.

The interaction of nonspatial visual inputs and motor signals may be mediated by either of two potential pathways: multiple corticocortical routes, no one of which is essential, and nonspatial inputs from IT that may converge, at the corticostriatal or striatopallidal level, with motor inputs from PMd and one or more oculomotor fields (such as SEF).

PHYSIOLOGY OF THE PREMOTOR CORTICAL AREAS

The phenomenology of neuronal discharge in relation to arm and eye movements has been well documented for each of the areas examined during conditional motor learning. In very brief outline, the striatum, PMd, SEF, and FEF have many common neurophysiological properties. Neuronal activity in FEF (Bruce and Goldberg, 1985; Schall, 1991a), SEF (Schall, 1993a,b), and PMd (Caminiti, Johnson, Burnod, Galli, and Ferraina, 1990; Caminiti, Johnson, Galli, Ferraina, and Burnod, 1991) correlates with both the amplitude (Bruce and Goldberg, 1985; Fu, Suarez, and Ebner, 1993) and direction (Caminiti et al., 1990; di Pellegrino and Wise, 1993) of effector movement. The coarse "directional tuning" resembles that in other cortical areas, such as the primary motor cortex. Cells modulate their discharge in temporal correlation with a variety of events. In any individual neuron, modulation may occur (1) before a temporally predictable sensory event (Bruce and Goldberg, 1985; Vaadia, Kurata, and Wise, 1988); (2) after one in the manner of a "sensory" response; (3) during a period of motor preparation; (4) before a movement (Weinrich and Wise, 1982; Alexander and Crutcher, 1990; Crutcher and Alexander, 1990; Fu et al., 1993); or (5) after a movement during the maintenance of steady posture (Bizzi, 1968; Alexander and Crutcher, 1990; Caminiti et al., 1990; Crutcher and Alexander, 1990).

These five basic patterns of neuronal activity have been observed repeatedly and have been subjected to hypothesis testing in various experimental tasks. Every conceivable combination of these patterns has been observed in individual neurons, and every combination of increased and decreased activity occurs as well. In addition, it has been shown more recently that directional "tuning" differs among these five activity patterns, even in the same neuron (di Pellegrino and Wise, 1993; Caminiti, Johnson, and Ferraina, personal communication). Activity after an instruction stimulus may be maximal for a movement directed up and to the left from the current posture, whereas the premovement modulation is greatest for a movement directed up and to the right. Thus, it has been a common (though controversial) practice to treat each activity pattern separately for the sake of hypothesis testing and other analysis.

It has been shown for PMd that the premovement activity occurs when the subject moves its limbs in total darkness without being reinforced for that movement (Wise, Weinrich, and Mauritz, 1986). Thus, at least a portion of that signal can be accepted as "motor," but this conclusion could not be applied without further testing to the activity that follows a sensory stimulus.

Careful behavioral designs have shown that the poststimulus activity, too, has at least a component that reflects the motor (or "instructional") significance of a sensory event (di Pellegrino and Wise, 1993; Boussaud and Wise, 1993). Examinations of the evolution of neuronal discharge during conditional motor learning have been conducted in this context.

EVOLUTION OF NEURONAL ACTIVITY DURING CONDITIONAL MOTOR LEARNING

For the visual and auditory cortex, several investigators have described systematic changes in neuronal response to repeated stimulus presentations (e.g., Diamond and Weinberger, 1989; Rolls, Baylis, Hasselmo, and Nalwa, 1989; Edeline, Pham, and Weinberger, 1993; Miller, Li, and Desimone, 1991, 1993; Miller and Desimone, 1994). In some sense, stimulus discrimination must precede conditional oculomotor learning. However, conditional motor learning can be distinguished from sensory discrimination learning in that the former involves the flexible association of stimuli with various actions. In this chapter, we will focus on our laboratory work published in the past few years (Mitz, Godschalk, and Wise, 1991; Chen and Wise, 1995a,b). However, the reader should be aware of and compare the future reports from W. Schultz' laboratory in Fribourg, Switzerland on evolution of striatal activity during comparable tasks (Tremblay, Hollerman, and Schultz, 1994).

Systematic studies of the evolution of neuronal discharge during conditional motor learning have been undertaken for PMd (Mitz et al., 1991; Germain and Lamarre, 1993), SEF and FEF of the frontal cortex (Chen and Wise, 1995a,b), and for the striatum (Tremblay et al., 1994). A few scattered observations have been made in the prefrontal areas as well (Niki, Sugita, and Watanabe, 1990). Two different general approaches have been employed. With the exception of the report by Germain and Lamarre (1993), the aforementioned studies have involved the examination of recorded neuronal activity as a monkey learned and solved novel conditional motor problems by trial and error. By contrast, Germain and Lamarre studied premotor cortical activity before versus after monkeys learned a two-problem conditional motor association. (In this chapter, the former approach will be emphasized.) Even under that umbrella, there have been some significant variations in the specific experimental designs. The most pertinent of these is the choice of effector system. Studies of PMd and striatum have focused on limb movements, whereas those of the FEF and SEF employed saccadic eye movements as the motor act of the conditional motor association.

Mitz et al. (1991) reported that cells in PMd systematically change their task-related activity during the learning of novel stimulus-response associations. In those experiments, a monkey learned which one of four limb responses (consisting of a joystick movement in one of three directions or the withholding of a response) was instructed by an initially novel visual stimulus. In the experiments of Chen and Wise, monkeys were conditioned to make one of four saccadic eye movements. Thus, Mitz et al. studied conditional *skeleto-motor* learning, whereas Chen and Wise studied conditional *oculomotor* learning. Although there were other differences in the experimental design, most of the salient features of the experiments were the same. In each case, the monkeys were extensively conditioned before recordings began, so that they could learn novel conditional motor associations within a time span (typically 15–30 minutes) in which we could reliably monitor the activity of cortical neurons.

In the conditional oculomotor task, the monkey began each trial by fixating a spot at the center of a video monitor (figure 12.2). Also presented on the screen were four potential saccade targets, each 7 degrees in visual angle from the fixation spot. These four targets were located left, right, up, and down, relative to the central fixation point. At the fixation spot appeared a complex visual instruction stimulus consisting of various combination of colored bars, annuli, and rectangles. These stimuli remained on the video screen for 500 ms, after which the monkey maintained steady fixation for a variable and unpredictable "instructed delay period" of 1.5 to 3.5 s. When the fixation spot disappeared, the monkey was required to make a saccadic eye movement

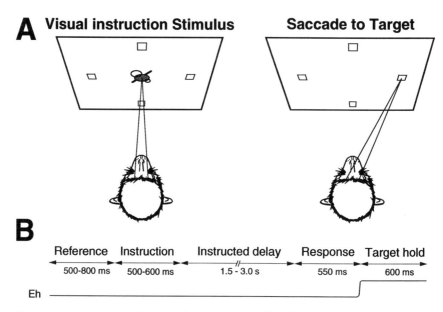

Figure 12.2 Experimental design for the conditional oculomotor learning task of Chen and Wise (1995a,b). A. The monkey fixates the center of a video screen, where a complex visual stimulus appears. B. After an instructed delay period, in which the stimulus is replaced by a fixation spot for a randomly varied time, that spot is removed. From that moment, the monkey has 550 ms to saccade to one of four targets (open squares) and hold fixation on it for 600 ms. Each stimulus instructs a movement to one of the four targets. Some stimuli were familiar to the monkey, others were novel. Eh, horizontal eye position. (Reprinted with permission from LL Chen, SP Wise, Neuronal activity in the supplementary eye field during acquisition of conditional oculomotor associations. J Neurophysiol 73:1101–1121.)

to one of the four saccade targets, according to the learned conditional association for each instruction stimulus. The monkey had to acquire the saccade target window within 550 ms and maintain fixation at the target for 600 ms to receive a fluid reward.

In a given block of trials, there were typically two types of instruction stimulus presented: familiar and novel. There were four *familiar* stimuli that the monkey had seen since the earliest stages of training. One of these familiar, or well-learned, stimuli was associated with each of the four possible saccadic eye movement targets (i.e., one familiar stimulus instructed an upward saccade, a different familiar cue dictated a rightward saccade, and so forth). Usually intermixed in the same block of trials were one, two, or three *novel* instruction stimuli. As with the familiar stimuli, each of these cues was associated with only one of the four possible responses for each trial. Because the monkey was allowed to make only one response on each trial and the monkey had never before seen the novel cue, there would be no reliable information in that cue to direct the response. However, the monkey was conditioned to execute a saccadic eye movement to one of the targets regardless of the familiarity of the cue. Thus the initial presentations of a novel instruction stimulus, the monkey appeared to select one of the four possible responses randomly. If that response was unrewarded, the monkey was less likely to select the same response (or target) the next time the same novel stimulus appeared but otherwise seemed to select randomly among the three remaining possibilities. If the response was rewarded, the monkey began to learn the appropriate stimulus-response association and typically attained performance in excess of 90 percent correct with only five to ten presentations of a given novel stimulus.

In what follows it must be emphasized that we will discuss neuronal activity for correctly executed trials only. Because of the monkeys' extensive training, there was no difference in fixation stability during the instructed delay period or during the period of holding fixation at the target. There was also no difference in the reaction times for responses to novel stimuli versus familiar ones, among saccades in the different directions, or with learning (i.e., as the monkey gained experience with an initially novel stimulus). Because of our experimental design and the stereotyped nature of the saccades, we can be confident that from the first time the monkey selected the "correct" response to a novel instruction stimulus (when the monkey was generally performing at chance levels) until its last several appearances (when the monkey nearly always selected the correct response) the stimulus was the same in all spatial coordinate systems and in all nonspatial properties. Furthermore, the movement was for all practical purposes identical. Thus, there can be no explanation of significant changes in activity during conditional motor learning in terms of simple sensory responses or in terms of motor skill learning as usually construed.

One of the principal results of our study is illustrated in figure 12.3. It shows one neuron's phasic discharge during correctly executed trials, plotted

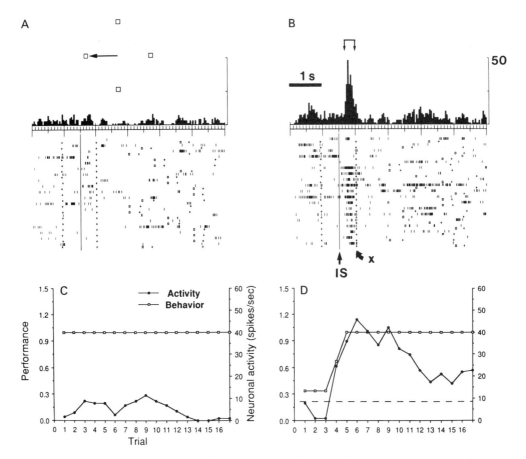

Figure 12.3 Learning-dependent activity of an SEF cell during conditional motor learning in a monkey. A, B. Raster and histogram displays for trials in which an instruction stimulus (IS) instructed a leftward saccade. The display shows only trials correctly performed in response to a familiar IS (A, C) or an initially novel stimulus (B, D). Thus, for all rows of each raster display (A, B), the stimulus and the motor response are identical. The first correct trial is shown at the top, the last at the bottom. Arrows at top (in B) show the region quantified for plotting (in C, D). C, D. Three-point moving averages of postcue activity (filled circles) and performance (open squares). Note in D that the first several correctly executed trials occur among several incorrect responses. On those trials, the cell is relatively inactive after the foveally presented instruction stimulus (solid vertical line in B [IS]). As the monkey learns the instructional significance of the initially novel stimulus, the cell discharges vigorously after the onset of the IS and before its offset (plus sign to the right of the IS line in B [x]). Activity scales are in impulses per second. Performance scale in C and D shows proportion of correct responses per three trials.

as a function of the order in which trials of exactly that kind occurred. Because these trials were intermixed with error trials and trials that involved different novel and familiar stimuli, it is impossible to determine from this illustration how many trials of other kinds might have intervened between successive trials shown in figure 12.3. However, note that trial types were randomly selected during a block of trials, and the monkey was required to solve from one to three novel conditional motor problems while performing

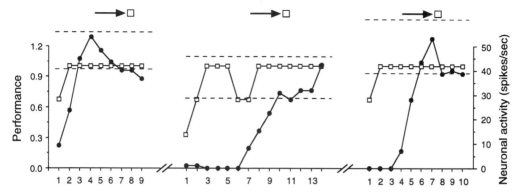

Figure 12.4 Repeated presentations of novel stimuli for an SEF cell in a monkey. In separate blocks of trials, the monkey learned that three different, initially novel stimuli instructed a rightward saccade. Format as in figure 12.3C, D.

in accord with four previously learned problems in a set of five to seven problems. The bottom part of figure 12.3 plots postcue activity during correctly executed trials along with the animal's learning curve. Clearly, the first few correct responses were made in a period when several incorrect responses were also selected. In the figure, the curve with open circles shows the monkey's improvement in selecting the correct response. The increase in neuronal modulation that parallels this conditional motor learning has been termed *learning-dependent activity*, and it has been observed in both PMd for conditional skeletomotor learning (Mitz et al., 1991; Germain and Lamarre, 1993) and for SEF for conditional oculomotor learning (Chen and Wise, 1995a,b). Learning-dependent activity is less commonly observed in FEF (Chen and Wise, 1995b), at least in the large-saccade region from which Chen and Wise recorded neuronal activity. Similar observations have been reported in abstract form for the striatum (Tremblay et al., 1994).

This learning-dependent activity can be observed repeatedly for individual neurons. If, after learning one set of conditional motor problems, the monkey is presented with a new set of novel and familiar stimuli in a subsequent block of trials, the cell modulation will begin again at relatively low levels and increase in close association with conditional motor learning. Figure 12.4 shows the activity of a cell for the original block, plus a second and third block of trials in which two new conditional oculomotor problems were solved for rightward saccades.

Learning-dependent activity occurs during all "epochs" or periods during a trial. Cells that show immediate postcue activity (illustrated in figure 12.3) may show learning dependency, and cells with delay-period, presaccadic, and postsaccadic activity may do so as well. A given neuron may show learning-dependent activity in one task period but not another, though its modulation significantly differs from reference (background) levels in both periods. Averaging all of one class of SEF cells from our sample across the whole trial, figure 12.5 shows the population histogram for activity around the presentation

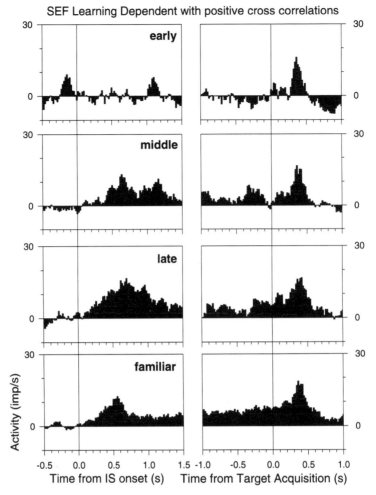

Figure 12.5 Population histogram for one class of learning-dependent SEF cells that showed significant time trends in discharge rate during conditional oculomotor learning. The histograms compare activity early, middle, and late in the learning process with activity on familiar-IS trials. The data for the familiar stimuli were recorded virtually simultaneously with the novel ISs for the relevant direction and task period. Data are aligned on the onset of the instruction stimulus in the left columns and target acquisition in the right columns. The mean activity in the reference period is subtracted from each bin and each neuron contributes to the population histogram in proportion to its maximal activity. The left column shows 0.5 s of activity before and 1.5 s of activity after the onset of the IS. The right column shows 1.0 s before and 1.0 s after target acquisition. (Reproduced with permission).

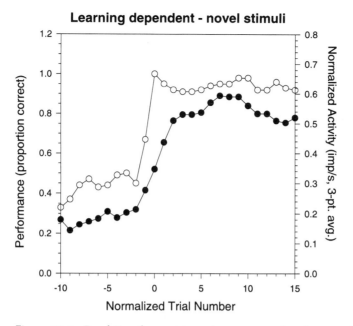

Figure 12.6 Population three-point moving averages of performance (open circles) from learning-dependent SEF cells exposed to novel instruction stimuli. Data are aligned on the first occurrence of a three consecutive correct responses. The average neuronal activity (filled circles) was computed with the same temporal alignment, using a three-point moving average of activity in the relevant task period for the relevant saccade direction. The activity of each cell was then normalized by dividing it by the maximal discharge rate for any trial, averaged over that task period.

of the instruction stimulus (left panels) and that around the acquisition of the target (right panels). In this average, all cells contribute in relation to their maximal activity. The top row shows the activity during the first few correctly executed presentations of the stimulus. Recall that all data are from correctly executed trials only. Activity during the preinstruction period is subtracted from the average, so some bins may have negative activity values. Note that for the early trials, average activity varies little from background except for the periods before the instruction stimulus and prior to the reward. By contrast, during middle and late phases of learning, the activity increases in all parts of the trial. This activity pattern can be compared to that for the familiar stimuli at the bottom of figure 12.5. Typical of the single-cell data, the depth of modulation during the later phases of learning exceeds that for familiar stimuli instructing the same response.

The time-course of increases in learning-dependent activity closely follows the animal's improvement in performance. Figure 12.6 shows the learning and activity-change curves for one class of SEF cells. Note that early in learning (compare figure 12.5, early, to the left part of figure 12.6), the activity of the population is relatively low, as is the proportion of correct responses. Later, both measures increase in close correlation. Because the stimuli and the

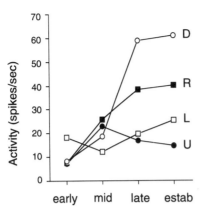

Figure 12.7 Evolution of directional preferences during conditional motor learning. Data from one SEF cell. Activity for each saccade target, down (D), right (R), left (L), and up (U) from center, during the first few correctly executed trials (early), middle trials (mid), later trials (late), when the monkey first began performing nearly perfectly, and trials during a subsequent period when the conditional motor association was more established (estab).

responses (in aggregate) are identical in all trials, these data show that SEF neurons reflect neither the properties of the instruction stimulus per se nor the saccadic eye movement. Instead, these data provide strong support for the hypothesis that SEF activity reflects the selection of action on the basis of arbitrary stimulus-response associations (i.e., conditional motor learning).

Learning-dependent changes may occur in cells with directional preferences (figure 12.7) and in neurons that lack directionality. The directional selectivity of the cell activity is especially significant to the interpretation of these results. Reward association and, over the course of learning, the frequency and expectation of reward is similar for all saccade directions and all instruction stimuli. However, for directionally selective cells, the evolution of activity differs for different saccade directions (figure 12.7), thus ruling out these and other nonspecific factors as correlates of the activity. Most cells show directional selectivity during some phase of learning (Wise and Chen, 1995). However, directionally nonselective cells may well reflect computations of reward anticipation, frequency, or expectancy. This possibility will require further investigation.

Not all of the evolution during learning is of the learning-dependent class. A different pattern of change was observed, one which Chen and Wise (1995a) termed *learning-selective* (figure 12.8). Note that there is little or no activity modulation illustrated in figure 12.8, left. These are the trials in which the familiar stimulus instructed the rightward saccade. It was the hallmark feature of learning-selective activity that the cells were nearly unmodulated when familiar stimuli instructed saccades in any direction. In intermixed trials, when a novel stimulus instructed the same saccadic eye movement, the cell discharged vigorously at first (see figure 12.8, right) but responded progressively less intensely as the monkey learned the novel stimulus-response asso-

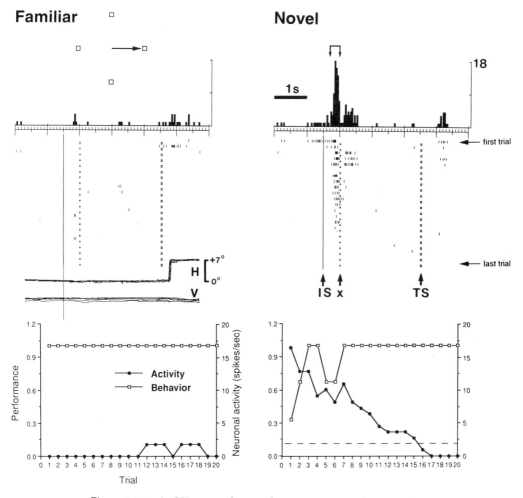

Figure 12.8 An SEF neuron showing decreases in activity during conditional motor learning (i.e., learning-selective activity). A, C. Activity for familiar-stimulus trials when the stimulus instructed a rightward saccade. B, D. Postcue activity when an initially novel stimulus instructed saccades to the right. Format as figure 12.3. H, horizontal eye position; V, vertical eye position; IS, instruction stimulus onset; x, IS offset; TS, trigger (or "go") stimulus.

ciation. The population average of this class of activity is shown in figure 12.9. Note that, unlike the cell in figure 12.8, not all of the learning-selective cells completely ceased modulation during the time that we could maintain isolation of the individual neurons. However, after a period of initial increase (correlating with the most rapid learning), these cells become less active. Chen and Wise (1995a) speculated that this activity would, like the learning-dependent cells, converge on that seen in trials with familiar stimuli instructing the same action—in this case, no modulation, were it possible to monitor the cells' activity indefinitely. Comparison of figures 12.6 and 12.9 highlights the fact that the changes in the learning-selective population precede those in the learning-dependent one. The increase in the learning-selective

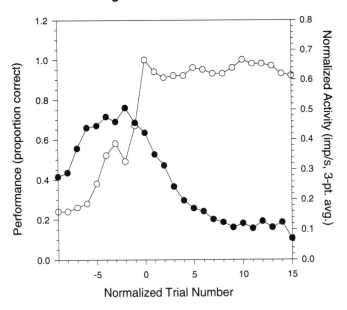

Learning selective - novel stimuli

Figure 12.9 Activity of a population of learning-selective cells exposed to novel stimuli, similar to that illustrated in figure 12.8, in the format of figure 12.6.

population from normalized trials −9 to −5 occurs when the learning-dependent population shows relatively little modulation. Thereafter, from normalized trials −2 or −3 until trial 4 or 5, the two activity classes show roughly inverse changes. These observations support the idea that SEF may contain a mechanism for guiding action based on both learned conditional associations (learning-dependent activity) and trial-and-error responses (learning-selective activity) that precede consolidated conditional motor behavior.

Only preliminary reports (Tremblay et al., 1994) are available for striatal activity during conditional motor learning, but it appears that changes similar to learning-dependent and learning-selective activity occur in those neurons as well. The task employed by W. Schultz and his colleagues was a delayed, go–no-go conditional motor association, with an additional, go-type trial consisting of an unrewarded movement. Action was triggered by the appearance of a red square. There was one familiar instruction stimulus for each of these three trial types. Schultz and his colleagues compared activity between the familiar and novel visual instructions for a population of cells located in the anterior caudate nucleus and the putamen rostral to the anterior commissure. Striatal activity was studied in the usual task periods, including immediately after the instruction cue, immediately after the triggering (go–no-go) cue, after liquid reward delivery, before an expected trigger, during the instructed delay period, before an expected reward, and before the next expected instruction stimulus. As the animals learned novel stimulus-response associations, Schultz and his colleagues found (1) reduced specificity of responses, (2) changes in the "strength of trial-specific activity in the initial learning trials, which progressively returned to the pattern observed for [familiar-stimulus] trials with experience," and (3) more radical changes. As an example of specificity changes, a neuron that was only active during "go" trials when the animal responded to familiar stimuli would show activity for 25 "no-go" trials in addition to "go" trials during learning. This result resembles that for the directionality of SEF neurons (Wise and Chen, 1995). Those neurons, too, might show less directional specificity during the various phases of learning (see figure 12.7). As an example of changes in modulation depth, Schultz (personal communication) reported that occasionally task-related changes would take a few trials to occur despite correct performance, much as was reported for both PMd and SEF. Putting these two learning-related phenomena together, we observe that a neuron could be unmodulated in the first few trials with novel instruction stimulus, then show a nonspecific behavioral relationship that after many trials would become as selective as that following familiar stimuli. This pattern, which resembles the learning-dependent activity in SEF and PMd, was most commonly observed in the period immediately after the instruction stimulus (Tremblay et al., 1994). As an example of radical changes, Schultz (personal communication) reported discharge modulations consisting of both increases and decreases of activity when there was very little modulation during familiar-stimulus trials, much like the learning-selective cells in SEF.

CONNECTIONIST MODELS OF CONDITIONAL MOTOR LEARNING

Recently, neural network models of conditional motor learning have been developed for both skeletomotor (Fagg and Arbib, 1992) and oculomotor (Dominey et al., 1995) behavior. These models posit that changes in the weight of synapses conveying nonspatial visual information lead to a given response being selected, in a winner-take-all manner, after an initially random response is reinforced. The model works by linking the nonspatial visual information with hidden-layer ("voting") units that induce motor output for a given direction. The performance of these networks resembles learning-related behavior, especially in their failure to produce any pattern in response selection during an initial trial-and-error period (Mitz et al., 1991; Chen and Wise, 1995a). The learning-dependent activity seen in the SEF and the striatum (Tremblay et al., 1994; W Schultz, personal communication) resembles that of certain hidden units in the model of Dominey et al. (1995). In the model's cells, as training proceeds, a novel instruction stimulus evokes an increasingly similar "response" as that seen after well-learned cues associated with the same saccade. Likewise, there appears to be an analog to learning-selective activity. Some hidden units, linked to an "incorrect" saccade, initially respond to highly effective input from "TT cells." As learning proceeds, the nonspatial aspects of the visual stimulus decreasingly activates those hidden units.

CONCLUSION

Motor learning, as traditionally defined (see chapters 6 and 19), consists of the mastery of movement sequences and other motor-command patterns: in a phrase, skill acquisition (see also chapters 13 and 14). A broader view of motor learning includes adaptive plasticity (see chapters 2 and 4), which subserves the accurate orientation of eyes, limbs, and body toward or otherwise in relation to stimuli in space. This more open view of motor learning includes classically conditioned (Pavlovian) reflexes (see chapters 5, 7, and 8) as well. An intricate neural machinery, much of it in the spinal cord, brainstem, and cerebellum, underlies those kinds of motor learning. However, limited to such skills, conditioned reflexes, and adaptations, the behavior of advanced mammals such as ourselves would be scarcely recognizable. We can learn to respond with any learned movement to any environmental context that can be detected and discriminated from another, and we can choose among spatial, nonspatial, and temporal aspects of environmental stimuli to guide action. This chapter has focused on the hypothesized role of the premotor cortex and basal ganglia in these higher motor functions, some of which have been termed *conditional motor learning*.

Conditional motor learning represents a sophisticated, flexible, and intelligent behavior, one characteristic of advanced mammals. As Passingham (1987, p 67) noted nearly a decade ago, "[W]hile the monkey's knowledge is impressive the same cannot be said of our knowledge of how the monkey does [these tasks]. We know something of the visual and of the motor mechanisms involved, but we are profoundly ignorant of the means by which the motor mechanisms receive their instructions about what it is appropriate to do." In the interim, we have learned that a vast network of cells, including at least the striatum, PMd, and SEF, show discharge modulation that evolves during conditional motor learning. Many of these cells have activity that correlates with eye or limb movement direction, and the evolution of their discharge rates correlates very closely with the monkey's acquisition of stimulus-response association (i.e., the solution of the conditional motor problem posed by the experimenter). Future work is needed to determine the cellular mechanisms underlying these changes and the mechanisms by which these changes may cause the selection of appropriate action.

REFERENCES

Alexander GE, Crutcher MD (1990). Preparation for movement: Neural representations of intended direction in three motor areas of the monkey. J Neurophysiol 64:133–150.

Bizzi E (1968). Discharge of frontal eye field neurons during saccadic and following eye movements in unanesthetized monkeys. Exp Brain Res 6:69–80.

Boussaoud D, Wise SP (1993). Primate frontal cortex: Effects of stimulus and movement. Exp Brain Res 95:28–40.

Boussaoud D, di Pellegrino G, Wise SP (1996). Frontal lobe mechanisms subserving vision for action vs. vision for perception. Behav Brain Res 72:1–15.

Bruce CJ, Goldberg ME (1985). Primate frontal eye fields: I. Single neurons discharging before saccades. J Neurophysiol 53:603–635.

Caminiti R, Johnson PB, Burnod Y, Galli C, Ferraina S (1990). Shift of preferred directions of premotor cortical cells with arm movements performed across the workspace. Exp Brain Res 83:228–232.

Caminiti R, Johnson PB, Galli C, Ferraina S, Burnod Y (1991). Making arm movements within different parts of space: The premotor and motor cortical representation of a coordinate system for reaching to visual targets. J Neurosci 11:1182–1197.

Canavan AGM, Nixon PD, Passingham RE (1989). Motor learning in monkeys (*Macaca fascicularis*) with lesions in motor thalamus. Exp Brain Res 77:113–126.

Chen LL, Wise SP (1995a). Neuronal activity in the supplementary eye field during acquisition of conditional oculomotor associations. J Neurophysiol 73:1101–1121.

Chen LL, Wise SP (1995b). Supplementary eye field contrasted with the frontal eye field during acquisition of conditional oculomotor associations. J Neurophysiol 73:1122–1134.

Chen Y-C, Thaler D, Nixon PD, Stern C, Passingham RE (1995). The functions of the medial premotor cortex (SMA): II. The timing and selection of learned movements. Exp Brain Res 102:461–473.

Crowne DP, Dawson KA, Richardson CM (1988). Unilateral periarcuate and posterior parietal lesions impair conditional position discrimination learning in the monkey. Neuropsychologia 27:1119–1127.

Crutcher MD, Alexander GE (1990). Movement-related neuronal activity selectively coding either direction or muscle pattern in three motor areas of the monkey. J Neurophysiol 64:151–163.

Deiber M-P, Passingham RE, Colebatch JG, Friston KJ, Nixon PD, Frackowiak PSJ (1991). Cortical areas and the selection of movement: A study with positron emission tomography. Exp Brain Res 84:393–402.

Diamond DM, Weinberger NM (1989). Role of context in the expression of learning-induced plasticity of single neurons in auditory cortex. Behav Neurosci 103:471–494.

di Pellegrino G, Wise SP (1993). Visuospatial vs. visuomotor activity in the premotor and prefrontal cortex of a primate. J Neurosci 13:1227–1243.

Dominey P, Arbib M, Joseph JP (in press). A model of corticostriatal plasticity for learning oculomotor associations and sequences. J Cogni Neurosci 7:311–336.

Eacott MJ, Gaffan D (1992). Inferotemporal-frontal disconnection: The uncinate fascicle and visual associative learning in monkeys. Eur J Neurosci 4:1320–1332.

Edeline J-M, Pham P, Weinberger NM (1993). Rapid development of learning-induced receptive field plasticity in the auditory cortex. Behav Neurosci 107:539–551.

Fagg AH, Arbib MA (1992). A model of primate visual-motor conditional learning. J Adap Behav 1:3–37.

Fu Q-G, Suarez JI, Ebner TJ (1993). Neuronal specification of direction and distance during reaching movements in the superior precentral premotor area and primary motor cortex of monkeys. J Neurophysiol 70:2097–2116.

Gaffan D (1994). Role of the amygdala in picture discrimination learning with 24-h intervals. Exp Brain Res 99:423–430.

Gaffan D, Harrison S (1988). Inferotemporal-frontal disconnection and fornix transection in visuomotor conditional learning by monkeys. Behav Brain Res 31:149–163.

Gaffan D, Harrison S (1989). A comparison of the effects of fornix transection and sulcus principalis ablation upon spatial learning by monkeys. Behav Brain Res 31:207–220.

Gaffan D, Murray EA (1990). Amygdalar interaction with the mediodorsal nucleus of the thalamus and the ventromedial prefrontal cortex in stimulus—reward associative learning in the monkey. J Neurosci 10:3479–3493.

Germain L, Lamarre Y (1993). Neuronal activity in the motor and premotor cortices before and after learning the associations between auditory stimuli and motor responses. Brain Res 611: 175–179.

Halsband U, Freund HJ (1990). Premotor cortex and conditional motor learning in man. Brain 113:207–222.

Halsband U, Passingham RE (1982). The role of premotor and parietal cortex in the direction of action. Brain Res 240:368–372.

Halsband U, Passingham RE (1985). Premotor cortex and the conditions for a movement in monkeys. Behav Brain Res 18:269–277.

Hein A (1974). Prerequisite for development of visually guided reaching in the kitten. Brain Res 71:259–263.

Held R, Bauer JA (1974). Development of sensorially-guided reaching in infant monkeys. Brain Res 71:265–271.

Hoover JE, Strick PL (1993). Multiple output channels in the basal ganglia. Science 259:819–821.

Jenkins IH, Brooks DJ, Nixon PD, Frackowiak RSJ, Passingham RE (1994). Motor sequence learning: A study with positron emission tomography. J Neurosci 14:3775–3790.

Kurata K, Hoffman DS (1994). Differential effects of muscimol microinjection into dorsal and ventral aspects of the premotor cortex of monkeys. J Neurophysiol 71:1151–1164.

Lynch JC, Hoover JE, Strick PL (1994). Input to the primate frontal eye field from the substantia nigra, superior colliculus, and dentate nucleus demonstrated by transneuronal transport. Exp Brain Res 100:181–186.

Marsden CD, Obeso JA (1994). The functions of the basal ganglia and the paradox of stereotaxic surgery in Parkinson's disease. Brain 117:877–897.

Miller EK, Desimone R (1994). Parallel neuronal mechanisms for short-term memory. Science 263:520–552.

Miller EK, Li L, Desimone R (1991). A neural mechanism for working and recognition memory in inferior temporal cortex. Science 254:1377–1379.

Miller EK, Li L, Desimone R (1993). Activity of neurons in anterior inferior temporal cortex during a short-term memory task. J Neurosci 13:1460–1478.

Mitz AR, Godschalk M, Wise SP (1991). Learning-dependent neuronal activity in the premotor cortex of rhesus monkeys. J Neurosci 11:1855–1872.

Murray EA, Wise SP (1995). Effects of hippocampectomy and amygdalectomy on conditional motor learning in macaque monkeys. Soc Neurosci Abstr 21:1494.

Niki H, Sugita S, Watanabe M (1990). Modifications of the activity of primate frontal neurons during learning of a go/no-go discrimination and its reversal. In E Iwai, M Mishkin (eds), Vision, Memory and Temporal Lobe. New York: Elsevier, pp 295–304.

Parthasarathy HB, Schall JD, Graybiel AM (1992). Distributed but convergent ordering of corticostriatal projections: Analysis of the frontal eye field and the supplementary eye field in the macaque monkey. J Neurosci 12:4468–4488.

Passingham RE (1985a). Premotor cortex: Sensory cues and movement. Behav Brain Res 18:175–185.

Passingham RE (1985b). Cortical mechanisms and cues for action. Philos Trans R Soc Lond B Biol Sci 308:101–111.

Passingham RE (1987). From where does the motor cortex get its instruction? In SP Wise (ed), Higher Brain Functions. New York: Wiley, pp 67–97.

Passingham RE (1988). Premotor cortex and preparation for movement. Exp Brain Res 70:590–596.

Passingham RE (1989). Premotor cortex and the retrieval of movement. Brain Behav Evol 33:189–192.

Passingham RE (1993). The Frontal Lobes and Voluntary Action. Oxford: Oxford University Press.

Passingham RE, Myers C, Rawlins N, Lightfoot V, Fearn S (1988). Premotor cortex in the rat. Behav Neurosci 102:101–109.

Petrides M (1982). Motor conditional associative-learning after selective prefrontal lesions in the monkey. Behav Brain Res 5:407–413.

Petrides M (1986). The effect of periarcuate lesions in the monkey on the performance of symmetrically and asymmetrically reinforced visual and auditory go, no-go tasks. J Neurosci 6:2054–2063.

Petrides M (1987). Conditional learning and the primate frontal cortex. In E Perecman (ed), The Frontal Lobes Revisited. New York: IRBN Press, pp 91–108.

Rolls ET, Baylis GC, Hasselmo ME, Nalwa V (1989). The effect of learning on the face selective responses of neurons in the cortex in the superior temporal sulcus of the monkey. Exp Brain Res 76:153–164.

Rupniak NMJ, Gaffan D (1987). Monkey hippocampus and learning about spatially directed movements. J Neurosci 7:2331–2337.

Saint-Cyr JA, Ungerleider LG, Desimone R (1990). Organization of visual cortical inputs to the striatum and subsequent outputs to the pallido-nigral complex in the monkey. J Comp Neurol 298:129–156.

Schall JD (1991a). Neuronal activity related to visually guided saccades in the frontal eye fields of rhesus monkeys: Comparison with supplementary eye fields. J Neurophysiol 66:559–579.

Schall JD (1991b). Neuronal activity related to visually guided saccadic eye movements in the supplementary motor area of rhesus monkeys. J Neurophysiol 66:530–558.

Schall JD, Morel A, Kaas JH (1993). Topography of supplementary eye field afferents to frontal eye field in macaque: Implications for mapping between saccade coordinate systems. Vis Neurosci 10:385–393.

Selemon LD, Goldman-Rakic PS (1985). Longitudinal topography and interdigitation of corticostriatal projections in the rhesus monkey. J Neurosci 5:776–794.

Stanton GB, Goldberg ME, Bruce CJ (1988). Frontal eye field efferents in the macaque monkey: I. Subcortical pathways and topography of striatal and thalamic terminal fields. J Comp Neurol 271:473–492.

Teuber H-L (1972). Unity and diversity of frontal lobe function. Acta Neurobiol Exp (Warsz) 32:615–656.

Thach WT, Goodkin HP, Keating JG (1992). The cerebellum and the adaptive coordination of movement. Annu Rev Neurosci 15:403–442.

Thaler D, Chen Y-C, Nixon PD, Stern C, Passingham RE (1995). The functions of the medial premotor cortex (SMA): I. Simple learned movements. Exp Brain Res 102:445–460.

Tremblay L, Hollerman J, Schultz W (1994). Neuronal activity in primate striatum neurons during learning. Soc Neurosci Abstr 20:780.

Vaadia E, Kurata K, Wise SP (1988). Neuronal activity preceding directional and nondirectional cues in the premotor cortex of rhesus monkeys. Somatosens Mot Res 6:207–230.

Webster MJ, Bachevalier J, Ungerleider LG (1993). Subcortical connections of inferior temporal areas TE and TEO in macaque monkeys. J Comp Neurol 335:73–91.

Webster MJ, Bachevalier J, Ungerleider LG (1994). Connections of inferior temporal areas TEO and TE with parietal and frontal cortex in macaque monkeys. Cereb Cortex 5:470–483.

Weinrich M, Wise SP (1982). The premotor cortex of the monkey. J Neurosci 2:1329–1345.

Wise SP (1984). Nonprimary motor cortex and its role in the cerebral control of movement. In G Edelman, WE Gall, WM Cowan (eds), Dynamic Aspects of Neocortical Function. New York: John Wiley, pp 525–555.

Wise SP, Chen LL (1995). Evolution of preferred directions in the supplementary eye field during conditional oculomotor learning. Soc Neurosci Abstr 21:517.

Wise SP, di Pellegrino G, Boussaoud D (1996). The premotor cortex and nonstandard sensorimotor mapping. Can J Physiol Pharmacol (in press).

Wise SP, Weinrich M, Mauritz K-H (1986). Movement-related activity in the premotor cortex of rhesus macaques. Prog Brain Res 64:117–131.

Yeterian EH, Hoesen GWV (1978). Cortico-striate projections in the rhesus monkey: The organization of certain cortico-caudate connections. Brain Res 139:43–63.

IV Complex Movements and Motor Sequences

13 Adaptation and Skill Learning: Evidence for Different Neural Substrates

Mark Hallett, Alvaro Pascual-Leone, and
Helge Topka

There are at least two broad categories of human knowledge: declarative and procedural. Declarative knowledge refers to facts and includes all information about which we think and that we communicate verbally. Procedural knowledge refers to sequential behavior and usually relates to motor performance. There is much less known about motor (or procedural) learning than that known about declarative learning. It *is* clear that the processes in the brain are separate, and motor memory may be more robust than declarative memory.

Motor learning itself is a complex phenomenon with a number of different components. One aspect can be defined as a change in motor performance with practice. Other aspects would involve increasing the repertoire of motor behavior and maintenance of a new behavior over a period of time. Even in the context of only a change in motor performance, there are likely to be several different phenomena. We distinguish between adaptation and skill learning (Sanes, Dimitrov, and Hallett, 1990). It is probably easiest to make this distinction by referring to the concept of *operating characteristic*. An operating characteristic describes a set of movements that relate different movement variables to one another. It describes the current state of capability of the system. Generally, a change in one variable will affect another. The best-known operating characteristic of motor performance is Fitts's law, which relates the speed and accuracy of movement (Fitts, 1954). Movement from point A to point B can be made at various speeds, and each speed is associated with an accuracy. Slower speeds are more accurate, faster speeds less accurate. Another operating characteristic would be the gain associated with a visuomotor tracking task. For a particular visual stimulus, there is an associated movement. With a change in gain, the appropriate movement might be smaller or larger.

Motor adaptation learning can be defined as a change in motor performance without a change in the operating characteristic. In a point-to-point movement, a faster movement with predictable increase in inaccuracy is a change in performance but not a change in operating characteristic. This is not necessarily just a trivial change in performance. Learning the new speed may require considerable practice but, if associated with an increase in inaccuracy, it does not indicate a new capability of the motor system. Likewise, a change in visuomotor gain by itself does not indicate anything more than a change in the point of working on the operating characteristic.

Motor skill learning can be defined as a change in motor performance with a change in the operating characteristic. It indicates a new capability of the motor system. If a point-to-point movement is made both faster and with greater accuracy, there is an apparent violation of Fitts's law, in that there is a new operating characteristic. In many circumstances, this characteristic would be recognized clearly as a new skill. Skill learning probably cannot stand alone if separated from adaptation learning. In satisfying a new motor requirement, it is not enough to achieve a new operating characteristic; it would likely be necessary as well to find the correct place on the operating characteristic to work.

In some circumstances, the distinction between adaptation and skill learning may be analogous to the distinction made by Brooks between "what to do" and "how to do" (Brooks, Kennedy, and Ross, 1983). In learning a new complex movement, the first task is to understand the requirements of the task and to develop a strategy or gross kinematic plan that has at least an appropriate form of response (the "what to do"). The second task is to refine the plan to produce a better performance (the "how to do"). The new skill would likely be the setting up of a new motor plan including a unique sequence of actions, whereas the refinement of the behavior would likely be achieved by adaptation.

Therefore, when assessing a situation for motor learning of the type characterized by a change in performance with practice, it is important to see whether there is a change in the operating characteristic. In some circumstances, the learning will not demonstrate such a change and can be considered mainly adaptation learning. In other circumstances, when the operating characteristic is changed, the situation may be dominated by skill learning, but it is likely that adaptation learning is also occurring.

Thus far, we have offered some theoretical definitions. These terms might be used somewhat differently by others, but these definitions seem useful in our work. We will now show that it is possible to use these terms to describe different experimental paradigms and that by doing so, we come to the conclusion that adaptation and skill learning use different neural substrates.

ADAPTATION LEARNING

Perhaps the classic example of adaptation learning is the change in gain of the vestibuloocular reflex (VOR). *The gain of the VOR* refers to the magnitude of eye movement resulting from head movement. The gain can change dependent on environmental circumstances. The amount of eye movement for a specific head movement depends on the working point of the operating characteristic, which is defined by the gain. Selecting the appropriate gain is learning, but there is no apparent skill acquired when the gain changes. VOR adaptation requires participation of the cerebellum and associated brainstem structures (Lisberger, 1988; see also chapter 2).

Eyeblink conditioning is recognized as a form of motor learning and could be argued to fit the definition proposed here for adaptation learning. Blinking of the eyelid to a conditioned stimulus either may occur or may not. Whether blinking will occur (and how much) could be described by a single operating characteristic. At any given time, the amount of "conditioning" could be the working point on the operating characteristic. In animal studies, eyeblink conditioning seems to require the cerebellum, at least for the expression and timing of the response (Thompson, 1990; see also chapter 5). We have studied eyeblink conditioning in normal subjects and in patients with cerebellar lesions to see if the intact cerebellum is required for eyeblink conditioning in humans (Topka, Valls-Solé, Massaquoi, and Hallett, 1993). We employed a classical delay-conditioning paradigm in five patients with pure cerebellar cortical atrophy and in seven patients with olivopontocerebellar atrophy. The results were compared with those obtained in a group of neurologically healthy volunteers matched with the patients according to age and gender. The two groups of patients experienced similar abnormalities in the acquisition of the conditioned response and produced fewer conditioned responses than in the control subjects in any given block of trials. Many of the patients' conditioned responses were inappropriately timed with respect to the conditioned stimulus. Such results have also been found by others (Lye, O'Boyle, Ramsden, Schady, 1988).

Adaptation to lateral displacement of vision as produced by prism glasses is a method for assessing learning of a visuomotor task (Weiner, Hallett, and Funkenstein, 1983; see also chapter 10). Pointing to a target is a clear example of the visual system directing the motor system. When prism glasses are used, at first there is a mismatch between where an object is seen and where the pointing is directed. With experience, normal human subjects adjust to this and begin to point correctly. This correct pointing can be a product either of a true change in the visuomotor coordination or of an intellectual decision to point in a direction different from that in which the object appears to be so as to correct the movement. When the glasses are removed, typically the subject initially points in the direction opposite that at the time the glasses were put on. In the naive subject, this is an excellent measure of true change in the visuomotor task because there is no reason for making any intellectual decision to point in any direction other than that in which the object appears to be. With additional experience, the subjects return to correct performance again. This type of motor learning fits well the definition of adaptation. With a stimulus, pointing could be anywhere. Choosing the correct visuomotor coordination to fit the current environmental situation is a type of adaptation learning. Patients with cerebellar damage show poor or no adaptation (figure 13.1) (Weiner et al., 1983). Note that on trial 26 in figure 13.1 (the first trial after the prisms are removed), cerebellar patients point

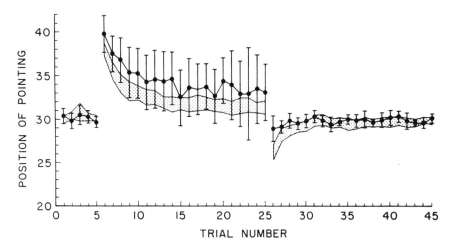

Figure 13.1 Pointing behavior of normal control subjects compared with that of patients with cerebellar lesions on 45 trials. Trials 6 to 25 were performed with prism glasses that shifted vision to the right. The shaded area indicates the normal range (mean ± 2 standard errors). The filled circles (mean) and error bars (± 2 standard errors) reflect patient data. (Reprinted from Weiner et al., 1983, with permission of the publisher, *Neurology*.)

almost exactly as they did on trial 5, before the experience with the prism glasses. Thus, no adaptation can be observed in this patient group. Patients with damage elsewhere in the brain (including basal ganglia and different regions of cortex) and patients with verbal memory deficits all show appropriate adaptation.

Another paradigm that can test adaptation learning is a task with a change in the visuomotor gain. An example is making movements of the elbow by matching targets on a computer screen. A change in the elbow gain with respect to the screen display will be followed by a change in amount of movement needed to match the targets. This simple gain change nicely fits the definition of adaptation motor learning. In the normal circumstance after a gain change, there would be an error that would would be reduced gradually with continued practice. Recently we compared a group of 10 normal subjects and a group of 10 patients with cerebellar damage from degenerative diseases (Deuschl, Toro, Zeffiro, and Hallett, 1993). By fitting to a curve the amplitudes of successive movements during the learning, we measured their rate of adaptation. Patients showed much slower learning than did the normal controls.

All these studies show that the cerebellum appears to play a part in adaptation learning. The cerebellum is traditionally thought to play an important role in motor coordination. Adaptation, "how" to make the movement, and refinement of behavior all may be thought of as improving coordination. Adaptation learning might be considered as an aspect of coordination.

Hallett, Pascual-Leone, and Topka

SKILL LEARNING

Such complex multijoint arm movement tasks as throwing a ball or playing the piano typically are considered to be skills. The ability to sequence all the component movements correctly, smoothly, and in an appropriate time is clearly difficult and appears to increase the behavioral repertoire. As such tasks are learned, they can be accomplished both more quickly and more accurately. This violates Fitts's law and establishes a new operating characteristic. Hence, by our definition, such learning would be skill learning.

In our first attempt to study skill learning, we asked subjects to trace polygons both with direct vision and while watching their performance with a mirror (Sanes et al., 1990). We asked the subjects to trace the figures as quickly and as accurately as possible. Pursuing a possible role of the cerebellum in skill learning, we compared normal control subjects to patients with cerebellar degeneration. In the direct vision task with the number of trials studied, both groups of subjects became faster but deteriorated in accuracy. Hence the performance was in keeping with Fitts's law, and we were not able to show that there was any skill learning. When doing the task with the mirror, normal subjects improved both time and accuracy, thereby showing that they had developed new skill. Patients with cerebellar cortical atrophy were deficient in this task, and we concluded that the cerebellum might play a role in skill learning as well as in adaptation learning. There were a number of problems of interpretation of the mirror experiment. First, patients with olivo-pontocerebellar atrophy were not abnormal and, in fact, performed faster than normal subjects from the beginning. We interpreted this finding as possibly due to a deficient visuomotor coordination in those patients, giving rise to less mismatch in the visual and proprioceptive guides that confuse normal subjects. Second, there is clearly an important adaptation component to the task, as there was an altered visuomotor transformation. Thus, an abnormality might be due to the important adaptation component.

In a second attempt to study skill learning, we asked 15 normal control subjects and 18 patients with cerebellar degenerations to perform on a data tablet multijoint arm movements generating a trajectory connecting five via points in a given sequence (Topka, Massaquoi, Zeffiro, and Hallett, 1991). Subjects were asked to increase their accuracy but to maintain their movement time constant. If they became more accurate in the same time, their increased accuracy would indicate a new operating characteristic and the development of skill learning. The subjects performed 100 trials with a movement time of approximately 3,500 ms (relatively slowly) and then did another 100 trials as fast as possible. In the slower task, both groups were successful in keeping time, and both improved relative accuracy at about the same rate. In the faster task, normal subjects performed more rapidly than the patients, yet they improved at a faster rate than the patients. A difference in learning rate with the faster task was confirmed by comparing a few normal subjects and patients doing the faster task first (before the slower task). These results made some facts clear: First, patients with cerebellar damage were able to learn new skills (according our definition). Second, their ability to learn appeared to be speed-related because it was worse when high speed was required. The coordination deficits of cerebellar patients also speed-dependent (Hallett and Massaquoi, 1993). They do much better with slow movements than with fast; correspondingly, their ability to refine movement variables needed for an adaptation component would likely be better with slow movements than with fast. We again come to the conclusion that the deficits of the cerebellar patients in this task could be related to an adaptation component.

Accepting the given that patients with cerebellar damage are able to learn a new skill, we turned our attention elsewhere to identify mechanisms related to skill learning. The cerebral motor cortex is clearly involved in movement, and we decided to examine it. We had already been looking at the plasticity of the motor cortex in a number of circumstances (Hallett et al., 1993). Using transcranial magnetic stimulation (TMS), it is possible to map the degree and extent of excitability of individual muscles on the scalp surface. The motor cortex region for muscles proximal to an amputation increase in size presumably at the expense of the cortical regions now de-efferented. Some of this change can occur within minutes, as demonstrated with a blood pressure cuff at the elbow used to create a "rapid, reversible amputation." Additionally, increased use of muscles will give rise to an increase in size of their representation. For example, the representation size of the first dorsal interosseous muscle is increased in blind subjects who read Braille, presumably as a result of extensive use of that muscle in the reading process (Pascual-Leone et al., 1993a).

We mapped the cortical motor areas targeting the forearm finger flexor and extensor muscles in normal subjects learning a one-handed, five-finger exercise on an electronic piano (Pascual-Leone et al., 1993b). The task was metronome-paced so that improvement in accuracy should identify skill learning. The piano was connected by a MIDI interface to a personal computer for quantification of times of key presses. Subjects practiced the task for 2 hr daily. They improved both in ability to keep accurate time with the metronome and in reduction of errors. Over the course of the 5 days, the cortical areas increased in size (figure 13.2). This indicates, at least, the association of a motor cortex change with skill learning.

It is not unreasonable to consider the motor cortex as a relevant site for motor skill learning. Clearly it is involved in movement, and cortical cells have complex patterns of connectivity including variable influences on multiple muscles within a body part. Long-term potentiation has been demonstrated in the motor cortex (Iriki, Pavlides, Keller, and Asanuma, 1989).

FUNCTIONAL IMAGING

Using blood flow as a marker for neuronal activity, it has been possible to image areas of the brain that are active during different tasks. Positron emis-

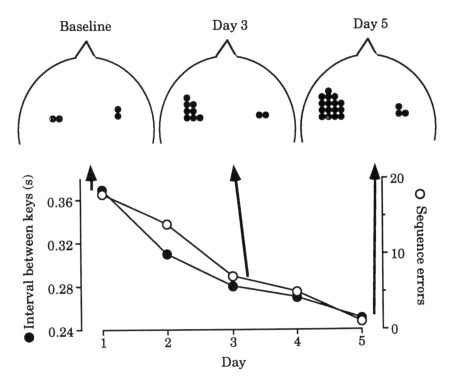

Figure 13.2 (Bottom) Performance of a representative subject in the right-handed five-finger movement exercise over the course of 5 days. Interval between keys should be 0.25 s because the subject was being paced by a metronome at that rate. Sequence errors indicate any key pressed in the incorrect order. (Top) Maps of cortical output for the right and left finger flexor muscles in the same subject at baseline and after 3 and 5 days. The dots mark the scalp positions from which the TMS induced motor-evoked potentials in the target muscle with a probability of equal to or greater than 60 percent. (Reprinted from Pascual-Leone et al., 1994b, with permission.)

sion tomography (PET) with blood flow methods has been the standard; more recently introduced is functional magnetic resonance imaging (fMRI) using contrast based on deoxyhemoglobin. In movement tasks, a variety of brain regions have been demonstrated to be active depending on the task. The primary motor cortex is almost always activated to some extent though, because of resolution, it has been often difficult to separate primary motor cortex from premotor cortex and primary sensory cortex. A number of studies have been done with motor learning (see chapter 11). The results have been somewhat confusing because techniques and experimental paradigms have differed.

Seitz and Roland (1992) studied learning of a complex finger tapping sequence and the data were reanalyzed subsequently by Schlaug, Knorr, and Seitz (1994). In all subjects, the only region that was consistently active with learning the task was the contralateral sensorimotor region. Unfortunately, learning was accompanied by an increase in movement frequency, which also causes an increase in contralateral sensorimotor region (Sadato et al., 1996). Friston, Frith, Passingham, Liddle, and Frackowiak (1992) studied practice of simple movements and the only change seen with learning was a decrease of activity in the cerebellum.

Grafton et al. (1992; Grafton, Woods, and Tyszka, 1994) have studied learning of a pursuit rotor task. The task is to keep a stylus on a target moving on a rotating disc. The experiment is appealing because motor behavior is continuous, but with practice the ability to stay on target is much improved. One problem, however, is that the motor strategy and patterns of muscle activation well may change during the learning. These studies show a clear activation of the contralateral sensorimotor region during learning. Other regions are active as well, including the supplementary motor area (SMA), the thalamus, the contralateral cingulate area, the ipsilateral anterior cerebellum, and the precuneate cortex.

Other motor learning tasks have been studied, but the tasks have been complicated, and whether the findings can be interpreted to isolate motor learning as such is unclear. Kawashima, Roland, and O'Sullivan, (1994) have studied pointing to a series of seven targets in the dark. The targets were circles of differing diameter, and the subject had to scan the targets and then plan a trajectory touching the circles in order of increasing size. Behavioral data from this study do show improvement with practice. The study was done with high resolution, and it was claimed that specific fields within contralateral primary motor cortex and premotor cortex were activated with learning. Jenkins, Brooks, Nixon, Frackowiak, and Passingham (1994) studied learning of a sequence of keypresses by trial and error using auditory feedback. This behavior was compared with a sequence of keypresses that was already learned. They found equal activation of primary motor cortex with both tasks. More active with learning were the prefrontal, premotor, and parietal cortices and the cerebellum, all bilaterally.

A recent study using fMRI focused attention on the contralateral primary motor cortex and used the experimental paradigm of finger tapping sequences (Karni et al., 1994). Two sequences were compared: one that was in the process of being learned and a second that was already learned. Though the learned sequence could have been performed faster, both sequences were performed at the same rate paced by an auditory stimulus. Hence, motor activity is well-matched. As the motor task was learned, more motor cortex area was activated. Within the same session, they also noted that repetitions of the same sequence at first activated a progressively smaller region of motor cortex, but as a sequence was learned, the region of motor cortex became progressively larger.

Clearly, much more work is needed in the area of functional imaging of motor learning, but it is already clear that many areas are involved (probably depending in large part on the details of the experimental paradigm). Additionally, it does appear that the contralateral primary motor cortex is involved even when the amount of movement is properly controlled.

SEQUENCE LEARNING WITH THE SERIAL REACTION TIME TEST

There has been a good deal of attention paid to the serial reaction time test (SRTT) as a paradigm to study motor learning of sequences (Nissen and Bullemer, 1987; Pascual-Leone, Grafman, and Hallett [1995]). The ability to carry out sequences of motor actions is clearly a critical part of most complex tasks, and the SRTT should be able to separate specific aspects of the learning. The task is a choice-reaction time with typically four possible responses. The responses can be carried out by keypresses with four different fingers. A visual stimulus indicates which is the appropriate response. The completion of one response triggers the next stimulus. Each movement is simple and separate from the others so that the movement aspect of this task is different (and easier) than other tasks considered previously, such as finger tapping or piano playing. The trick in this task is that, unknown to the naive subject, the stimuli are a repeating sequence. With practice at this task, the responses get faster even though the subject has no conscious recognition that the sequence is repetitive. This is called *implicit learning*. With continuing practice and improvement, the subject recognizes that there is a sequence but may not be able to specify what it is. Now knowledge is becoming explicit. With even more practice, the sequence can be specified, and it has become declarative as well as procedural. Performance gets even better at this stage, but the subject's strategy can change because the stimuli can be anticipated.

Thus, the SRTT appears to assess processes relating to the sequencing of motor behavior, factoring out elements of motor coordination. As such, it might be considered a test of some components of motor skill learning.

We have looked at the intermanual transfer of implicit learning in the SRTT (Wachs, Pascual-Leone, Grafman, and Hallett 1994). After a few blocks of training with one hand, subsequent blocks were done with the other hand. Four groups of normal subjects were studied each with one condition: (1) random sequence, (2) a new sequence, (3) parallel image of the original sequence, and (4) mirror image of the original sequence. Only group 4 showed a carryover effect from the original learning. This result suggests that what is stored as implicit learning is a specific sequence of motor outputs and not a spatial pattern.

Implicit learning is impaired in patients with cerebellar degenerations, Parkinson's disease, Huntington's disease, and progressive supranuclear palsy (Pascual-Leone et al., 1993c; Pascual-Leone, Grafman, and Hallett, 1995; Pascual-Leone, Wassermann, Grafman, and Hallett, in press). Patients with cerebellar degenerations were particularly severely affected. Implicit learning is preserved in patients with temporal lobe lesions and patients with short-term declarative memory disturbances, such as most patients with Alzheimer's disease. We have demonstrated recently that transient disruption of the dorsolateral prefrontal cortex with repetitive TMS will impair implicit learning in the SRTT (Pascual-Leone et al., in press).

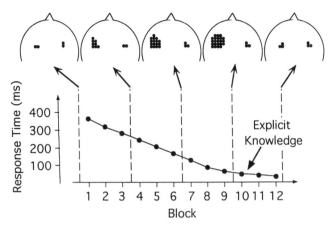

Figure 13.3 Modulation of motor cortical outputs in the course of procedural learning in the SRTT. The graph shows the median response time in each block of the SRTT in a representative subject performing with the right hand. The schematic representations of the head plot the number of scalp positions that, when stimulated with focal TMS (single pulse, 110 percent of subject's baseline motor threshold intensity), evoke motor potentials in the contralateral forearm finger flexors equal to or greater than 60 percent of the subject's maximal baseline amplitude. Several TMS maps are shown for different time points during the SRTT. Note that the increasing size of the cortical output maps to the forearm finger flexor muscles of the hand used in the task during the first several blocks of the SRTT, and the rapid return to baseline following development of complete explicit knowledge of the sequence. (Reprinted from Pascual-Leone et al., 1995a, with permission.)

In relation to the question of the involvement of the primary motor cortex in implicit learning, we mapped the motor cortex with TMS contralateral to the hands of normal subjects performing the SRTT (Pascual-Leone, Grafman, and Hallett, 1994a; Pascual-Leone, Grafman, and Hallett, 1994b). Mapping was done at intervals while the subjects were at rest between blocks of the SRTT. The map gradually enlarged during the implicit and explicit learning phases, but as soon as explicit learning was achieved, the map size returned to baseline (figure 13.3). This suggests an important role for primary motor cortex in both learning phases.

Learning during the SRTT has been studied using PET (Grafton, Hazeltine, and Ivry 1995). Two situations were imaged. In one, there was a second, distracting task to be done at the same time as the SRTT. Such distraction does not interfere with implicit learning but makes explicit learning much less likely. Hence, regions that were active are likely to reflect implicit learning. In a second experiment, there was no other task, and subjects were scanned in the explicit learning phase. In the implicit learning situation, there was activation of the contralateral primary motor cortex, SMA, and the putamen. Involvement of the basal ganglia is consistent with the patient data described above. In the explicit learning situation, there was activation of the ipsilateral dorsolateral prefrontal cortex and premotor cortex and of the parietal cortex bilaterally. This suggests that different structures are active in implicit and explicit learning.

In summary of the studies of the SRTT, it appears that multiple structures in the brain are involved at various stages, but there is a dissociation at least for some structures that are important to declarative learning. There seems to be good evidence of involvement of cortical structures (including the primary motor cortex), the basal ganglia, and the cerebellum.

CONCLUSION

Motor learning is a complex phenomenon with many components. Depending on the particular task, different anatomical structures are involved. It would be an oversimplification to say that only one part of the brain is involved with any task; it is more likely that a network is functional. On the other hand, it is possible to identify some aspects where particular structures play a major role: The cerebellum takes the principal part in adaptation learning. On the other hand, in skill learning, the cerebellar role is smaller, and cortical structures including the motor cortex are important. Skill learning has many facets and likely engages large portions of the brain. To the extent that sequencing is important, the cerebellum appears to have an important role.

From a clinical point of view, patients with cerebellar damage show ataxia characterized by incoordination of movement and failure to fine-tune a motor performance. Various types of neocortical damage may lead to the clinical deficit of apraxia, characterized by an inability to carry out learned movements in the presence of the elemental motor capability to carry out that movement. This might be interpreted as a gross deficiency of skilled motor memories. Such a consideration adds weight to the idea that the cerebral cortex plays an important role in skill learning.

REFERENCES

Brooks VB, Kennedy PR, Ross HG (1983). Movement programming depends on understanding of behavioral requirements. Physiol Behav 31:561–563.

Deuschl G, Toro C, Zeffiro T, Hallett M (1993). Adaptation of arm movement in cerebellar and olivary disease. Electroencephalogr Clin Neurophysiol 87:S67–S68.

Fitts PM (1954). The information capacity of the human motor system controlling the amplitude of movement. J Exp Psychol 47:381–391.

Friston KJ, Frith CD, Passingham RE, Liddle RF, Frackowiak RSJ (1992). Motor practice and neurophysiological adaptation in the cerebellum: A positron tomography study. Proc Roy Soc Lond Biol Sci 248:223–228.

Grafton ST, Hazeltine E, Ivry R (1995). Functional mapping of sequence learning in normal humans. J Cogn Neurosci 7:497–510.

Grafton ST, Mazziotta JC, Presty S, Friston KJ, Frackowiak RSJ, Phelps ME (1992). Functional anatomy of human procedural learning determined with regional cerebral blood blow and PET. J Neurosci 12:2542–2548.

Grafton ST, Woods RP, Tyszka M (1994). Functional imaging of procedural motor learning: Relating cerebral blood flow with individual subject performance. Hum Brain Map 1:221–234.

Hallett M, Cohen LG, Pascual-Leone A, Brasil-Neto J, Wassermann EM, Cammarota AN (1993). Plasticity of the human motor cortex. In AF Thilmann, DJ Burke, and WZ Rymer (eds), Spasticity: Mechanisms and Management. Berlin: Springer, pp 67–81.

Hallett M, Massaquoi S (1993). Physiologic studies of dysmetria in patients with cerebellar deficits. Can J Neurol Sci 20, Suppl 3:S83–S89.

Iriki A, Pavlides C, Keller A, Asanuma H (1989). Long-term potentiation of motor cortex. Science 245:1385–1387.

Jenkins IH, Brooks DJ, Nixon PD, Frackowiak RSJ, Passingham RE (1994). Motor sequence learning: A study with positron emission tomography. J Neurosci 14:3775–3790.

Karni A, Meyer G, Jezzard P, Adams M, Turner R, Ungerleider LG (1994). Where practice makes perfect: A fMRI study of long-term motor cortex plasticity associated with the acquisition of a motor skill. Soc Neurosci Abstr 20:1291.

Kawashima R, Roland PE, O'Sullivan BT (1994). Fields in human motor areas involved in preparation for reaching, actual reaching, and visuomotor learning: A positron emission tomography study. J Neurosci 14:3462–3474.

Lisberger SG (1988). The neural basis for learning of simple motor skills. Science 242:728–735.

Lye RH, O'Boyle DJ, Ramsden RT, Schady W (1988). Effects of a unilateral cerebellar lesion on the acquisition of eyeblink-conditioning in man. J Physiol (Lond) 403:58.

Nissen MJ, Bullemer P (1987). Attentional requirements of learning: Evidence from performance measures. Cogn Psychol 19:1–32.

Pascual-Leone A, Cammarota A, Wassermann EM, Brasil-Neto JP, Cohen LG, Hallett M (1993a). Modulation of motor cortical outputs to the reading hand of Braille readers. Ann Neurol 34:33–37.

Pascual-Leone A, Cohen LG, Dang N, Brasil-Neto JP, Cammarotta A, Hallett M (1993b). Acquisition of fine motor skills in humans is associated with the modulation of cortical motor outputs. Neurology 43 (Suppl 2):A157.

Pascual-Leone A, Grafman J, Clark K, Stewart M, Massaquoi S, Lou J-S, Hallett M (1993c). Procedural learning in Parkinson's disease and cerebellar degeneration. Ann Neurol 34:594–602.

Pascual-Leone A, Grafman J, Hallett M (1994a). Modulation of cortical motor output maps during development of implicit and explicit knowledge. Science 263:1287–1289.

Pascual-Leone A, Grafman J, Hallett M (1994b). Transcranial magnetic stimulation in the study of human cognitive function. In M Sugishita (ed), New Horizons in Neuropsychology. Amsterdam: Elsevier, pp 93–100.

Pascual-Leone A, Grafman J, Hallett M (1995). Procedural learning and prefrontal cortex. In J Grafman, KJ Holyoak, F Boller (eds), Structure and Function of the Human Prefrontal Cortex. New York: New York Academy of Sciences pp 61–70.

Pascual-Leone A, Wassermann EM, Grafman J, Hallett M (in press). The role of the dorsolateral frontal lobe in implicit procedural learning. Exp Brain Res.

Sadato N, Ibañez V, Deiber M-P, Campbell G, Leonardo M, Hallett M (1996). Frequency-dependent changes of regional cerebral blood flow during finger movements. J Cereb Blood Flow Metab 16:23–33.

Sanes JN, Dimitrov B, Hallett M (1990). Motor learning in patients with cerebellar dysfunction. Brain 113:103–120.

Schlaug G, Knorr U, Seitz RJ (1994). Inter-subject variability of cerebral activations in acquiring a motor skill: A study with positron emission tomography. Exp Brain Res 98:523–534.

Seitz RJ, Roland PE (1992). Learning of sequential finger movements in man: A combined kinematic and positron emission tomography (PET) study. Eur J Neurosci 4:154–165.

Thompson RF (1990). Neural mechanisms of classical conditioning in mammals. Philos Trans R Soc Lond B Biol Sci 329:161–170.

Topka H, Massaquoi SG, Zeffiro T, Hallett M (1991). Learning of arm trajectory formation in patients with cerebellar deficits. Soc Neurosci Abstr 17:1381.

Topka H, Valls-Solé J, Massaquoi S, Hallett M (1993). Deficit in classical conditioning in patients with cerebellar degeneration. Brain 116:961–969.

Wachs J, Pascual-Leone A, Grafman J, Hallett M (1994). Intermanual transfer of implicit knowledge of sequential finger movements. Neurology 44 Suppl 2:A329.

Weiner MJ, Hallett M, Funkenstein HH (1983). Adaptation to lateral displacement of vision in patients with lesions of the central nervous system. Neurology 33:766–772.

14 Learning of Sequential Procedures in Monkeys

Okihide Hikosaka, Shigehiro Miyachi,
Kae Miyashita, and Miya K. Rand

We perform an immense variety of learned actions such as writing words with a pencil, riding a bicycle, typing a keyboard, and playing the piano. When we first learn such actions, we focus our attention entirely on carrying them out, but after they are repeated, the actions become nearly automatic. It is such an attentive-to-automatic process that allows us to acquire a vast behavioral repertoire (Fitts, 1964); otherwise, our attentive mental capacity would be exhausted, and we would be unable to acquire a new action. These relatively automatic actions have been termed *procedural memory* to contrast with other kinds (Anderson, 1982; Tulving, 1985).

As we learn a new action, our brain creates a neural code or memory for carrying it out. However, little is known about the nature, localization, structure, dynamics, and mechanism of that memory. Where is the memory stored? Is it in the cerebral cortex, the basal ganglia, or the cerebellum? What kind of structure does it have? Is it a series of sequential neural connections? Is it a distributed neural network, or does it have a hierarchical organization? How does the neural network change its activity so as to produce sequential changes in the action? Which brain areas are necessary for creating the memory, and how is it done? Is such a learning mechanism different from the mechanism for memory storage? Are there different stages in learning to which different brain regions contribute?

It has been difficult to answer any of these questions for at least three reasons: time scale, variety, and structure. First, it takes a long time to acquire this type of memory—procedural memory—unlike other kinds of memory (such as declarative memory) (Fitts, 1964). In short-term memory tasks, such as the delayed nonmatching-to-sample task, the subject remembers whatever is presented as a sample stimulus and compares that memory with subsequent test stimuli. Single-cell activity correlated with the memory of selective items has been recorded in different cortical areas (e.g., Miyashita and Chang, 1988; Funahashi, Bruce, and Goldman-Rakic, 1989; Fuster, 1990). In contrast, it is usually impractical to follow the long-lasting process of procedural learning while continuing to record single-cell activity. In addition, it generally is thought that once acquired, the procedural memory remains robust even if the subject stops performing the procedure (Kolers, 1976). Such an irreversible nature of procedural memory tends to restrict further experimental manipulation because in principle we cannot repeat examination of procedural learning by using the same procedure. We would then need to have the subject learn different procedures, but that leads to the second difficulty: lack of variation.

For declarative memory, for example, one could present many different pictures, including some that the subject has never observed (Miyashita and Chang, 1988). For motor learning using simple stimulus-response (SR) paradigms, one can change the magnitude of the sensory stimulus to a novel value (Gilbert and Thach, 1977) or change the gain of the SR relationship (Optican, 1985; Ojakangas and Ebner, 1992; Oohira and Zee, 1992), thus effectively presenting new situations for repeated examination. Such a manipulation is (or at least has been) very difficult for procedural learning; the animal subject can learn a couple of different procedures but not more (Brooks, Reed, and Eastman, 1978; Sasaki and Gemba, 1982; Canavan, Nixon, and Passingham, 1989; Sakamoto, Arissian, and Asanuma, 1989). One might still be able to record single-cell activity related to learning (e.g., Mitz, Godschalk, and Wise, 1991; see also chapter 12), but it remains difficult to examine whether the activity is selective for the procedural content of the memory by studying a cell's activity as the animal learns many different procedures.

The third difficulty arises from the structure of procedural memory. Any behavioral procedure is more or less sequential. Thus it is not sufficient to locate the site of its stored neural code; of equal or more importance is the question of how the sequence is implemented. A picture as a stimulus for declarative memory may be dealt with as an independent item and therefore can be correlated with the strength of neural activity. For procedural memory, such a simple one-to-one correlation would not be valid. We need to obtain some hint of the structure of procedural memory.

How can we examine the neural mechanism underlying the procedural learning? It is essential to devise a behavioral paradigm by which we can examine the process of learning and, most importantly, do so repeatedly. Furthermore, that paradigm must be fairly easy so that an animal subject would try it willingly.

A HYPOTHETICAL PROCESS OF PROCEDURAL LEARNING

Before discussing our experimental results, we will consider a working hypothesis (figure 14.1C). For learning, we need to store temporarily the information regarding the action that has been done and to evaluate it (short-term memory). By repeating this procedure, the information would gradually be stored as a long-term memory. Well-learned procedures then would be retrieved from the long-term memory storage.

A critical point here is our postulate that the temporary storage mechanism and the permanent (or long-term) storage mechanism are independent

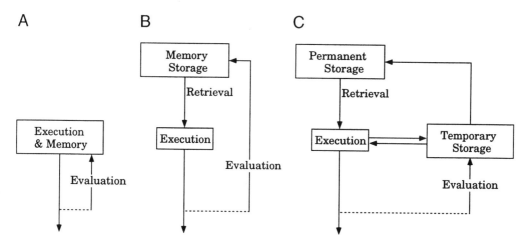

A

Execution
& Memory

Evaluation

B

Memory
Storage

Retrieval

Execution

Evaluation

C

Permanent
Storage

Retrieval

Execution

Temporary
Storage

Evaluation

Figure 14.1 Hypothetical processes of procedural learning. A, B, and C show different concepts of such learning.

(figure 14.1C). However, there is no reason to believe that this is so. It is possible that the same brain area(s) may store both the short-term and the long-term memory (figure 14.1B). Furthermore, there might be no mechanism that is specialized for memory storage (figure 14.1A); in this case, an execution mechanism itself might also store the memory.

In principle, our experimental design will be able to differentiate between these possiblities, especially if the results favor the separate mechanisms (figure 14.1C). Therefore, the first objective of our experiments is to indicate whether the hypothesis schematized in figure 14.1C is correct. Our discussion will proceed on the basis of this hypothesis: When we learn a new procedure, a neural system involving the temporary storage mechanism is activated. On the other hand, when we perform a well-learned procedure, another system involving the permanent storage mechanism is activated.

To differentiate between the learning mechanism and the memory mechanism, we need a behavioral paradigm that allows us to examine new procedures repeatedly. These procedures would preferably be similar or equivalent in terms of their structures. They all must be relatively easy to learn so that the animal subject can have both a number of well-learned procedures and (in addition) the opportunity to learn new ones. Such a variety of learned procedures would allow us to examine the structures of underlying memories by changing the structures of the procedures.

With such an urgent need in mind, we devised a behavioral paradigm, which we will call the *2 × 5 task* (figure 14.2) (Hikosaka, Rand, Miyachi, and Miyashita, 1995). This is a sequential hand movement task consisting of 10 button presses with many different variations. Because only two stimuli are presented as a set at a time, the subject is required only to press the two in a correct (predetermined) order; yet, after performing five consecutive

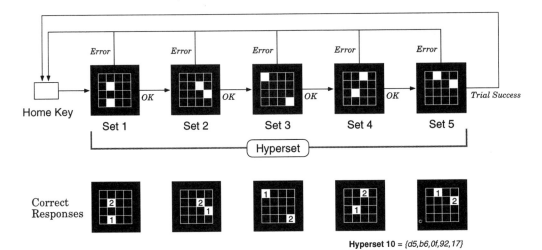

Figure 14.2 Procedure of 2 × 5 task. Figure shows distinction between sets and hypersets. Top row stimuli presented to the subject. Bottom row: correct responses.

sets, the subject is led to complete all 10 button presses (which we call the *hyperset*) successfully. The task has a hierarchical structure (set and hyperset) similar to our daily learned actions (Anderson, 1982). It also provides the situation appropriate for the manipulation of structural changes. Two monkeys conditioned to perform the 2 × 5 task have learned (with no serious difficulty), more than 100 different hypersets, some of which have been learned sufficiently to qualify as skills or habits.

A NEW TASK TO EXAMINE PROCEDURAL LEARNING

In front of a subject (in this case a Japanese monkey) is a panel on which 16 LED buttons are arranged in a 4 × 4 matrix. Beneath the panel is another button called the *home key*. If the monkey presses the home key, 2 of the 16 LED buttons are illuminated simultaneously. The monkey has to press them in a correct (predetermined) order, which it has to learn by trial-and-error. This two-key sequence is called a *set*. If it is successful, a second set is illuminated, requiring the monkey also to press this pair of LEDs in a predetermined order. A total of five sets is presented in a fixed order for completion of a trial, which we call a *hyperset*. When the monkey presses a wrong button, the trial is aborted and the monkey has to start again from the home key as a new trial.

One block of experiments is terminated when the monkey has performed 10 or 20 trials successfully for a particular hyperset, and another hyperset is used for another block of experiments.

A major advantage of the 2 × 5 task is that new hypersets can be generated practically without limit. Because the number of possible combinations for a

Hikosaka et al.

Number of completed sets

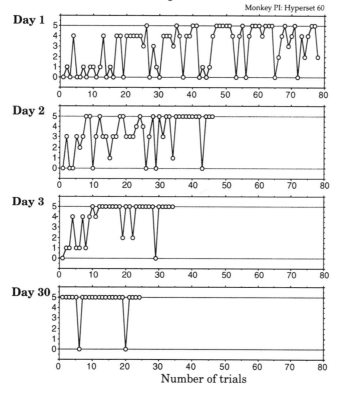

Monkey PI: Hyperset 60

Number of trials

Figure 14.3 Learning of a hyperset across trials. The change in the number of completed sets (ordinate) across trials (abscissa) for hyperset 60 (monkey PI) is compared between the first (Day 1), second (Day 2), third (Day 3), and thirtieth (Day 30) days of practice of this hyperset.

set is $_{16}P_2$, the number of possible combinations for a hyperset is $(_{16}P_2)^5$, which amounts to approximately 7.96×10^{11}, an astronomical value.

Some of the hypersets were chosen as learned hypersets and were examined daily. Besides being exposed to the learned hypersets, the monkey experienced many *new* hypersets, each of which was learned just once (one block).

A Short-Term Process of Learning

Figure 14.3 shows the process of learning for a particular hyperset, hyperset 60. For each trial on this hyperset, the number of successful sets performed is plotted. When this hyperset was presented for the first time (day 1), the monkey at first made errors mostly at the first or second set. Each time the monkey failed, the same hyperset was started over. The number of completed sets started increasing gradually, indicating that the monkey was learning (by trial-and-error) the order of button press for the initial consecutive sets. The monkey completed the whole hyperset (five sets) first at the twenty-sixth

Learning of Sequential Procedures

trial. The monkey then became able to complete the hyperset more often, indicating that learning occurred for the whole sequence of this hyperset. The time spent in this process was less than 5 min.

On day 2, the monkey failed at the initial several trials, but the performance improved faster than on day 1 and became nearly complete after the thirtieth trial. On day 3, the near-complete performance was reached by the twelfth trial. On day 30, the monkey failed only twice before completing 20 successful trials.

To evaluate the progress of learning across days, we set a criterion of 10 completely successful trials and defined two parameters: the number of trials to criterion and the total performance time.

A Long-Term Process of Learning

Using the two parameters, we show how learning proceeded over the days of practice (figure 14.4). The number of trials to criterion decreased rapidly over

A. Number of trials to criterion (10 success trials)

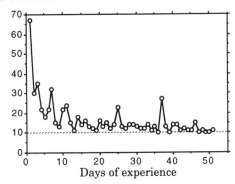

B. Performance time (sec) (first 10 success trials)

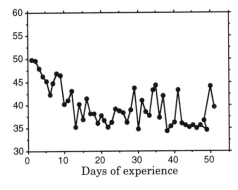

Figure 14.4 Learning of procedure and speed across days. A. The procedural learning is measured by the number of trials to criterion (10 successful trials) B. The speed of performance is measured by the total performance time for the initial 10 successful trials. The data were obtained for hyperset 60 (monkey PI).

the first few days and more gradually afterward until approximately about day 30, approaching the minimum value of 10. The total performance time decreased more gradually and kept on shortening even after day 30.

In this manner, we trained two monkeys to learn many hypersets. Figure 14.5 shows the time schedule for monkey PI. During the period of learning, the monkey performed the hypersets as the daily routine, one block for each hyperset. For most of the hypersets, the monkey was allowed to use only one hand. For example, hypersets 60, 88, and 176 were for the left hand only; 61, 89, and 175 were for the right hand only.

Different hypersets were started at different stages. For example, the monkey started learning hypersets 60 and 61 in September 1992, and continued to learn until recently. Other hypersets, such as 88 and 176 were started thereafter. Despite the difference in the monkey's experience, the process of learning these hypersets was similar.

In summary, although the performance of previously started hypersets had become nearly perfect, the monkey had to start over for newly introduced

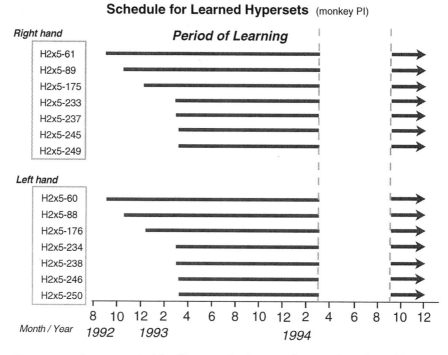

Figure 14.5 Long-term schedule of learning. The duration of practice for 14 learned hypersets for monkey PI are indicated by solid lines with respect to the chronological date. Half of the hypersets were performed by the right hand only; the others by the left hand only. During the period of learning, the monkey performed the hypersets as the daily routine, one block (until 20 successful trials were completed) for each hyperset. In addition to the learned hypersets, the monkey experienced 285 new hypersets, each of which was learned just once (one block) with the right hand or the left hand. The monkey did not perform any of the learned or new hypersets during a 6-mo period starting from March 1994, and resumed the 2 × 5 task in September 1994.

hypersets. In other words, what the monkey acquired was the ability to perform individual sequences, not general strategic improvements.

With daily practice, monkey PI became able to perform all of the 28 hypersets (examples are shown in figure 14.5) almost perfectly. We call these *learned hypersets*. In addition, the monkey experienced 932 hypersets only once (i.e., for one block), which we call *new hypersets*. Monkey BO had a similar repertoire of learned and new hypersets.

The purpose of new hypersets was to examine the monkey's ability to learn new procedures, which may well change according to the monkey's experience with the 2×5 task in general. Even though we stop riding a bicycle for a long time, we can ride the bicycle again without much difficulty. Our monkeys also had a chance to take a rest for 6 mo away from the 2×5 task (figure 14.5). We questioned whether they would remember any of the learned hypersets after the interruption.

Long-Term Retention of Procedural Memory

In figure 14.6, we compared monkey PI's performance, (i.e., the number of errors) on the 14 learned hypersets (shown in figure 14.5) just before the interruption with that after the first the interruption. The number of errors for these hypersets before the interruption was less than one on the average. The median number of errors after the interruption was also one. Both hypersets were performed nearly completely, which contrasted with the high frequency of errors when the same hypersets were performed for the first time (day 1).

Furthermore, performance on learned hypersets was much better than that for new and different hypersets, which were examined during the corresponding periods. This result excluded the possibility that the monkey became better in general at performing the 2×5 task. Instead, the memory for individual sequences was maintained for a long time without practice—not for just 1 motor sequence but for 14 different sequences.

Role of Saccadic Eye Movements in Learning

We found that eye movement plays an important role in learning the 2×5 task (Miyashita et al., submitted for publication). As already explained, if the monkey pressed the two illuminated LED buttons in a correct order, the two lights turned off sequentially. As expected, we found that the monkey looked at the button it was going to press and, on pressing, made a saccade to the next button.

In this paradigm, there is a time gap (150–300 ms) between the sets, during which no button was illuminated. The manner in which the monkey spent this period depended on the level of learning. We found that, as learning proceeded, anticipatory saccades appeared during the gap period. Figure 14.7 shows two-dimensional trajectories of saccades that occurred during the performance of hyperset 175, set 3 by monkey PI. Figure 14.7A

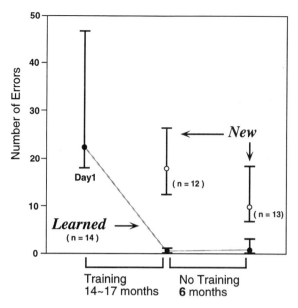

Figure 14.6 Long-term retention of procedural memory in monkey PI. The number of errors made before reaching a criterion (10 successful trials) for 14 learned hypersets is compared between three conditions: (1) the first experiment for each of the hypersets (Day 1), (2) the last experiments before an interruption (6 mo) of 2 × 5 task, and (3) the first experiments after the interruption. The duration of practice before the interruption varied between 14 and 17 mo, because the hypersets were started at different times. For each of these conditions, the median value as well as a percentile range (25–75 percent) is shown based on the data obtained for the 14 hypersets. For comparison are shown the median numbers of errors for new hypersets obtained during the periods just before (n = 12) and just after (n = 13) the interruption.

shows saccades that started just *before* the two target LEDs were illuminated; figure 14.7B shows saccades that occurred just *after* the target onset.

On the first day, the monkey made saccades to the first target *after* the target LEDs were illuminated. On day 25 (after sufficient learning), the saccades to the target occurred *before* the target onset. The posttarget saccades were directed to the second target. The saccades on day 1 were guided by visual inputs, whereas the saccades on day 25 were guided by memory. The memory in this case was procedural memory, which was specific to the individual sequence of hyperset 175. In fact, the ratio of anticipatory saccades increased with the long-term process of learning: That is, the ratio of anticipatory saccades indicates how robust the procedural memory had become.

Hand movements also became anticipatory. On pressing target 2 of set 2, the hand started moving toward target 1 of set 3. When the two targets of set 3 were illuminated, the hand was close to target 1. Of course, the gaze had already reached the target. The anticipatory eye and hand movements might contribute to the process in which the retrieval of a memory becomes more automatic.

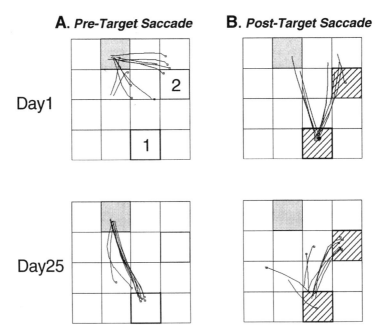

A. *Pre-Target Saccade*   **B.** *Post-Target Saccade*

Day1

Day25

(Monkey PI, Hyperset 175 Set 3)

Figure 14.7 Eye movements became anticipatory as learning proceeded. A, B. Trajectories of saccades that started just before and after, respectively, the onset of the illumination of the two target LEDs (1 and 2). The end of each saccade is indicated by a small square. The illumination of the target LEDs is indicated by hatching. The eye-movement records of the initial 10 successful trials of hyperset 175 (set 3) are superimposed. After releasing the second target of the previous set (set 2, shadowed square), the monkey PI pressed the first target of the current set (set 3, target 1). On the first day (day 1), the targeting of saccades (those directed to target 1) started after its illumination (posttarget saccades); on day 25, they started before target onset (day 25, pretarget saccades).

POSSIBLE BASAL GANGLIA CONTRIBUTION TO PROCEDURAL LEARNING

These behavioral experiments have provided us with means to investigate the neural mechanism underlying procedural memory and learning. Consider the model in figure 14.1C. When the monkey learns to perform a hyperset for the first time, the mechanism for temporary storage and evaluation of information functions. When the monkey performs a well-learned hyperset, the mechanism for permanent storage and retrieval of information functions. Tentatively we will call these mechanisms the *learning mechanism* and the *memory mechanism*, respectively.

We made a prediction based on these schemes (figure 14.8). If the learning mechanism did not function, new hypersets would not be learned, though already-learned hypersets would be performed normally. On the other hand, if the memory mechanism did not function, learned hypersets would not be performed, but new hypersets would be learned normally.

Predictions

Dysfunction of	Performance in	
	Learned Hypersets	New Hypersets
Learning mechanism	No change	↓
Memory mechanism	↓	No change

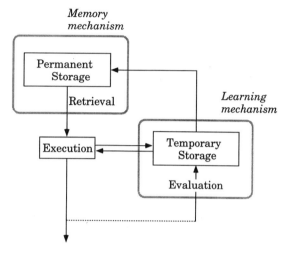

Figure 14.8 The learning mechanism and the memory mechanism can be dissociated by the differential performances in learned hypersets and new hypersets, provided that one of the mechanisms is inactivated selectively.

To establish localized dysfunction experimentally, we injected muscimol, a GABA agonist, to block neural functions locally in the basal ganglia. Figure 14.9 shows injection sites plotted on magnetic resonance images. The injections were classified into four groups based on their effects: group 1, the anterior striatum, including the head of the caudate, nucleus accumbens, and the anterior part of the putamen; group 2, the posterior part of the caudate; group 3, the posterior part of the putamen; and group 4, the anterior part of the globus pallidus. In most cases, the injections were bilateral, in two to four locations. For control experiments, we injected saline into these areas.

We analyzed the following parameters: number of errors, number of anticipatory saccades for one block of experiments, simple reaction time, choice reaction time, saccadic velocity, and latency of home-key release.

The performance with saline injections was as expected, normal. The mean number of errors before completing 10 successful trials was just 0.36 errors for learned hypersets and 18.9 errors for new hypersets. Muscimol injections into the anterior striatum produced significant effects: The number of errors

A: Anterior striatum

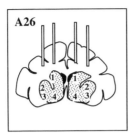

B: Caudate body

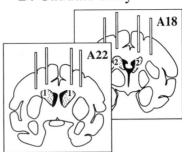

C: Putamen

D: Pallidum(anterior)

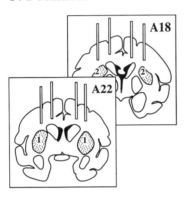
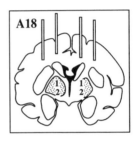

Figure 14.9 Sites of muscimol injections in the basal ganglia. A total of 12 guide tubes were implanted at three rostrocaudal levels (approximately at A26, A22, and A18, according to stereotaxic coordinates). The four guide tubes at each level were aimed at the caudate and putamen on both sides of the brain. The contours of subcortical structures are drawn on the basis of magnetic resonance images: Shaded areas indicate the (A) anterior striatum, (B) body of the caudate nucleus, (C) posterior putamen, and (D) anterior globus pallidus. Numbers (1–4) indicate the estimated locations of the injections. Most injections were bilateral (two locations) at symmetrical positions.

increased for both the learned hypersets (mean: 2.53; $p < .01$) and new hypersets (mean: 37.7; $p < .01$). This result suggests that the anterior striatum contributes to the memory mechanism as well as the learning mechanism.

In contrast, the muscimol injections into the posterior putamen and the anterior pallidum produced selective effects. After the putamen injections, the number of errors increased for learned hypersets (mean: 3.11; $p < .0001$), but not for new hypersets (mean: 20.9; $p > .05$). This suggests that the posterior putamen is part of the memory mechanism, not the learning mechanism. In contrast, after anterior pallidal injections, the number of errors increased for new hypersets (mean: 39.7; $p < .01$), not for learned hypersets (mean: 0.65; $p > .05$), suggesting that this area is part of the learning mechanism, not the memory mechanism.

As we showed before, the number of anticipatory saccades indicates the strength of procedural memory. In fact, in the case of saline injections, the number of anticipatory saccades was much greater in learned hypersets (mean: 15.3) than in new hypersets (mean: 3.39). As for muscimol injections, onlys those into the posterior putamen led to a significant decrease in the number of anticipatory saccades (mean: 9.36; $p < .0001$). This result again suggests that the posterior putamen is involved in the memory mechanism.

This hypothesis was supported by examining choice reaction time and simple reaction time. For each set, two LED buttons were illuminated, and the monkey chose one of them and pressed it. This left only one illuminated button to press. Thus, the time required for pressing the first button can be regarded as *choice reaction time*, whereas the time for pressing the second button can be regarded as *simple reaction time*.

As expected, the simple reaction time was virtually the same between learned hypersets and new hypersets. In contrast, the choice reaction time was much greater for new hypersets than for learned hypersets. We calculated the difference between these reaction times for each hyperset, and we call that difference the *time for choice*. If the time for choice is small, it indicates that the memory is strong.

In saline-control experiments, the mean time for choice was 428.9 ms for new hypersets, whereas it was only 18.9 ms for learned hypersets. A significant increase in this value for learned hypersets was observed after injections into the putamen (mean: 102.7 ms; $p < .0001$) and the anterior striatum (mean: 80.8 ms; $p < .01$), supporting the idea that these structures are part of the memory mechansism.

The results of muscimol injections enabled us to observe: (1) local functional blockade of the anterior striatum led to deficient performances in learned hypersets as well as in new hypersets, (2) blockade of the posterior putamen led to a selective deficit for learned hypersets, (3) blockade of the anterior pallidum led to a selective deficit for new hypersets, and (4) blockade of the posterior caudate nucleus produced no significant changes.

CONCLUSIONS

The selective deficits, such as those observed by the posterior putamen injections, suggest that the learning and memory mechanisms may indeed be separate. Furthermore, different regions in the basal ganglia appear to contribute to these mechanisms differentially.

The posterior part of the putamen may be part of the memory mechanism. There are at least two possibilities: First, long-term memories are stored in the putamen. Second, long-term memories are retrieved through the putamen. However, what remains unknown is the manner in which the memory information is sent out of the basal ganglia.

In contrast, the anterior part of the globus pallidus may be part of the learning mechanism, which carries short-term or temporary memories. In view of the known anatomical connections, the information might be provided by the anterior striatum.

However, our results suggest that the anterior striatum is also necessary for the memory mechanism. As to why that should be, our current hypothesis is that short-term memories are probably necessary even for the performance of learned hypersets; otherwise, any error would not be corrected. Additionally, the anterior striatum might be the source of the information of short-term memory.

We think, however, that these basal ganglia mechanisms are only part of a greater system, perhaps including the frontal cortical areas and the cerebellum.

REFERENCES

Anderson JR (1982). Acquisition of cognitive skill. Psychol Rev 89:369–406.

Brooks VB, Reed DJ, Eastman MJ (1978). Learning of pursuit visuo-motor tracking by monkeys. Physiol Behav 21:887–892.

Canavan AGM, Nixon PD, Passingham RE (1989). Motor learning in monkeys (Macaca fascicularis) with lesions in motor thalamus. Exp Brain Res 77:113–126.

Fitts PM (1964). Perceptural-motor skill learning. In AW MeHou (ed), Categories of Human Learning. New York: Academic, pp 243–285.

Funahashi S, Bruce CJ, Goldman-Rakic PS (1989). Mnemonic coding of visual space in the monkey's dorsolateral prefrontal cortex. J Neurophysiol 61:331–349.

Fuster JM (1990). Inferotemporal units in selective visual attention and short-term memory. J Neurophysiol 64:681–697.

Gilbert PFC, Thach WT (1977). Purkinje cell activity during motor learning. Brain Res 128: 309–328.

Hikosaka O, Rand MK, Miyachi S, Miyashita K (1995) Learning of sequential movements in the monkey: I. Process of learning and retention of memory. J Neurophysiol 74:1652–1661.

Kolers PA (1976). Reading a year later. J Exp Psychol: Hum Learn Mem 2:554–565.

Mitz AR, Godschalk M, Wise SP (1991). Learning-dependent neuronal activity in the premotor cortex: Activity during the acquisition of conditional motor associations. J Neurosci 11:1855–1872.

Miyashita Y, Chang HS (1988). Neuronal correlates of pictorial short-term memory in the primate temporal cortex. Nature 331:68–70.

Miyashita K, Rand MK, Miyachi S, Hikosaka O. Anticipatory saccades in sequential procedural learning in monkeys. J Neurophysiol (submitted for publication).

Ojakangas CL, Ebner TJ (1992). Purkinje cell complex and simple spike changes during a voluntary arm movement learning task in the monkey. J Neurophysiol 68:2222–2236.

Oohira A, Zee DS (1992). Disconjugate ocular motor adaptation in rhesus monkey. Vision Res 32:489–497.

Optican LM (1985). Adaptive properties of the saccadic system. In A Berthoz, G Melvill-Jones (eds), Adaptive Mechanisms in Gaze Control: Facts and Theories. Amsterdam: Elsevier, pp 71–79.

Sakamoto T, Arissian K, Asanuma H (1989). Functional role of the sensory cortex in learning motor skills in cats. Brain Res 503:258–264.

Sasaki K, Gemba H (1982). Development and change of cortical field potentials during learning processes of visually initiated hand movements in the monkey. Exp Brain Res 48:429–437.

Tulving E (1985). How many memory systems are there? Am Psychol 40:385–398.

15 The Role of the Cerebellum in the Acquisition of Complex Volitional Forelimb Movements

James R. Bloedel, Vlastislav Bracha, Yury Shimansky, and Matthew S. Milak

It is not known precisely what role is played by the cerebellum in the acquisition of voluntary behaviors involving complex, goal-directed movements. Most hypotheses pertaining to this question have been derived from investigations of behaviors requiring comparatively simple neural substrates for their execution. In vertebrates, these behaviors include primarily the conditioning of a variety of reflexes evoked by aversive stimuli (Welsh and Harvey, 1992; Bloedel and Bracha, 1995; see also chapter 5 for reviews) and the adaptation of the vestibuloocular reflex (Miles and Lisberger, 1981; Ito, 1984, 1993; Lisberger, 1988; Peterson, Baker, and Houk, 1991; see also chapter 2). Several discussions of these findings have proposed the cerebellum as a necessary and sufficient site for the storage of plastic changes underlying the modification of these behaviors (see Thompson and Krupa, 1994, for review). Perhaps as a result of this emphasis, discussions also have proposed a possible role for the cerebellum in storing the engrams required to recall volitional, complex motor sequences (see Stein and Glickstein, 1992, and Thach, Goodkin, and Keating, 1992).

However, the acquisition of volitional movements includes aspects of information processing that are not believed to play a role (or at least as significant a role) in the modification of vestibular or withdrawal reflexes. Most goal-directed movements clearly involve cognitive functions, sometimes in several aspects of the task. These functions can include motor planning and the conceptualization of specific movement sequences required to meet the task's objectives. In addition, the successful performance of most volitional tasks used in operant conditioning paradigms is related to achieving an objective in the terminal phase of the movement (such as contacting a target or manipulating a device). Although the reflexes that were investigated using classical conditioning paradigms consist of a characteristic pattern of motor activity and are directed toward a specific objective, these movements generally do not require precise end-point control. For example, withdrawal reflexes are organized to remove a body part from an offending stimulus quickly. Eyeblink reflexes are organized to close the eyes rapidly, protecting the cornea from any impending aversive stimulus. In these tasks, the effectiveness of the movement is based on the rapidity of its execution rather than on its terminal accuracy. The requirement of terminal accuracy during voluntary movements (together with the multiple degrees of freedom of the extremity) necessitates the selection of a coordination scheme or strategy with which the movement can be performed efficiently enough to attain its objective.

These unique features of volitional movements often are overlooked in studies examining and discussing the cerebellum's role in their acquisition. Most previous investigations of this issue have focused on examining the learning of motor tasks by human subjects. Such examinations either compared the capacity of cerebellar patients with normal controls to learn certain motor behaviors (see chapters 10 and 13) or examined changes in activation patterns related to the cerebellum during the learning and performance of specific movements (see chapter 11). One of the tests (employing a visuomotor task) required subjects to throw darts at a target while wearing prism glasses that laterally displaced the perceived target location. Compared with control subjects, cerebellar patients were unable to adapt their motor performance adequately enough to compensate for the errant visual cues regarding target location (Weiner, Hallett, and Funkenstein, 1983; Thach et a., 1992; See also chapters 10 and 13). In another study, Sanes, Dimitrov, and Hallett (1990) compared the performance of cerebellar patients and normal subjects in the performance of a mirror drawing task. In addition to contrasting these two groups based on a standard training task, they compared their capacity to draw the mirror image of a visualized template. These investigators concluded that there was a substantial difference in the capacity of these two groups to learn and perform the mirror-image tracing task.

However, this conclusion was based on a comparison of the absolute measures of motor performance in the two groups. Because of the significant motor deficit in cerebellar patients, differences in absolute levels of performance between these patients and normal subjects (measured by performance errors) would be expected even if some degree of improved performance was achieved by the cerebellar patients. For this reason, Timmann et al. (1994) recently compared the rate at which cerebellar patients and normal subjects learned a complex visuomotor task. All subjects were required to learn the shape of an irregularly shaped image, mentally rotate it 90 degrees, and draw it from memory in the rotated position. Cerebellar patients and normal subjects acquired this task at the same rate even though there was a substantial difference in the absolute level of performance between the two groups. Thus, assessing the *rate* of acquisition revealed that cerebellar patients have a substantial capacity to improve performance through practice.

Several imaging studies also have implicated the cerebellum in the learning of complex motor tasks. These studies demonstrated that activation of cerebellar structures can occur while a new motor task is being learned (Friston, Frith, Passingham, Liddle, and Frackowiak, 1992; Flament, Ellermann, Ugurbil, and Ebner, 1994; Jenkins, Brooks, Nixon, Frackowiak, and Passingham, 1994;

Seitz et al., 1994). One of these experiments specifically implicated the dentate nucleus in this process (Seitz et al., 1994). A special role for the dentate nucleus in the learning of complex movements was further suggested by functional magnetic resonance imaging studies (Kim, Ugurbil, and Strick, 1994). These investigators demonstrated that dentate nucleus activation occurred during a series of movements made by the subject in attempting to solve a complex puzzle but failed to occur with the same movements in the absence of any learning. Consequently, this activation pattern was dependent on the combined effort generated both to solve the puzzle and to produce the sequence of movements.

CURRENT EXPERIMENTS

To understand the general concepts underlying the cerebellum's role in the acquisition of different motor tasks, our laboratory complemented studies of the cerebellum's contribution to the acquisition and performance of conditioned reflexes (Bracha, Stewart, and Bloedel, 1993; Bracha, Webster, Winters, Irwin, and Bloedel, 1994; Bloedel and Bracha, 1995; see also chapter 8) with experiments using cats as experimental models to investigate the cerebellum's role in the learning of complex, goal-directed forelimb movements. Proceeding on the hypothesis that the cerebellum's role in such learning was related primarily to task acquisition and the coordination of the movement to be learned, we undertook investigations (1) to determine whether the inactivation of any of the ipsilateral cerebellar nuclei affects the recall of a previously learned complex forelimb movement; (2) to assess the nature of the acquisition process during the inactivation of the ipsilateral interposed and dentate nuclei; and (3) to examine the acquisition-related changes in the modulation of cerebellar nuclear neurons.

The paradigm developed to address these three issues required a cat to learn to perform a task in which a vertical manipulandum was moved through a pattern of two to three consecutive, straight grooves located in a horizontal Plexiglas template. At the sound of a tone, the cat reached for the vertical bar and attempted to negotiate the template. If the reward zone was reached within 3 s, a food reward was presented on a planchet located on the upper end of the manipulandum. The implementation of this task made it possible to examine issues related to both acquisition and retention of this behavior. In studies of the acquisition process, the animal was required to learn a specific template during temporary nuclear inactivation or while the activity of multiple nuclear neurons was being recorded. The cerebellum's role in retention was examined by requiring the animal to learn a specific template and then assessing the effect of cerebellar nuclear inactivation on the cat's capacity to recall the movement pattern required to complete the task.

In all three experiments reviewed here, electromyogram (EMG) electrodes were implanted in five muscles in the performing forelimb and three muscles in the contralateral forelimb. Velcro patches also were applied over the shoulder, elbow, and wrist joints and at two locations on the paw of the performing forelimb. During each experimental session, infrared emitting diodes (IREDs) were secured to these Velcro patches so as to measure the kinematics of the cats' movements with an Optotrak system. Data collection ensured the temporal relationship between the kinematic measurements, the EMG recordings, the movement through the template, and the unitary activity recorded from nuclear neurons. The manipulandum and the template groove were instrumented to permit the measurement of reaction time, reach-duration, and the movement durations through the various segments of the template.

Effects of Cerebellar Lesions on the Retention and Performance of a Previously Learned, Operantly Conditioned Task

The first series of experiments assessed how inactivating individual cerebellar nuclei would affect retention of the previously learned template. We hypothesized that inactivating the neurons in the fastigial, interposed, or dentate nuclei would not affect the cat's capacity to recall and execute the template within the duration of the trial despite the expected ataxia characterizing the animal's movements.

Animals were trained initially to perform an inverted L template with the right forelimb, a template requiring a medial-to-lateral movement followed by an anterior-to-posterior longer movement to the reward zone. Each cat was trained to perform this task until the mean values of all temporal measurements characterizing the movement were consistent from day to day and until the trial-to-trial variability was minimal. (These measurements included reach duration, time required to execute the first limb of the template, time required to execute the second limb of the template, and total movement time). Once this level of performance was achieved, guide tubes for injection needles were implanted directed towards the fastigial nucleus, the anterior interposed, the posterior interposed, and the dentate nucleus. The tubes were directed toward the center of each nucleus with their tips located approximately 2.5 mm above center.

Following recovery from the implantation procedure, the effects of a 1-μl injection of muscimol (800 ng/μl) were assessed at successive sites located 0.5 mm apart along a track through each nucleus. The kinematic measurements determined the depth at which the maximal effect on the movement occurred. No more than one injection was made on any given day. All sites designated as optimal injection sites were marked at the completion of the experiment.

The muscimol microinjections into each of the cerebellar nuclei produced quantifiably distinguishable (but qualitatively similar) deficits in the performance of the previously learned task. Injections in the interposed nuclei produced a dramatic, tremorlike, ataxic movement just as the bar was to be contacted by the paw. In contrast, the most striking deficit following the inactivation of the dentate nucleus was the incoordination exhibited while executing the movement through the template. The deficits following fastigial nuclear inactivation often included ataxia of both the reach and the template component of the task.

Most significant for the issues addressed in this chapter is the fact that the cat was able to recall and perform the task following the inactivation of any of the ipsilateral cerebellar nuclei. All cats included in this study were capable of performing the task within the required 3-s time-window despite the injection-produced ataxia. The effect of the microinjections on retention was quantified by determining the number or percent of successful trials over consecutive blocks of 20 trials following the injection. These data did not reveal a decreased task retention associated with the injection of either the fastigial or the interposed nuclei. Interestingly, microinjections in the dentate nucleus produced a somewhat different effect in two of five animals. Although the percent of *conditioned responses*, defined as a successful completion of a given trial within 3 s, was unaffected by dentate inactivation in three cats; in the other two, the percent of conditioned responding became somewhat erratic, decreasing to 40 to 60 percent in some blocks. Because these blocks with a lower percent response were interspersed with those showing response at criterion (90 percent successful trials over 20 successive trials) or near criterion levels, these modest changes following dentate microinjections likely reflect a performance deficit rather than a direct effect on retention. This suggestion is consistent with the fact that the principal abnormality following the injection of this nucleus was the failure to maintain grasp of the bar as the template was executed.

The effect on the performance of a previously learned template also was determined by injections *simultaneously* into the interposed and dentate nuclei via three different cannulae in order to ensure that the negative effects on retention in these previous experiments were not in some way due to the fact that only single nuclei were injected. As shown on the right of figure 15.1, these multiple injections produced only a transient effect on the animal's performance. In the initial block of 10 trials, the animal was unable to execute at criterion level. This capacity was regained quickly in this animal after 20 trials. The percent of successful trials during these first two blocks was increased when the criterion for performance was extended from a trial length of 3 s to 6 s. This suggests that the transcient decrease was related to the profound ataxia produced by the nuclear inactivation. Clearly the animal could recall the general pattern of the movement that must be executed to complete the task. After the first 20 trials, the animal readapted and again could execute the task within 3 s.

In summary, the data in these experiments strongly suggest that the retention of this type of operantly conditioning task is unaffected following injection of either the interposed or fastigial nuclei.

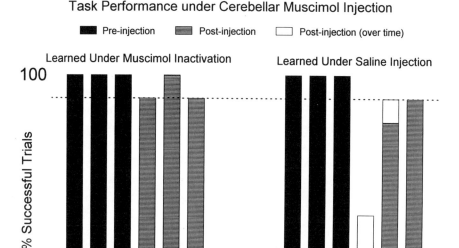

Figure 15.1 Effects of inactivating the dentate and interposed nuclei simultaneously on the capacity to recall and perform the template task described in the text. The percent of successful pre- and postinjection trials are shown for data from two animals, one that had an initial period of learning under muscimol inactivation (left plot) and one that originally learned to perform the template task under saline injection and consequently was not required previously to perform this task with the cerebellar nuclei inactivated (right plot). Percent of successful trials indicates the percent of trials in each block completed within the usual trial duration (3 s). The plots on the right show the postinjection data calculated both on the basis of performing the template within the required 3 s (hatched bars) and performing the task within an extended 6-s period (overtime). The dashed horizontal line indicates criterion performance.

Temporary Inactivation of the Ipsilateral Cerebellar Nuclei and Acquisition of an Operantly Conditioned Complex Forelimb Movement

The next series of experiments examined specifically the role of the cerebellum in the acquisition of the previously described forelimb task. The cerebellum was implicated strongly in some aspect of the acquisition of these tasks on the basis of previous studies investigating its role in modifying other types of motor behaviors (most notably the adaptation of the vestibuloocular reflex [VOR] and the classical conditioning of the eyeblink reflex). Adaptation of the VOR has been reported to be absent (Robinson, 1976; Cohen, Cohen, Raphan, and Waespe, 1992) or impaired (Pastor, De la Cruz, and Baker, 1994) following ablation of the cerebellum. In addition, though the eyeblink reflex can be classically conditioned in decerebrate, decerebellate rabbits (Kelly, Zuo, and Bloedel, 1990), lesions of the cerebellum in intact rabbits either block the acquisition process (Krupa, Thompson, and Thompson, 1993; Nordholm

Thompson, Dersarkissian, and Thompson, 1993) or the expression of the conditioned response (Welsh and Harvey, 1991; see also chapter 6). Perhaps more pertinent to the retention of voluntary movements, the experiments presented in the previous section demonstrated clearly that inactivating the cerebellar nuclei does not eliminate the retention of the task (i.e., it could be recalled and executed in most trials following the microinjection of muscimol). Based on these observations, we hypothesized that in the learning of these complex forelimb movements, the cerebellum's role may be related more substantially to the acquisition of the behavior than to providing the storage site for the engram established as the task is practiced. To explore this possibility, experiments were undertaken to examine the capacity of cats to learn the previously described template task during the inactivation of the ipsilateral interposed and dentate nuclei.

Cats were trained initially to reach for the manipulandum bar and move it through a single anterior-posterior groove to a target zone within a 3-s period. Once the animals' performance became optimal (based on measurements of the temporal features of the movement), guide tubes were implanted directed toward the center of the posterior interposed, anterior interposed, and dentate nuclei ipsilateral to the limb trained to perform the task. The placement of EMG electrodes and IREDs was identical to that described in the previous section. Next, by assessing the movement abnormalities associated with the execution of the straight groove template, the optimal injection site (the site at which the injection of 1 μl of muscimol exerted its maximal effect) was determined as previously described.

The cats were separated into two groups: (1) those evaluated for the effects of injecting simultaneously 1 μl of muscimol at each of the optimal nuclear injection sites and (2) those assessed for the effects of simultaneous 1-μl injections of buffered saline into each nucleus. Because of the difficulty of obtaining animals that attempted the execution of new templates while the ipsilateral dentate and interposed nuclei are inactivated, the experiments were limited to three animals in each group.

The protocol employed for investigating the acquisition and subsequent performance of the template task was the same for each animal, regardless of muscimol or buffered saline microinjections. In brief, on successive days the animals were required to learn to execute a two-limb template in which the first limb required a medial-to-lateral movement and the second an anterior-to-posterior movement. The trials began with the angle between the limbs of the template at 110 degrees. Once the task was executed to criterion (completion of the template within 3 s in 18 of 20 consecutive trials), the angle was decreased, and the training was repeated. The angle was decreased consecutively by 10 degrees in the first step and by 5 degrees on each successive step. This process was repeated until determination of the smallest angle the cats could execute. An animal was considered to have reached maximum performance when it could no longer master a template at a specific angle over 40 successive trials. On occasion, an additional 20 trials were run at the same template angle after criterion was attained to ensure that the animal had in fact mastered the specific template. In addition, occasionally it was necessary to increase the angle of the template for several trials (i.e., make the task easier) when the animal clearly encountered appreciable difficulty. Without this modification, the animal could become frustrated and stop working for the food reward well before attaining its maximum performance level.

After determination of the most difficult template the animal could acquire, each animal was retrained on the same series of templates in the absence of any cerebellar nuclear injection. The purpose of this part of the protocol was twofold: to determine whether the animal retained the capacity to perform the template in the absence of nuclear inactivation and to determine any differences in execution when performing the task with an operational cerebellum for the first time. The same protocol for characterizing the original learning curve determined retention, any additional learning or relearning that occurred during the retraining, and the most difficult angle that could be performed after retraining.

Once the animal had learned to perform the task in the absence of any injection, the effects on the recall of the template task caused by inactivating the interposed and dentate nuclei simultaneously were evaluated. Using the most difficult template the cat had previously learned, this part of the experiment determined whether the animal was capable of recalling and performing the task during cerebellar nuclear inactivation after having been retrained on the task with a fully functional cerebellum. These results were presented in the previous section.

One of the most critical results in this experiment is that all cats with inactivated output of the interposed and dentate nuclei during learning were able to acquire the ability to execute reasonably difficult templates with the two grooves at least at 90 degrees. A learning curve for one of the animals in the study is shown in figure 15.2. Equally interesting, animals that had first learned the task under muscimol were incapable initially of performing the task when tested without injection and had to "relearn" it over an acquisition period in which the percent successes improved progressively until the task was executed adequately on every trial. The plot in figure 15.2 illustrates the performance of one cat during retraining after it had already learned the task while the nuclei were inactivated. Notice that the animal's performance on the templates with larger angles was quite poor initially and that considerable practice was necessary to attain again a performance level of 85 to 90 percent (0 degrees and −5 degrees), even though some savings may have occurred based on the number of days required for reacquisition of the behavior. Thus, even though the animal had learned to perform the task reasonably well while the nuclei were inactivated, a relearning of the task occurred when the cerebellum was capable of participating in the process. In contrast, no comparable reacquisition period was observed in the saline-conditioned control subjects. Rather, the control animals continued to perform the task as proficiently as they did at the conclusion of the initial period of learning.

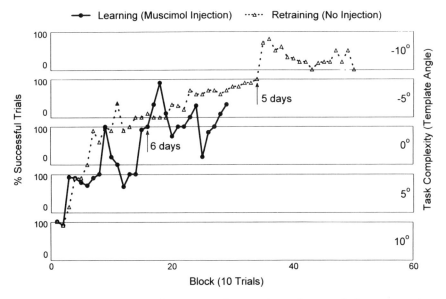

Figure 15.2 Learning curves characterizing the acquisition of progressively more complex templates under two conditions: when the animal first attempted to learn the task with the cerebellar nuclei inactivated (solid lines, filled circles), and when the uninjected animal was retrained on the task after first acquiring it during nuclear inactivation (dashed lines, open triangles). The plot consists of a succession of learning curves, each characterizing the percent of successive trials (1–100%, left axis) as a function of the required blocks of trials for each angle (right axis). The arrows indicate the day of training on which the maximum level of performance was attained for each condition, defined as the day on which criterion on the template with the smallest angle was reached.

Third, as predicted from the experiments presented in the first section, the injection of the dentate and interposed nuclei with muscimol after retraining did not affect the retention of the task in any of the animals in either experimental group. Furthermore, a comparison of the data plotted on the left and right in figure 15.1 suggests that task acquisition under muscimol is different from that occurring in the uninjected animal. Notice that inactivation-produced ataxia resulted in some missed trials early after the injection of animals that had not performed the task previously under muscimol (right plots, figure 12.1). However, no comparable effect was produced in animals that previously had learned the task with inactivated nuclei, even when they had intervening experience performing the behavior in the absence of any injection (preinjection condition, left plots, figure 15.1).

This series of experiments demonstrates that (1) cats with inactivated interposed and dentate nuclei are capable of learning a complex forelimb movement and performing it at a level of complexity near but not quite that demonstrated by normal cats, and (2) the task is "reacquired" when the normal animal is retrained on the template it had learned previously during cerebellar nuclear inactivation. Furthermore, as already presented in the previous section, the simultaneous inactivation of the dentate and interposed nuclei does not block the performance of a previously learned template.

Modulation of Cerebellar Nuclear Neurons During Task Acquisition

The foregoing experiments suggest that, although the acquisition of tasks involving complex, volitional forelimb movements is possible without the cerebellum, the acquisition process employed under this condition differs from that employed in learning the task with a functional cerebellum. This possibility may reflect a specific, active role for the cerebellum in the acquisition of this type of motor behavior. We hypothesized that this role may relate to the establishment of an effective, efficient strategy for executing the desired task and the reinforcement of that strategy as it is practiced. To obtain insights into whether this view may be correct, we performed experiments in which we recorded the modulation of multiple single units located in various cerebellar nuclei of cats during the learning of novel templates and related this activity to specific features of the acquisition process.

In these experiments (Milak, Bracha, and Bloedel, 1995), after the cat learned the single-groove task described earlier, a recording system was implanted consisting of six bundles of four microwires (24 μm in diameter). Each bundle of microwires passed through a positioned guide tube directed at a specific cerebellar nuclear region: the anterior and posterior parts of the fastigial nucleus, the anterior and posterior interposed nuclei, and the anterior and posterior portions of the dentate nucleus. The microwire bundles were connected to individual manipulators that permitted the isolation of neurons and changes in recording position as required by the protocol. The implantation of the EMG electrodes and the attachment of the Velcro strips for securing IREDS were identical to that described for the experiments in the previous sections.

Just prior to initiating a learning session, on average 6 to 12 nuclear neurons were isolated, and the template was changed to a two- to three-limb template to which the animal had not been exposed previously. Next, the cat was required to negotiate the template by moving the manipulandum through the grooves to the reward zone. Throughout each learning session, measurements were made of the EMG of several forelimb muscles, the kinematics of the ipsilateral forelimb movements, and the temporal characteristics of the different components of the task. In addition, the unitary activity from each channel was digitized and stored for subsequent data analysis.

Data were processed by constructing histograms characterizing each neuron's responses over the various stages of the learning process. This was done by sorting trials based on the extent to which the movement to be learned was performed successfully. The categories into which the trials were sorted were based on characteristics of the kinematics and different temporal characteristics of the movement. These categories included the first 10 attempts at performing the trials, the first 10 successful trials, the first 10 times the task was performed successfully on consecutive trials, the first 10 times that the manipulandum was moved through the template smoothly (defined as one primary peak on the velocity profile for the specific component of the movement), the first 10 trials performed within a specific range of movement times, and 10 well-practiced trials, defined as trials executed near the end of the recording period (at a time when the animal performed the task very well). Once the trials were sorted, histograms were constructed by aligning trials on such specific features of the task as bar contact, paw liftoff, and the time at which various corners of the template were reached by the manipulandum. For the response of the cells related most dramatically to a feature of the movement, a response window was selected, and the amplitude of the response component was measured in histograms characterizing the responses at successive stages of the acquisition process.

The plots in figure 15.3 illustrate the primary finding in these experiments. Approximately 90 percent of the neurons recorded within the cerebellar nuclei underwent a characteristic and statistically significant ($p < .05$) change in the amplitude of their event-related modulation during the acquisition period. The amplitude of these cells' responses increased up to the time the movement sequence required to execute the task successfully was first performed reasonably well. This usually corresponded to either the trials in which the task was first performed over successive trials or the first trials in which the task was executed smoothly. In addition, as the task continued to be practiced, the response amplitude progressively decreased but usually did not disappear.

This trend in the amplitude of the event-related modulation of cerebellar nuclear neurons was found to be related to the various stages of the acquisition process rather than to a change in some kinematic feature of the movement. A specific attempt was made to examine the correlation between measurements such as movement velocity and the modulation amplitude of the cells, and no consistent relationship was found. The trend in modulation amplitude over the time-course of acquisition also is not likely due to the anxiety or stress of performing the task, because these factors would be expected to be greatest when the task was first encountered, which was not the time at which the modulation amplitude was greatest. Consequently, the data suggest that the cerebellum is involved actively in neuronal interactions related to the acquisition process and particularly the component of the process occurring when the strategy for performing the movement becomes established.

Altered Kinematics of Movements Learned During Cerebellar Inactivation

If the acquisition-related function of the cerebellum involves establishing and possibly reinforcing a highly effective and efficient strategy for performing a

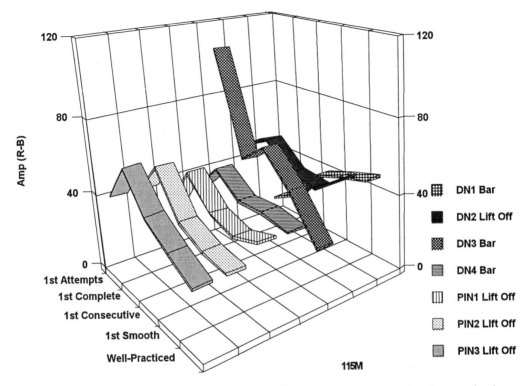

Figure 15.3 Ribbon plots illustrating the changes in the amplitudes of event-related responses over the time-course of acquiring the template task described in the text. All the neurons in this set were recorded simultaneously, and their location is indicated in the key. PIN = posterior interposed nucleus; DN = dentate nucleus. The feature of the behavior with which the response was correlated is also indicated in the key. Response amplitudes (Amp) are expressed as response (R) minus background (B) discharge rate. The categories used to sort the histograms from which these measurements were made are indicated on the graph. (Reprinted from Milak et al., 1995, with permission.)

novel voluntary behavior, the absence of this cerebellar contribution could be reflected in the variability of motor patterns with which the movement is executed, even after it has been learned well enough to be performed on consecutive trials. To evaluate this possibility, the kinematics of the movements acquired with and without the cerebellar nuclei inactivated were compared. Measurements of the lateral deviation of the reach from a straight-line trajectory and the angle of deviation from this straight line as the movement was initiated were appreciably more variable when the task was learned with the cerebellum inactivated. When the task was acquired by control animals in the absence of nuclear inactivation, the variability of these measurements was substantially less.

The variability in movement kinematics when the task was learned during nuclear inactivation is very apparent in the three trials shown in figure 15.4. These trials were obtained from the period during acquisition in which the

Nuclear Inactivation

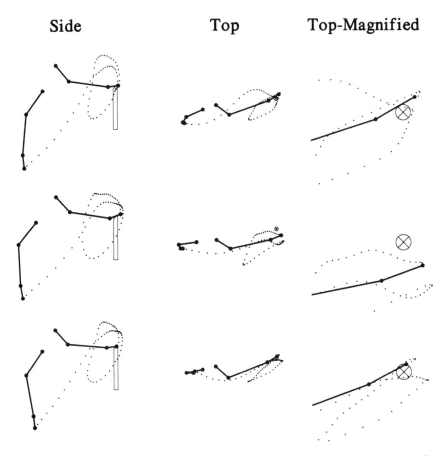

Figure 15.4 Effects of simultaneous inactivation of the dentate and interposed nuclei on the motor patterns employed by a cat learning to perform the template task. This figure focuses on the component of the movement performed by the animal just prior to moving the manipulandum through the template, the component in which the cat prepares to move the handle from left to right. Three views are shown for each of three different trials, with the traces of each trial shown in separate rows. All trials were taken from the period during which the animal began to perform the task reasonably well over consecutive trials. The top magnified view illustrates the position of the IREDs and trajectories in a view of the distal extremity in the vicinity of the bar (shown by the crossed circle). The lines indicate the position of the stick figures at the beginning and end of this phase of the movement. The location of the individual IREDs are indicated by the filled circles along the lines (shoulder, elbow, wrist, and paw dorsum). The dotted line indicates the trajectory of the paw IRED from the beginning to the end of the movement's time course.

task was executed successfully over consecutive trials. Notice the differences in reaching and grasping characterized by the trajectories and the positions of the stick figures across the trials. Not only was the reach variable; the grasping of the bar was inconsistent from trial to trial. In the first and third trials, the bar was grasped with the limb on the side of the bar ipsilateral to the same extremity. After forming a grasp, the manipulandum was "pulled" through the first limb of the template. In contrast, in the second (middle) trial, the reaching limb passed on the opposite side of the mani-pulandum, and the paw "pushed" the device through this part of the tem-plate. Thus, even though the animal had acquired the capacity to perform the task on successive trials, the variability of the execution was extensive. This variability could not be ascribed only to the ataxia exhibited by the cat, because this degree of variability in performance was never seen when the animals' capacity to execute the task was tested during muscimol inactivation of the nuclei after the task had been learned. In contrast, when the task was learned by a naive animal during saline injection or relearned by an animal during the retraining period after first acquiring it with the nuclei inactivated, this type of variability was not seen. Figure 15.5 illustrates three trials per-formed just after the retraining period by the same animal whose movements are shown in figure 15.4. Notice the substantial decrease in the variability of these movements when the task was relearned in the absence of nuclear inactivation. The same consistent performance was observed for the naive saline control cats during the late acquisition period after the animals were capable of performing the task on consecutive trials.

IMPLICATIONS REGARDING ACQUISITION AND STORAGE

Our previously reviewed studies demonstrate that though cats were capable of learning a complex forelimb task with the ipsilateral interposed and dentate nuclei inactivated, the performance of the acquired movement was quite different from that observed following task acquisition in normal cats. These differences included a greater variability in the measurements characterizing the movements and in the use of different motor patterns to execute the task across successive trials. In fact, as shown in figures 15.4 and 15.5, when an animal was retrained on the task in the absence of any injection after first acquiring it during cerebellar nuclear inactivation, it adopted a different, very consistent strategy for performing the task. Significantly, the variability in motor performance observed during the later stages of acquisition while the nuclei were inactivated (see figure 15.4) did not reflect only the ataxia asso-ciated with lesions of these structures, because evaluation of the effects of muscimol on the performance of a previously learned template did not reveal this degree of variability.

The multiple single-unit data also are consistent with a special involvement of the cerebellum in the acquisition process. The increase in the amplitude of the task-related modulation of cerebellar nuclear neurons at the time the

Intact Cerebellum

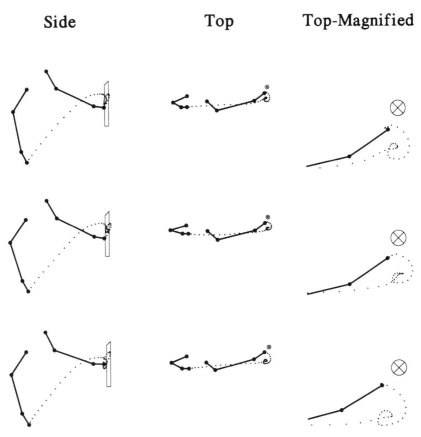

Side Top Top-Magnified

Figure 15.5 Characteristics of the same movement shown in figure 15.4 performed by the same cat in the absence of cerebellar nuclear inactivation after the retraining period. These three trials (shown in separate rows) show the consistency of this animal's performance during the late reacquisition period (see text for explanation). The consistency in the way the task is performed is identical to that of control animals acquiring the task for the first time. The nature of the stick figures and the trajectory of the paw are as described in the legend of figure 15.4. This cat consistently performed this part of the task in a movement with two components (a reach followed by a small additional movement during which it grasps the bar). Not all cats displayed this particular nuance at the final stage of the reaching movement; however, some cats did use strategies of this type as they learned to perform the task.

required motor sequence is first performed reasonably well may reflect a change in neuronal activity critical for establishing or specifying an optimal strategy for the task's performance and for reinforcing interactions required for establishing modifications in synaptic efficacy that likely accompany the learning process. Interestingly, the trend in the modulation of these cells during acquisition is consistent with the acquisition-related activation of cerebellar structures observed using positron emission tomography (Friston et al., 1992; Jenkins et al., 1994; Seitz et al., 1994; see also chapter) or functional magnetic resonance imaging (Flament et al., 1994) when human subjects are required to learn to perform novel volitional movements. This trend is also comparable to that of the occurrence of complex spike responses of Purkinje cells during the acquisition of a scaling task (Ojakangas and Ebner, 1992).

Elucidation of the specific nature of the information processing to which the cerebellar output contributes will require additional experiments. However, the time-course of these changes in modulation is not consistent with that expected based on theories regarding the mechanisms for establishing intracerebellar memory engrams related to the acquisition of motor skills (Marr, 1969; Albus, 1972; Gilbert and Thach, 1977; Ito, 1984). According to these views, the greatest modulation of cerebellar neuronal activity would be expected to be either directly or inversely proportional to the error signals reflecting the difference between the intended and the actual performance characteristics of the task, depending on the specific theory being considered. In the experiments reported here, the amplitude of the modulation first increased as the performance errors decreased. Furthermore, once the task could be performed reasonably well and any error signal was decreased substantially, the amplitude of modulation continued to decrease. Clearly, neither a simple direct or inverse relationship exists between the error signal and the magnitude of the nuclear cells' task-related modulation. Furthermore, in an experiment directly testing the Marr-Albus hypothesis using a paradigm requiring the learning of a complex, volitional upper-extremity movement in monkeys, Ebner et al. (see chapter 11) failed to show the relationship between the simple- and complex-spike activity during acquisition predicted by this theory. One of the strongest arguments against the acquisition-related change in modulation amplitude reflecting the establishment of memory traces within the cerebellum is derived from one of the other findings in our experiments. The microinjection of muscimol into the cerebellar nuclei either individually (Milak, Bracha, Kolb, and McAlduff, 1992) or simultaneously (Shimansky, Wang, Bloedel, and Bracha, 1994; figure 15.1) did not suppress the recall of the motor sequence required to execute the template task. Thus, it seems unlikely that the memory traces for the template-guided movement reside in the cerebellum.

HYPOTHESIS REGARDING CEREBELLAR INVOLVEMENT IN THE ACQUISITION OF COMPLEX VOLITIONAL FORELIMB MOVEMENTS

Based on the preceding observations, we propose that the cerebellum participates in the learning of complex volitional tasks in at least two ways: First, the cerebellum likely participates in the coordination of the movement sequence required to accomplish the task's objective. This postulate is far from controversial, because this structure's role in coordinating novel, goal-directed movements is well-known (see Gilman, Bloedel, and Lechtenberg,

1981 and Thach et al., 1992 for reviews). Specifically, we contend that the cerebellum is preferentially involved in certain projections capable of executing the desired movement and that this involvement enhances the coordination of initial movements employing this substrate. Furthermore, as a consequence of continued practice, the specific strategy or motor pattern mediated by this substrate becomes the strategy employed in the learned behavior when the task is recalled. Stated differently, this set of interactions provides a specific mechanism for determining which among the possible motor patterns or strategies available for performing the task is selected for execution as the behavior is learned. The selected strategy includes not only the organization of the phasic movements of the extremity but also the interactions required for motor planning and motor set (Hore and Vilis, 1984; Kim et al., 1994).

Second, we propose that the cerebellum contributes to the reinforcement required for the establishment of engrams generated as the task is learned. This proposal is not inconsistent with the finding that the template task can be learned while the cerebellar interposed and dentate nuclei are inactivated. Clearly, memory traces required for recalling specific motor sequences can be established in the absence of the cerebellum. However, our findings indicate that the way in which the task is performed is highly variable trial by trial when it is acquired in the absence of functional dentate and interposed nuclei. We further propose that these fluctuations in task performance reflect the failure of the motor control system first to coordinate optimally one or a few possible motor patterns and second to reinforce this strategy as the task is practiced. Even without the cerebellum, the animal is cognitively aware of the task's solution and, on the basis of this knowledge, can execute a movement which achieves the task's objective. However, the system fails to select adequately a relatively uniform motor pattern for this purpose. The importance of the cerebellum to the selection and reinforcement of a strategy for executing the behavior is emphasized by the fact that the system actually relearns the task when given the opportunity to execute it with the cerebellum, even though it had learned to perform it previously in the absence of this structure.

A diagram illustrating some of these concepts is shown in figure 15.6. According to this scheme, the structures responsible for formulating a motor plan can implement one of a subset of substrates (S1–S3), each of which can achieve the objectives of the task but with different motor patterns. Even in the performance of novel movements, a subset of all possible substrates is selected based on several factors that include previous experience and the extent to which the new task relates to previously learned behaviors. The online action of the cerebellum affects the activity more substantially in some of these pathways than others (S2 in this example). Through this set of interactions, the cerebellum increases the level of coordination with which that motor pattern can be executed, ensuring that this substrate can accomplish the objectives of the planned behavior more effectively than motor patterns mediated through other substrates (S1 and S3). The substrate most

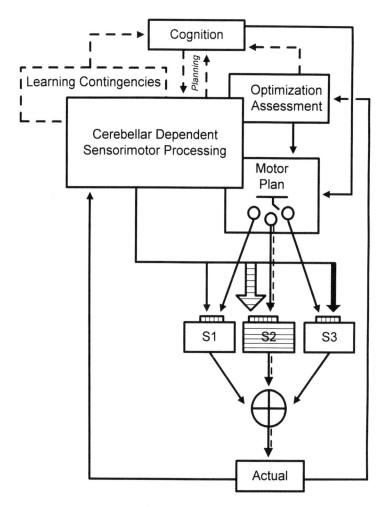

Figure 15.6 Conceptual scheme regarding the hypothetical role the cerebellum may play in the acquisition of complex, volitional forelimb movements. S1–3 = substrates.

affected by the cerebellar output undoubtedly will be task-dependent or, at the very least, dependent on certain contingencies of the task.

When a specific task is to be learned (dashed lines), additional interactions involving the cerebellum occur for selecting, performing, and improving the desired behavior. The multiple single-unit data presented earlier support the view that the cerebellum participates actively in this acquisition process. The involvement of the cerebellum in later stages of task acquisition also is supported by other recent imaging studies previously mentioned (Flament et al., 1994; Jenkins et al., 1994; Seitz et al., 1994). Our hypothesis is that the preferential interactions of the cerebellum within a specific substrate (S2) (and within structures responsible for the motor plan) assist in optimizing the task's performance, resulting in turn in the reinforcement of those pathways by which the behavior can be regulated and performed most effectively. As

Bloedel et al.

a consequence, plastic changes may be established in this projection as the task is first performed repetitively, and may be reinforced through the continued involvement of the cerebellum as the task continues to be practiced. Interestingly, if these changes in modulation amplitude reflect the cerebellum's participation in this type of process, all or a part of the movement sequence required to execute the task may be specified through these interactions, rather than only the component of the movement considered to be novel. Though not emphasized earlier in the description of the data, often the increased modulation amplitude of cerebellar nuclear neurons occurred in relation to task components *preceding* the learned movement through the template (e.g., reaching, paw liftoff, and bar contact) (Milak et al., 1995). Notice in figure 15.3 that the modulation of cells DN2 and PIN1–3 was primarily related to paw liftoff but yet underwent an increased modulation at the same time during the acquisition process as that which occurred for cells related to later components of the movement. The processes in which the cerebellum is involved also may include motor planning, as suggested by the data of Kim et al. (1994).

The diagram in figure 15.6 offers certain predictions regarding the consequence of cerebellar lesions on the acquisition process. Clearly, task acquisition can proceed without this structure through interactions responsible for cognitive aspects of the task, motor planning, and the assessment of the task's performance. However, notice that without the cerebellum, the on-line interactions responsible for optimizing the performance of the strategy mediated by S2 are not present. Consequently, although some basis for assessing the optimality of the task's performance remains, the differences in the effectiveness of the motor pattern mediated by each substrate are appreciably smaller than when the cerebellum is functional. A possible consequence is that the motor patterns used to perform a task acquired while the cerebellar nuclei are inactivated would be quite variable, a circumstance that definitely occurred in the experiments described above.

The preceding arguments require that plastic changes underlying the acquisition of volitional movements of the extremities take place outside the cerebellum, preferably at sites receiving converging inputs from simultaneously active cerebellar efferent projections and projections from other regions of the motor system. It should be emphasized that this contention does not exclude the possibility of plastic changes also occurring in the cerebellum, a possibility our experiments were not designed to analyze. However, the findings strongly suggest that the storage occurring at extracerebellar sites is at least adequate for recalling the motor sequence with which the task is executed. Animals either with individual cerebellar nuclei inactivated or with the ipsilateral interposed and dentate nuclei simultaneously inactivated still could recall the motor sequence required to execute the required task.

The location of extracerebellar sites supporting the plasticity established during the acquisition of the template task is not known. However, based on inferences drawn from the study of substrates required for the acquisition of other motor behaviors, the sites are likely to be in pathways responsible for the integration required for the execution of this specific type of task, as we previously proposed (Bloedel, Bracha, Kelly, and Wu, 1991). For example, there is now strong evidence that changes in synaptic efficacy occur at the level of the vestibular nuclei in the adaptation of the vestibuloocular reflex (Lisberger, Pavelko, and Broussard, 1994; Pastor et al., 1994). However, changes in synaptic efficacy established during the classical conditioning of the eyeblink reflex clearly involve different structures. Although plastic changes in the cerebellum are considered by some laboratories to be necessary and sufficient for the conditioning of this reflex (Krupa et al., 1993; Nordholm et al., 1993), sites serving this function either afferent (Bracha, Wu, Cartwright, and Bloedel, 1991) or efferent to the cerebellum (Berthier and Moore, 1980; Desmond and Moore, 1983; Rosenfield, Dovydaitis, and Moore, 1985) also are tenable based on current data regarding this system. Furthermore, this reflex can be conditioned in the absence of the cerebellum in the decerebrate rabbit (Kelly et al., 1990) and in the reduced brainstem preparation of the turtle (Keifer, 1993). In contrast, the classical conditioning of a different reflex system—the withdrawal reflex of the forelimb—may involve changes in synaptic efficacy in the thalamocortical system (Rispal-Padel and Meftah, 1992) and in the red nucleus (Murakami, Oda, and Tsukahara, 1988; Ito and Oda, 1994; Pananceau, Meftah, and Rispal-Padel, 1994). Significantly, the studies investigating the substrates supporting plastic changes related to the acquisition of the flexion withdrawal reflex indicate the involvement of *multiple* sites in establishing the required plastic changes. Based on these examples drawn from several different paradigms and behaviors, the plastic changes related to the acquisition of the template task employed in our experiments also are likely distributed among substrates involved in its execution.

The scheme in figure 15.6 also implies that the sites of the plastic changes are locations receiving convergent inputs from cerebellar efferents and other projections involved in mediating the behavior (Bloedel and Bracha, 1995). This principle is obeyed by the multiple sites currently believed to support the plastic changes in the conditioning of the forelimb flexion withdrawal reflex in the paradigm of Murakami et al. (1988), Rispal-Padel et al. (1994), and Ito and Oda (1994). This principle also applies to the plastic changes in the vestibular nuclei underlying VOR adaptation (Lisberger et al., 1994; Pastor et al., 1994).

CONCLUSION

Taken together, the findings in the literature and those from our laboratory strongly support at least three principles related to the sites at which plasticity is established during motor learning: (1) it occurs in task-specific pathways, (2) multiple locations can be involved, depending on the behavior, and (3) these sites often include the nuclei receiving converging projections from specific regions of the cerebellum and other fiber systems involved in the behavior. The importance of these convergent patterns in the control and acquisition of motor behaviors has been emphasized previously (Bloedel and Bracha, 1995). Additionally, it should be emphasized that none of the findings reported here has ruled out the possibility of plastic changes also occurring in the cerebellum. However, if intracerebellar engrams exist relative to the acquisition of the template task, they cannot be solely responsible for the recall of the task, at least across the conditions tested in our experiments. Consequently, based on the findings presented in this chapter and the available data on the substrates for adaptation and conditioning of various reflexes, we propose that the plastic changes established during the acquisition of complex, volitional motor behaviors are distributed over multiple sites that participate in regulating the required movement.

ACKNOWLEDGMENTS

These experiments were supported by National Institutes of Health grants R01 NS21958 and P01 NS30013. The authors also thank Shelley Webster, David Wunderlich, Kristina Irwin, and Richard Bauer for their help in the conduct of these experiments and data processing. We also thank Jan Carey for her help in preparing the manuscript.

REFERENCES

Albus JS (1971). A theory of cerebellar function. Math Biosci 10:25–61.

Berthier NE, Moore JW (1980). Disrupted conditioned inhibition of the rabbit nictitating membrane response following mesencephalic lesions. Physiol Behav 25:667–673.

Bloedel JR, Bracha V (1995). On the cerebellum, cutaneomuscular reflexes, movement control, and the elusive engrams of memory. Behav Brain Res 68:1–44.

Bloedel JR, Bracha V, Kelly TM, Wu J-Z (1991). Substrates for motor learning: Does the cerebellum do it all? In JR Wolpaw, JT Schmidt (eds), Activity-Driven Changes in Learning and Development. New York: New York Academy of Science, pp 305–318.

Bracha V, Stewart SL, Bloedel JR (1993). The temporary inactivation of the red nucleus affects performance of both conditioned and unconditioned nictitating membrane responses in the rabbit. Exp Brain Res 94:225–236.

Bracha V, Webster ML, Winters NK, Irwin KB, Bloedel JR (1994). Effects of muscimol inactivation of the cerebellar nucleus interpositus on the performance of the nictitating membrane response in the rabbit. Exp Brain Res 100:453–468.

Bracha V, Wu J-Z, Cartwright S, Bloedel JR (1991). Selective involvement of the spinal trigeminal nucleus in the conditioned nictitating membrane reflex of the rabbit. Brain Res 556: 317–320.

Cohen H, Cohen B, Raphan T, Waespe W (1992). Habituation and adaptation of the vestibuloocular reflex: A model of differential control by the vestibulocerebellum. Exp Brain Res 90:526–538.

Desmond JE, Moore JW (1983). A supratrigeminal region implicated in the classically conditioned nictitating membrane response. Brain Res Bull 10:765–773.

Flament D, Ellermann J, Ugurbil K, Ebner TJ (1994). Functional magnetic resonance imaging (fMRI) of cerebellar activation while learning to correct for visuomotor errors. Soc Neurosci Abstr 20:20.

Firston KJ, Frith CD, Passingham RE, Liddle PF, Frackowiak RSJ (1992). Motor practice and neurophysiological adaptation in the cerebellum: A positron tomography study. Proc R Soc Lond Biol Sci 248:223–228.

Gilbert PFC, Thach WT (1977). Purkinje cell activity during motor learning. Brain Res 128: 309–328.

Gilman S, Bloedel JR, Lechtenberg R (1981). Disorders of the Cerebellum. Philadelphia: Davis.

Hore J, Vilis T (1984). Loss of set in muscle responses to limb perturbations during cerebellar dysfunction. J Neurophysiol 51:1137–1148.

Ito M (1984). The Cerebellum and Neural Control. New York: Raven Press.

Ito M (1993). Cerebellar flocculus hypothesis. Nature 363:24–25.

Ito M, Oda Y (1994). Electrophysiological evidence for formation of new corticorubral synapses associated with classical conditioning in the cat. Exp Brain Res 99:277–288.

Jenkins IH, Brooks DJ, Nixon PD, Frackowiak RSJ, Passingham RE (1994). Motor sequence learning: A study with positron emission tomography. J Neurosci 14:3775–3790.

Keifer J (1993). The cerebellum and red nucleus are not required for classical conditioning of an in vitro model of the eye-blink reflex. Soc Neurosci Abstr 19:1001.

Kelly TM, Zuo C-C, Bloedel JR (1990). Classical conditioning of the eyeblink reflex in the decerebrate-decerebellate rabbit. Behav Brain Res 38:7–18.

Kim S-G, Urgurbil K, Strick PL (1994). Activation of a cerebellar output nucleus during cognitive processing. Science 265:949–951.

Krupa DJ, Thompson JK, Thompson RF (1993). Localization of a memory trace in the mammalian brain. Science 260:989–991.

Lisberger SG (1988). The neural basis for motor learning in the vestibulo-ocular reflex in monkeys. Trends Neurosci 11:147–152.

Lisberger SG, Pavelko TA, Broussard DM (1994). Neural basis for motor learning in the vestibuloocular reflex of primates. I. Changes in the responses of brain stem neurons. J Neurophysiol 72:928–953.

Marr D (1969). A theory of cerebellar cortex. J Physiol (Lond) 202:437–470.

Milak MS, Bracha V, Bloedel JR (1995). Relationship of simultaneously-recorded cerebellar nuclear neuron discharge to the acquisition of a complex, operantly conditioned forelimb movement in cats. Exp Brain Res 105:325–330.

Milak MS, Bracha V, Kolb F, McAlduff JD, Bloedel JR (1992). Selective effects of muscimol injections into cerebellar nuclei in cats performing both a locomotor and a reaching task. Soc Neurosci Abstr 18:1550.

Miles FA, Lisberger SG (1981). Plasticity in the vestibuloocular reflex: a new hypothesis. Annu Rev Neurosci 4:273–299.

Murakami F, Oda Y, Tsukahara N (1988). Synaptic plasticity in the red nucleus and learning. Behav Brain Res 28:175–179.

Nordholm AF, Thompson JK, Dersarkissian C, Thompson RF (1993). Lidocaine infusion in a critical region of cerebellum completely prevents learning of the conditioned eyeblink response. Behav Neurosci 107:882–886.

Ojakangas CL, Ebner TJ (1992). Purkinje cell complex and simple spike changes during a voluntary arm movement learning task in the monkey. J Neurophysiol 68:2222–2236.

Pannanceau M, Meftah EM, Rispal-Padel L (1994). Plasticity of the cerebello-rubral synapses during the conditioning of a forelimb motor response. Soc Neurosci Abstr 20:786.

Pastor AM, De la Cruz RR, Baker R (1994). Cerebellar role in adaptation of the goldfish vestibuloocular reflex. J Neurophysiol 72:1383–1394.

Peterson BW, Baker JF, Houk JC (1991). A model of adaptive control of vestibuloocular reflex based on properties of cross-axis adaptation. In JR Wolpaw, JT Schmidt (eds), Activity-Driven Changes in Learning and Development. New York: New York Academy of Sciences, pp 319–337.

Rispal-Padel L, Meftah E-M (1992). Changes in motor responses induced by cerebellar stimulation during classical forelimb flexion conditioning in cat. J Neurophysiol 68:908–926.

Robinson DA (1976). Adaptive gain control of vestibuloocular reflex by the cerebellum. J Neurophysiol 39:954–969.

Rosenfield M, Dovydaitis A, Moore JW (1985). Brachium conjunctivum and rubrobulbar tract: Brain stem projections of red nucleus essential for the conditioned nictitating membrane response. Physiol Behav 34:751–759.

Sanes JN, Dimitrov B, Hallett M (1990). Motor learning in patients with cerebellar dysfunction. Brain 113:103–120.

Seitz RJ, Canavan AGM, Yaguez L, Herzog H, Tellmann L, Knorr U, Huang Y, Homberg V (1994). Successive role of the cerebellum and premotor cortices in trajectorial learning. Neuroreport 5:2541–2544.

Shimansky Yu, Wang J-J, Bloedel JR, Bracha V (1994). Effects of inactivating the deep cerebellar nuclei on the learning of a complex forelimb movement. Soc Neurosci Abstr 20:21.

Stein JF, Glickstein M (1992). Role of the cerebellum in visual guidance of movement. Physiol Rev 72:967–1017.

Thach WT, Goodkin HP, Keating JG (1992). The cerebellum and the adaptive coordination of movement. Annu Rev Neurosci 15:403–442.

Thompson RF, Krupa DJ (1994). Organization of memory traces in the mammalian brain. Annu Rev Neurosci 17:519–549.

Timmann D, Shimansky Yu, Larson PS, Wunderlich DA, Stelmach GE, Bloedel JR (1994). Visuomotor learning in cerebellar patients. Soc Neurosci Abstr 20:21.

Weiner MJ, Hallett M, Funkenstein HH (1983). Adaptation to lateral displacement of vision in patients with lesions of the central nervous system. Neurology 33:766–772.

Welsh JP, Harvey JA (1991). Pavlovian conditioning in the rabbit during inactivation of the interpositus nucleus. J Physiol (Lond) 444:459–480.

Welsh JP, Harvey JA (1992). The role of the cerebellum in voluntary and reflexive movements: History and current status. In: RR Llinás, C Sotelo (eds), The Cerebellum Revisited. New York: Springer-Verlag, pp 301–334.

16 Sequential Hand and Finger Movements: Typing and Piano Playing

John F. Soechting, Andrew M. Gordon, and
Kevin C. Engel

We are very adept at using our hands and fingers to manipulate objects. The apparent ease with which we achieve such tasks as picking up a pen and then putting it to paper may obscure the actual challenges faced by the motor system in executing this task. In picking up the pen, typically all four fingers and the thumb make contact. This requires the proper orientation of the hand relative to the pen (Soechting and Flanders, 1993) and the shaping of the hand's posture so that its aperture is scaled appropriately to the pen's diameter (Jeannerod, 1984). At contact, the proper amount of force must be generated by each of the fingers, scaled to the object's texture and weight (Johansson and Cole, 1992). Each of these aspects of the task requires the coordination of a large number of degrees of freedom and, on its own, would appear to present considerable computational challenges. However, the next step appears to be more complicated yet.

For the pen to be used for writing, its orientation relative to the hand must be changed. In this process, contact forces in each of the fingers must vary dynamically. In fact, each of the fingers may periodically lose contact with the pen, and the points of contact may change over time. At this point, the pen is grasped firmly and writing may begin. Though little is known about how such a complex movement is controlled by the brain, it seems inconceivable that it is planned and executed as one unit from the initial grasp up to the time writing begins. It also seems inconceivable that the task can be executed in the absence of sensory information about the interaction of the hand with the environment (i.e., the contact forces) (Moberg, 1983). Instead, it would appear that the task can be understood better as consisting of a sequence of movements with sensory information affecting the execution of each element in the sequence and helping to determine the time at which each successive element is initiated.

Such a decomposition of a complex movement into an ordered sequence of simpler movements appears to be characteristic of a variety of motor tasks, such as tactile handling for object recognition, tool use, handwriting, and drawing (Schwartz, 1994; Soechting and Terzuolo, 1987a). In fact, it is tempting to speculate that all skilled, learned motor acts are built up from simpler elements. Accepting that speculation for the sake of discussion, two questions arise: (1) What are the simple elements and (2) how are they put together? A simple scheme for the organization of movement sequences would be that the elements are executed in a strictly serial order (i.e., the kinematics of one element would be unaffected by the element that came next). The generation of a movement sequence would then reduce to the problem of choosing the correct elements in the proper order, determining the time at which each elemental movement was initiated, and ensuring continuity of the movement from one element to the next.

Such a scheme appeared adequate to account for the kinematics of the arm during drawing movements executed in three-dimensional space (Soechting and Terzuolo, 1986, 1987b). During each elemental movement, the wrist approximated an elliptical arc generated by a sinusoidal modulation of the orientation angles (Soechting and Ross, 1984) of the arm. The plane of the hand's motion could change abruptly from one segment to the next (Soechting and Terzuolo, 1987a). In fact, this abrupt change in the plane of the motion led us to conclude that the motion was segmented. The force trajectory produced by subjects making three-dimensional drawing under isometric conditions exhibits a similar segmentation (Massey, Lurito, Pellizzer, and Georgopoulos, 1992; Pellizzer, Massey, Lurito, and Georgopoulos, 1992), suggesting that this effect was not due to the limb's inertial properties.

However, studies of another type of skilled movement suggest that such a simple serial ordering may not hold true in all cases. Researchers studying speech production have described the phenomenon termed *coarticulation*, in which the acoustic quality of one phoneme is altered by the subsequent phoneme, implying that the movements to produce two successive phonetic segments overlap (Kent and Adams, 1989). For example, the letter *s* in the word *soon* is generated with rounded lips, whereas they are not rounded when the letter *s* precedes an unrounded vowel, as in *seen*. Assuming each phoneme corresponds to an elemental movement, in speech it appears that the kinematics of the motor apparatus (vocal cords, tongue, jaw, and lips) for a particular element in a sequence are subject to modification by succeeding elements.

In this chapter, we describe some of our recent results on the generation of movement sequences of the hands and fingers. We have chosen two tasks that share some similarities but also exhibit differences in the task constraints: typing and piano playing. The timing of the key presses in typing has been well-studied, and this topic has been reviewed in detail by Viviani and Terzuolo (1983). Both tasks require the depression of a series of keys in a serial order, and it seems reasonable to associate a movement element with each key press. Both tasks require practice to attain proficiency and both require coordinated movements of all the fingers of both hands.

Aside from these similarities, there are major differences between the requirements of the two tasks. The most significant one is that piano playing imposes a rhythmic requirement on the timing of the key presses, whereas typing has no implicit timing requirements other than that the keys be struck in the proper order. There are other differences as well: In typing, the key is first struck with a force that need not be tightly regulated and then quickly released, whereas in piano playing, the speed with which the key is depressed influences the loudness of the tone and the key must remain depressed for a specified period of time. In contrast to typing, the piano-playing task requires subjects to press several keys at once, typically bimanually. In typing, there is a one-to-one association between the key and the finger used to strike the key, and typists are trained to begin movements from a stereotypical posture (the "home position"), to strike the key, and then to return back to the home position. In contrast, in piano playing there is no unique relation between the key and the finger used to depress it, and pianists are trained to "look ahead" (i.e., to anticipate the movements of the hand and fingers long before they are executed). Thus, one might expect to find the equivalent of "coarticulation" in the generation of movement sequences in piano playing.

In view of both the similarities and the differences between the demands of typing and piano playing, one can expect that studying the motion of the hands and fingers during these tasks should provide insights into the general question of how movement sequences are learned and controlled—how the large number of degrees of freedom of the hand is coordinated and the extent to which task constraints shape the kinematics. In fact, we found both similarities and differences in the hand movements for typing and piano playing.

RECORDING FINGER AND HAND MOTION

The methods used to characterize the motion of the hands and fingers during these tasks have been described in detail elsewhere (Flanders and Soechting, 1992). We used a video camera at a frame rate of 100 Hz interfaced to a personal computer to record bimanual hand movements, placing reflective markers proximally at the metacarpophalangeal (MCP) joint and at the distal interphalangeal (DIP) joint of each finger. An example of the results for typing is shown in figure 16.1. In this illustration, the proximal and distal markers on each finger of the right hand have been connected, as have the four proximal markers on the hand. The recording system provides a description of the hand's motion in the keyboard plane, but it ignores the component of motion perpendicular to this plane.

Thus, we did not attempt to describe in detail the motion at each of the joints of each finger. Instead, we used the four proximal markers to describe the motion of the hand (resulting from rotation at the shoulder, elbow, and wrist) and the motion of the four distal markers relative to the proximal markers to describe the finger motions. Wrist motion was characterized as a translation of the hand (along the x-axis in the direction of the rows of the typewriter keyboard and along the y-axis perpendicular to the rows) and a rotation of the wrist. Translations directed laterally and anteriorly are defined to be *positive*, as are rotations in the clockwise direction. For example, in figure 16.1 (top row), the wrist is rotated in the negative, counterclockwise

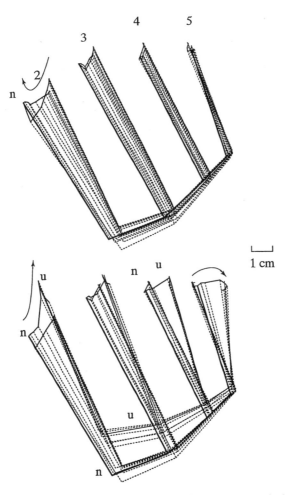

Figure 16.1 Motion of the hand and fingers in typing the letter *n* (top) and the combination *nu* (bottom). The location of markers placed at the MCP and DIP joints of the fingers of the right hand is shown at 100-ms intervals. The direction of the motion of the index finger (2) is indicated by the arrows. Points connected by solid lines denote the posture of the hand at the time the keys *n* and *u* are depressed. Data are averages of trials aligned on the time of the key press of the letter *n*.

direction. Two parameters describe the motion of each finger: the change in distance between proximal and distal markers, and the change in the orientation of each finger (measured relative to the *y*-direction). The fingers are numbered conventionally, starting with the thumb. Thus, in figure 16.1 (top row), the index finger (2) initially undergoes a negative, counterclockwise rotation, whereas the rotation of the middle (3) and ring fingers (4) is smaller.

For typing, we also recorded the key and the time at which each key was struck. Time was measured with a 1-ms resolution. In those experiments, we used a standard 101-key computer keyboard. For piano playing, we used an electronic keyboard interfaced to a personal computer, and we also recorded the time at which each key was released and the speed with which the key was depressed.

TYPING

During typing, key presses produced by *one hand* are executed in strictly serial fashion; the movement to the subsequent key press is not initiated until the first key has been pressed, and the kinematics of the first key press are unaffected by the particular key that is struck thereafter (Soechting and Flanders, 1992). The two hands move independently of each other and the movements executed by *alternating hands* overlap in time (Flanders and Soechting, 1992). Surprisingly, despite the hand's large number of degrees of freedom and the corresponding potential to execute a key press by a variety of movements, hand and finger movements during typing were highly stereotypical. Generally, all the fingers were in motion when a particular key was struck.

We came to these conclusions by asking subjects to type short phrases containing words that had a peculiar characteristic: all but one or two of the letters were typed with the left hand. For example, we used such words as *standard, banners, denuded,* and *canoes.* Thus we were able to study the kinematics of an isolated element in the sequence (i.e., the letter *n*) and pairs of elements (e.g., *no*) performed in their natural context. The top row in figure 16.1 shows a stick figure diagram of the motion of the right hand typing the letter *n*. The dashed lines indicate hand posture every 100 ms, with the motion proceeding in the direction of the arrow. The posture of the hand at the time the letter *n* is struck is indicated by heavier, solid lines.

The movement illustrated in figure 16.1 is the average of 21 trials, aligned on the time of key press. The lighter solid lines in figure 16.2 show the translation and rotation of the wrist for this average and the rotation and length of each of the fingers, plotted as a function of time. The lighter dashed lines denote the standard deviation of this average. The heavier solid and dashed lines in figure 16.2 denote the average and standard deviation of the average hand and finger motion to type the sequence *nu*, also aligned on the time of key press of the letter *n*. The stick figure plot for these same trials is shown in the lower plot of figure 16.1. Up to the time of keypress of the *n*, the kinematics of the hand and finger are statistically indistinguishable (Soechting and Flanders, 1992). Within 20 ms of the key press, the trajectories diverge, the hand returning to the home position in the case of the isolated letter *n* and proceeding toward the next letter when the combination *nu* is typed.

The results shown in figures 16.1 and 16.2 are representative of results obtained in all three subjects we studied and for all letter combinations. In particular, we did not find any instance in which the initial hand and finger movements were modified in anticipation of the next element in the movement sequence, either when the same finger was used to type both letters (as

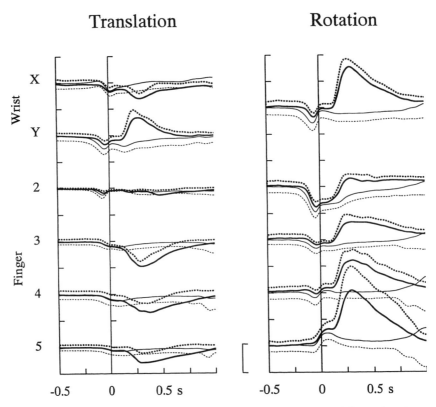

Figure 16.2 Hand and finger kinematics for the letter *n* (light traces) and the combination *nu* (heavier traces). Motion of the wrist is defined by the average translation of the four MCP markers in the *x*- (lateral) and *y*- (anterior) direction, and by the rotation of the wrist (right column). Motion of each finger is defined by the length between the MCP and DIP markers (left column), and the change in each finger's orientation relative to the anterior direction (right column). Averages (aligned on the time of key press of the letter *n*) are denoted by solid lines, and the dashed lines denote ± 1 SD. The calibration bar corresponds to 12.5 mm for translation and 10 degrees for rotation.

in the case illustrated) or when two different fingers of one hand were used. In all instances, motion toward the second target began within 20 ms of the first key press. Thus typing movements executed by one hand are executed in strictly serial fashion.

Each keystroke involves the coordinated motion of the hand and of all the fingers of the hand, including those that do not strike the key. For example, the letter *n* is struck by rotating the wrist in a counterclockwise direction, pivoting about the MCP joint of the little finger (figure 16.1). The index finger (2), used to strike the key, is initially abducted (figures 16.1 and 16.2), and the distance between MCP and DIP joints decreases. However, all the other fingers also flex and rotate. For example, fingers 3 and 4 are also rotated, by a lesser amount in the counterclockwise direction, whereas finger 5 is rotated in the clockwise direction. The pattern for a particular subject is highly repeatable, as evidenced by the small and constant standard deviations of each trace in figure 16.2. Because of the large number of degrees of freedom, the pattern of motion can be different for different subjects.

The fingers do not move independently of each other. To ascertain this, we (Fish and Soechting, 1992) asked typists to type a series of words in which each of the letters of the alphabet appeared once, and in which all of the other letters were typed with fingers of the opposite hand. We then computed pairwise correlation coefficients for the motions of the fingers. The motions of adjacent fingers tended to be highly and positively correlated, and the motions of nonadjacent fingers showed lesser degrees of correlation. Correlation coefficients for fingers 3 and 4 were higher on average than those for fingers 2 and 5, indicating a lesser degree of individuation of the movements of the middle and ring fingers. Finally, the extent to which the motion of pairs of fingers was correlated was less when one of the two fingers was used to strike the key. This indicates that the extent of coupling of finger movement is task-dependent and that the fingers can be moved more independently of each other when this is required by the task.

These results are consistent with observations by Schieber (1991) on finger movements in monkeys trained to make individuated finger flexions or extensions with each of their digits. In general, he also found that the remaining digits tended to move in parallel with the instructed digit. More recently, Schieber (1995) examined the patterning of muscle activation underlying these instructed individuated movements and found that each instructed movement was generated by combined activation of several muscles, many acting on more than one digit.

The results we have discussed thus far show that the motion of the hand in typing a letter represents a stereotyped pattern with a high degree of coupling of the motion of all fingers. Furthermore, this pattern is not altered to accommodate the production of subsequent keystrokes. However the two hands move independently of each other. Normally, the keystrokes for pairs of letters executed by alternating hands overlap in time. In fact, the time between key presses executed by alternating hands tends to be shorter than the time between key presses executed with the same hand (Terzuolo and Viviani, 1980; Viviani and Terzuolo, 1983). The motion of one hand (and of the fingers of that hand) does not influence the motion of the other hand. We (Flanders and Soechting, 1992) demonstrated this by asking subjects to type a set of words, each containing the same letter typed with the right hand (e.g., *h*) but surrounded by different letters typed with the other hand (e.g. *cashews*, *wretched*, and *bathwater*). The kinematics of the wrist and fingers were the same for the letter *h*, irrespective of the letters typed with the left hand. We also computed pairwise correlation coefficients between the motion of the corresponding fingers of each hand. The between-hands correlations were clustered around zero, and only 7.7 percent of the values exceeded the 95 percent-confidence limit for a correlation coefficient that did not differ from zero. (Thus the number of correlation coefficients deemed significant was about what one would expect by chance.)

So far, we have shown that each keystroke can be considered to be a discrete element in a movement sequence. Other results suggest that each keystroke itself may consist of three distinct components: an approach phase bringing the finger from the home position to a location above the key, striking the key, and a return phase bringing the hand back to the starting posture. Part of the evidence in favor of such a parcellation comes from experiments in which we (Angelaki and Soechting, 1993) intentionally varied the interval between successive key presses. Changing the rhythm of typing over a threefold interval affected the speed of the movements but in a nonuniform manner. In general, the velocity of the fingers at the time of key press did not vary with key press intervals, but the speed with which the hand approached the target did; the longer the interval between successive key presses, the longer was the time taken to approach the key. This observation suggests that the approach phase constitutes a distinct component of the overall movement.

Other evidence suggests that the return back to the home position also represents a distinct component. We have already shown (see figure 16.2) that this component is omitted when the next letter is typed with the same hand. We also found that this component sometimes may be suppressed when the next letter typed with the hand is the same as the one just typed, but there are intervening letters typed with the other hand (such as in the word *vengeance*). In such instances, subjects sometimes returned back to the home position after typing the first *n* and later repeated the entire movement to type the second *n*. However in other instances subjects were more economical, and the index finger remained poised over the *n* after the initial movement.

What determines the time at which each keystroke is initiated? When two successive keystrokes are performed with the same hand, the second one is initiated within 20 ms of the first key press (figure 16.2). When alternate hands are used, the movements overlap, and the second keystroke is initiated before the time of the first key press. Thus, tactile information generated by finger keyboard contact cannot be used as a cue for the initiation of the next element in the sequence. Nevertheless, it is possible that such cues could be used to initiate the movement after that. Alternatively, the initiation of each elemental movement could be internally triggered, based on the expected times of the key presses. Even so, tactile afferent information (and more generally, information about the successful execution of each element in the sequence) could be used to maintain the typing rhythm. Such a possibility is suggested by the observation of Terzuolo and Viviani (1980) that the normal pattern of key press intervals is disturbed when subjects do not make contact with the keyboard with the fingers of one hand by typing in air.

To investigate the role of tactile afferent information in the generation of finger movement sequences, we conducted a series of experiments in which we anesthetized the tip of the right index finger (Gordon and Soechting,

Soechting, Gordon, and Engel

1995). Subjects were still able to move the finger but no longer had any sensation of touch or pressure on its distal portion. We expected that if subjects did make use of tactile information as a cue to initiate elements in the movement sequence, we would find a disruption in the normal pattern of intervals between key presses. In particular, one would expect that one of the intervals (perhaps the second or third) following a key press with the anesthetized finger would be affected by being prolonged or shortened or by becoming more variable. One also would expect that suppression of information about the timing of key presses executed by the right index finger would lead to an increase in timing errors (i.e., transposition of typed letters).

To our surprise, movement timing was not affected by this intervention. All the intervals following a key press of the anesthetized finger were comparable to values obtained in the control condition prior to digital anesthesia. Two of the six subjects who were studied showed a uniform increase in typing rate after anesthesia, but this decrease in intervals was uniform for the six intervals following a key press of the index finger. (Subjects normally show variations in typing rate [Terzuolo and Viviani, 1980] with a uniform scaling of all intervals.) Furthermore, the variability in the intervals following a key press of the right index finger was uniform. Finally, the proportion of typing errors attributable to timing errors did not increase. Together, all these observations indicate that tactile afferent information is not essential for the properly timed initiation of each keystroke.

Tactile afferent information is important for movement accuracy and for the detection of errors, however. Following digital anesthesia, the probability of a misdirected movement of the anesthetized finger (i.e., one in which an adjacent key is struck) increased dramatically, as shown in the histogram on the left in figure 16.3. Averaged over the six subjects in this study, the frequency of aiming errors made by the right index finger increased about 10-fold, from approximately 0.5 percent to approximately 6 percent. The probability of aiming errors made by the other fingers showed little change. (The increase in the frequency of errors made with the right little finger may be anomalous because of the small sample size of key presses with that finger.) There was variability among individual subjects, some subjects' accuracy showing a much greater susceptibility to digital anesthesia than others. However, all subjects showed a statistically significant increase in misdirected movements of their right index finger.

When tactile cues were absent, subjects no longer recognized that they made errors with the anesthetized finger. Normally, the interval immediately following a mistyped letter is greatly prolonged (figure 16.3, right panel). Since typical interkey intervals range from 60 ms to 200 ms (Terzuolo and Viviani, 1980), this implies that subjects are able to recognize errors very quickly and that they are also able to interrupt quickly a successive movement. As can be seen in figure 16.3, the interkey intervals following an error made with the anesthetized index finger did not differ from normal. Other

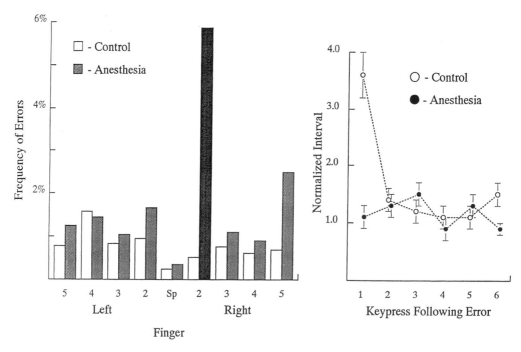

Figure 16.3 Effect of digital anesthesia of the right index finger on the frequency of errors made with each finger and on the intervals of key presses following an error made with the right index finger. The histogram on the left shows the probability of striking an adjacent key with each of the finger of the hand under control conditions and following digital anesthesia. The data are a composite of results from six subjects. On the right are shown the first six intervals between key presses following a typing error under control conditions and that following digital anesthesia. Key press intervals have been normalized with respect to the mean interval in correctly typed phrases. Normally, the first interval following an error is significantly prolonged. The prolongation is absent following digital anesthesia. Data are from one subject.

errors made by the same subjects in the same context did lead to a prolongation of the next interval. Therefore this finding suggests that subjects failed to recognize errors in the absence of tactile information.

Because information signaled by afferents from muscle stretch receptors should not have been affected by the digital anesthesia, the decrease in movement accuracy and the failure to recognize errors suggest that information from cutaneous afferents may contribute importantly to encoding the posture of the fingers. In our experimental situation, postural information may have been signaled by tactile afferents in a fairly simple way: The raised edge on the keys in the home row can be used potentially to standardize the starting posture of the movement. Thus increased variability in the starting posture could have contributed to a decrease in their accuracy of the movement. Some recent observations by Lackner and DiZio (1994) suggest that tactile afferents may encode postural information. In particular, they found that tactile cues at the end of an arm movement facilitated the adaptation to movement errors induced by Coriolis forces. We (Helms Tillery, Flanders, and Soechting, 1994) have suggested that tactile cues may be needed to potentiate information signaled by proprioceptors.

Before leaving the subject of typing, we should mention that it is a motor task involving sensory and cognitive as well as motor processes and that it is a skill that requires considerable practice for one to become proficient. When a typist types from a written text, as in our experiments, visual cortical areas are obviously engaged. Language areas are also involved in this task. For example, it is well-known (cf. Viviani and Terzuolo, 1983) that common words tend to be typed more quickly than less common words and that words that exist in a particular language are typed faster than are strings of letters which obey orthographic conventions of the language but have no meaning. Strings of letters that are unpronounceable are typed at an even slower rate. The patterning of typing intervals also suggests that the elemental keystrokes are grouped word by word, or for longer words, syllable by syllable.

One would expect other cortical areas, in addition to visual and language areas, to be involved as well. Ultimately, the task requires a sequence of movements directed at spatially defined goals, namely the keys on the keyboard. There is an association of a particular movement and a particular finger with each letter. Conceivably, this association could be direct, but it is also conceivable that there could be an intervening step: Each letter could be associated with a particular locus in space and, in turn, each spatial locus could be associated with a particular movement. We (Gordon, Casabona, and Soechting, 1994) have recently carried out some experiments aimed at distinguishing between these two possibilities.

LEARNING NEW TYPING SKILLS

We examined the changes in hand kinematics that occurred as subjects were required to learn a novel sequence of movements. In particular, we switched pairs of keys on the computer keyboard and examined the changes in timing of key presses and the patterns of finger movements as subjects adapted to the novel layout of the keyboard. As will be appreciated by anyone who has used a keyboard in a foreign country or a computer keyboard with a slightly different arrangement of keys, such a novel arrangement is learned relatively quickly. Initially, typing rate does decrease, primarily because there is a delay before the switched key is struck and a delay before the subsequent key is struck. All other intervals in a given word are unaffected. We also found a delay before the subject began to type words that contained a switched letter but not before words without switched letters. This particular observation supports an organization of typing at the word level, as well as at the level of individual letters, in agreement with conclusions from previous studies described above.

Whereas the key press of a switched letter was delayed, the kinematics of the keystroke were normal. In general, the time from a movement's initiation to the time of key press was the same as under control conditions, before the keys had been switched. Peak velocity of the movement was sometimes faster with the novel layout of the keyboard. Had the subjects actually learned a novel movement, we would have expected the movements to be initially performed much more slowly, with speed increasing as learning progressed. The fact that movement kinematics were essentially unchanged argues for a different interpretation of what is learned in this task; subjects learn to associate a new spatial locus with the key but maintain a constancy in the association between spatial locus and movement. Thus in this particular task, learning (or more precisely, relearning) appears to proceed at a fairly abstract level.

PIANO PLAYING

As mentioned earlier, though there are similarities between the tasks of typing and piano playing, there are also substantial differences in the requirements of these two motor tasks. Recently, we have begun to study piano playing to determine whether the sequential nature of the execution of finger movements of one hand in typing holds true for piano playing, as well. If in fact each keystroke in piano playing were executed sequentially and were found to be unaffected by the notes that followed, one would conclude that the strict sequential ordering of hand movements reflected a neural constraint, especially as pianists are explicitly trained to look and plan ahead. However, there does not appear to be such a neural constraint, because we have found instances in which a particular movement sequence is altered to facilitate the execution of subsequent elements.

Figure 16.4 provides one example of the task we presented to our subjects. In the two selections, the first four notes played with the right hand are identical diverging thereafter. The numbers above each note indicate the finger that is used to play that note. This example illustrates one of the characteristics of piano playing: there is no one-to-one correspondence between a particular note and the finger that plays it. In both examples, the fourth note (D) is the same, but it is played with the ring finger (4) in figure 16.4A and with the thumb (1) in figure 16.4B. (That is because the notes in part B are on an ascending scale, requiring a repositioning of the hand to maintain the continuity of the movement.) The notes played with the left hand are also different in the two examples. As was mentioned earlier, we showed that the two hands move independently of each other during typing. We assumed that this was also true for piano playing and consequently, we focused solely on the motion of the right hand.

Figures 16.5 and 16.6 show stick figure diagrams of the right hand for the two selections illustrated in figure 16.4. The motion of the hand for the first selection (part A) is shown in figure 16.5 and that for the second selection

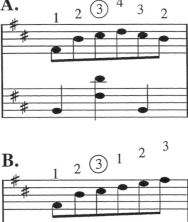

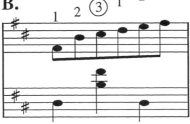

Figure 16.4 Examples of musical selections chosen to test serial ordering of finger movements during piano playing. In both selections (adopted from *Valse Mélancolique* by V Rebikoff), the first three notes for the right hand are identical and are played with the same fingers. Thereafter, there is a divergence. In A, the fourth note is played with the ring finger (4), whereas the thumb (1) is used in B.

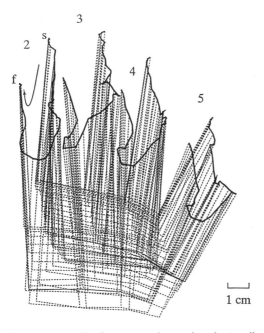

Figure 16.5 Hand motion in playing the selection illustrated in figure 16.4A. The posture of the right hand is illustrated every 50 ms, beginning with the posture at the time the first key is depressed. The direction of the movement is indicated by the arrows, progressing from s (start) to f (finish).

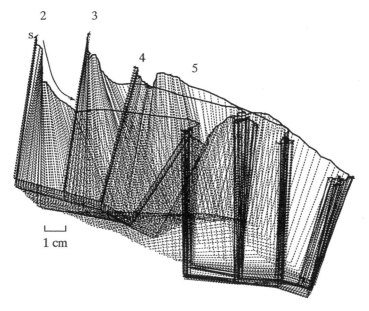

Figure 16.6 Hand motion in playing the selection illustrated in figure 16.4B. The data are from one trial by the same subject as studied in figure 16.5. Changes in posture every 10 ms are shown in this instance, beginning with the depression of the first key.

(part B) is shown in figure 16.6. The letter *s* indicates the start of the movement (the depression of the first key), and the motion progresses in the direction of the arrows. In figure 16.5, the hand is translated in a path that appears to be roughly elliptical in a clockwise progression, hand motion being directed initially proximally, then to the left, and finally distally. In figure 16.6, the motion is initially the same. This can best be appreciated by examining the path of the index finger DIP joint. In both figure 16.5 and figure 16.6, this point initially follows a curved path counterclockwise proximally and to the left. Then there is a translation of this point along an approximately straight line, directed proximally, after which the two paths diverge. In figure 16.5, the path continues proximally, looping to the left. In figure 16.6, the index finger DIP joint is translated to the right and proximally. In figure 16.6, it is clear that during this period the wrist undergoes a rotation in the counterclockwise direction. This is best observed by inspecting the lines connecting DIP and MCP joints on the index and middle fingers. This part of the movement ("crossing under") is preparatory to placing the thumb (1, not shown in the figures) in position to play the fourth note. Thereafter, the hand is rotated back in the clockwise direction and remains relatively stationary for a period of time.

The question now is, at what time, relative to the playing of each of the notes, do the two sets of movements begin to diverge? The answer to this question is provided in figure 16.7, which shows the averages and standard deviations of 15 trials for each of the two selections, aligned on the time of

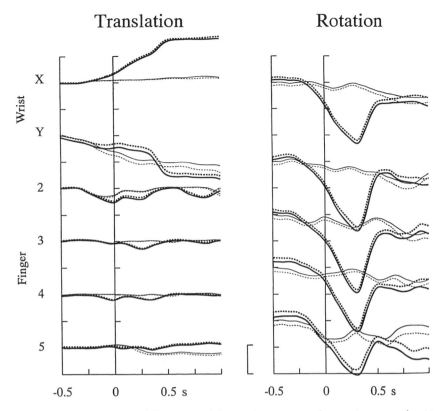

Figure 16.7 Kinematics of the wrist and fingers during piano playing. Averages of wrist and finger motion for the two selections illustrated in figure 16.4 are shown, aligned on the time of depression of the last common key (C#, played with the right middle finger). Lighter traces correspond to the selection in A, the heavier traces to the selection shown in B. Note that the two sets of traces begin to diverge about 200 ms before time 0. The data are plotted to the same scale as in figure 16.2, except for wrist translation (5.0 cm/division for x, 2.5 cm/division for y).

the depression of the last key (C#, circled in figure 16.4) that the two pieces have in common. The format of figure 16.7 is identical to that of figure 16.2. It is clear in figure 16.7 that the two sets of traces begin to diverge long before time 0. Both the translation of the wrist in the x- and y-direction and the rotation of the wrist and fingers differ substantially. In relation to the time at which each of the notes was played, the movements begin to diverge at about the time that the note prior to the last common note (i.e., B) is played.

This observation was true for all four subjects who played this selection. Three of the four subjects also showed such anticipatory modifications of the sequence of hand and finger movements for another pair of selections. For two other pieces, however, the finger and wrist motions were identical up to the time to depress the last key that the two selections had in common.

It is noteworthy that in piano playing, as in the case of typing, there is little trial-to-trial variability in the kinematics (see figure 16.7). Thus the movement sequences are assembled in a highly stereotypical fashion. It is also noteworthy that even when we did find anticipatory modifications of the trajectories of the hand and fingers, these modifications became evident only one note in advance. Thus, although there is look-ahead processing in the case of piano playing, such look-ahead processing generally does not appear to encompass the entire phrase.

CONCLUSIONS

In this chapter, we have focused on one principal topic—how sequences of hand and finger movements are assembled. We studied two different motor tasks—typing and piano playing—and found both similarities and differences in the results obtained by studying both these tasks. For typing, the sequence of hand and finger movements of one hand appears to be assembled in a strictly sequential manner; the demands of an upcoming movement do not alter the kinematics of the preceding movement. In some cases, the kinematics of piano playing also appear to conform to this rule. However, in other instances we found that the motion of the hand and finger for a given key press could be modified to facilitate an upcoming movement. In this regard, piano playing appears to be more similar to speech production than to typing.

Therefore coarticulation appears to be a general feature of the assembly of movement sequences, in the sense that the neural controller is not limited to a strict serial ordering of the individual elements comprising a movement sequence. Nevertheless, it would appear that unless the task actually demands anticipatory modification of movement elements, these elements are assembled in a serial fashion. Clearly, such a rule would provide for a simplification of the control problem, as there would be a one-to-one correspondence between elemental movements and task elements (such as keys in typing or piano playing). The number of possible movements would increase dramatically if the kinematics were to be determined by all possible pairwise combinations. For example in typing, 15 keys are struck with the fingers of the left hand (excluding numerical and function keys). If each keystroke were to depend on the upcoming key as well, this would lead to 15^2 or 225 possible keystrokes.

Why do subjects exhibit anticipatory modifications of their hand movements during piano playing and not during typing? One can only speculate on this question, but nevertheless it may be useful to consider some of the task differences and their possible importance. First, we should mention that differences in skill levels cannot account for the difference. Both our typists and piano players exhibited a range of proficiency on the tasks. Both highly skilled pianists and those who were not as proficient exhibited anticipatory modification of the finger movements in the example illustrated here. By the same token, we have never found an example of look-ahead processing in the typists we have studied.

Both typing and piano playing require a serial ordering of the depression of keys with the fingers. Piano playing also imposes rhythmic demands on the task; each key should be pressed at a specified time and should remain depressed for a time also specified. These temporal constraints are not present in typing. In fact, the intervals between key presses are highly nonuniform in typing (Terzuolo and Viviani, 1980), and some of this nonuniformity is attributable to biomechanical factors. Thus one possibility is that anticipatory modification of the kinematic elements in a sequence is invoked whenever there are temporal constraints on the performance. This could account for the differences between typing and piano playing, and it is also compatible with the coarticulation found in speech.

Though we have focused on the rules whereby a sequence of hand and finger movements are assembled, the study of typing and piano playing also can provide insights into a variety of other issues pertaining to the control and coordination of hand movements. These issues include, among others, (1) bimanual coordination of movements and the extent to which the two hands can move independently, (2) the extent to which movements of each finger can be controlled independently, (3) the role of sensory information in generating movement sequences, and most pertinent to the present volume, (4) the learning of skilled movements.

ACKNOWLEDGMENT

This work was supported by grants from the US Public Health Service NS-15018 and by the National Science Foundation BNS 90-21244. A. M. Gordon was supported by a National Research Service Award (NS-09509).

REFERENCES

Angelaki DE, Soechting JF (1993). Non-uniform temporal scaling of hand and finger kinematics during typing. Exp Brain Res 95:319–329.

Fish J, Soechting JF (1992). Synergistic finger movements in a skilled motor task. Exp Brain Res 91:327–334.

Flanders M, Soechting JF (1992). Kinematics of typing: Parallel control of the two hands. J Neurophysiol 67:1264–1274.

Gordon AM, Casabona A, Soechting JF (1994). The learning of novel finger movement sequences. J Neurophysiol 72:1596–1610.

Gordon AM, Soechting JF (1995). Use of tactile afferent information in sequential finger movements. Exp Brain Res 107:281–292.

Helms Tillery SI, Flanders M, Soechting JF (1994). Errors in kinesthetic transformations for hand apposition. Neuroreport 6:177–181.

Jeannerod M (1984). The timing of natural prehension movements. J Mot Behav 16:235–254.

Johansson RS, Cole KJ (1992). Sensory-motor coordination during grasping and manipulative actions. Curr Opin Neurobiol 2:815–823.

Kent RD, Adams SG (1989). The concept and measurement of coordination in speech disorders. In SA Wallace (ed), Perspectives on the Coordination of Movement. New York: North-Holland, pp 415–450.

Lackner JR, DiZio P (1994). Rapid adaptation to Coriolis force perturbations of arm trajectory. J Neurophysiol 72:299–313.

Massey JT, Lurito JT, Pellizzer G, Georgopoulos AP (1992). Three-dimensional drawings in isometric conditions: Relation between geometry and kinematics. Exp Brain Res 88:685–690.

Moberg E (1983). The role of cutaneous afferents in position sense, kinaesthesia and motor function of the hand. Brain 106:1–19.

Pellizzer G, Massey JT, Lurito JT, Georgopoulos AP (1992). Three-dimensional drawings in isometric conditions: Planar segmentation of force trajectory. Exp Brain Res 92:326–337.

Schieber MH (1991). Individuated finger movements of rhesus monkeys: A means of quantifying the independence of the digits. J Neurophysiol 65:1381–1391.

Schieber MH (1995). Muscular production of individuated finger movements: The roles of extrinsic finger muscles. J Neurosci 15:284–297.

Schwartz AB (1994). Direct cortical representation of drawing. Science 265:540–542.

Soechting JF, Flanders M (1992). Organization of sequential typing movements. J Neurophysiol 67:1275–1290.

Soechting JF, Flanders M (1993). Parallel, interdependent channels for location and orientation in sensorimotor transformations for reaching and grasping. J Neurophysiol 70:1137–1150.

Soechting JF, Ross B (1984). Psychophysical determination of coordinate representation of human arm orientation. Neuroscience 13:595–604.

Soechting JF, Terzuolo CA (1986). An algorithm for the generation of curvilinear wrist motion in an arbitrary plane in three-dimensional space. Neuroscience 19:1395–1405.

Soechting JF, Terzuolo CA (1987a). Organization of arm movements. Motion is segmented. Neuroscience 23:39–52.

Soechting JF, Terzuolo CA (1987b). Organization of arm movements in three-dimensional space. Wrist motion is piece-wise planar. Neuroscience 23:53–61.

Terzuolo CA, Viviani P (1980). Determinants and characteristics of motor patterns used for typing. Neuroscience 5:1085–1103.

Viviani P, Terzuolo C (1983). The organization and control of movement in handwriting and typing. In B Butterworth (ed), Language Production. London: Academic Press, vol 2, pp 103–146.

V   Perspectives of Motor Learning

17 Substrates and Mechanisms for Learning in Motor Cortex

John P. Donoghue, Grzegorz Hess, and Jerome N. Sanes

In this chapter, we discuss the evidence for involvement of primary motor cortex (MI) in various forms of learning. After defining motor learning, we will review the evidence that the MI contains anatomical and functional substrates to support learning-related changes in cell properties and in motor representation patterns. Here, we place particular emphasis on intrinsic horizontal connections in the cortex as a substrate for learning. At least three possible mechanisms to support learning-related restructuring of motor cortex have been identified. The first mechanism (which many agree is the major candidate to mediate learning) involves activity-dependent modification in synaptic efficacy, such as long-term potentiation (LTP) and its counterpart, long-term depression (LTD). We review recent work showing that most connections in MI can exhibit activity-dependent modification. However, the modification rules vary for each connection, perhaps reflecting local synaptic spatial and temporal contingencies. Generalized changes in neuronal excitability and morphologic restructuring appear to be two additional mechanisms by which learning-related changes may be expressed in MI. Together these results indicate that motor cortex contains neural machinery well-suited to participate in motor learning, but the precise conditions under which these systems are engaged remain to be determined.

FORMS OF LEARNING AND THE MOTOR CORTEX

Motor skill learning assumes many forms, as discussed elsewhere (see chapters 6, 13, and 19). For working definitions, we consider three types of learning relevant to the motor cortex: adaptation, skill learning, and conditional associations. Briefly, *adaptation* can be considered a reciprocal exchange of one behavior for another, as in exchanging speed for accuracy (Fitts, 1954) or in the reciprocal modification of motor output in response to gain changes in sensory input, such as that needed to maintain static gaze in the vestibulo-ocular reflex (Lisberger, 1988). These types of reciprocal changes may have relationships to adaptive gain control. *Skill learning* entails nonreciprocal modifications of output variables, such as speed and accuracy (Adams, 1987;

Atkeson, 1989) or modifications in muscle activity patterns (Dugas and Marteniuk, 1989). Hallett et al. (chapter 13) describe this as a change in the "operating characteristic" of the system. In our view, skill learning would include typing and instrument control musical or otherwise (Gordon, Casabona, and Soechting, 1994; Jaric, Corcos, Gottlieb, Ilic, and Latash, 1994; see also chapter 16). Necessarily, this form of learning involves the formation of novel temporal sequences of muscle activity and the reconstruction of existing muscle control architectures, a form of movement fractionation. Indeed, skill learning often involves changes in the timing and patterning of muscle activity accompanied by improved speed and accuracy without concomitant deterioration in other performance measures (Pew, 1966; Schmidt, 1976). *Conditional associations* generally entail acquiring new relationships among events, for example, between arbitrary sensory cues and already learned motor responses (e.g., Halsband and Freund, 1990; Mitz, Godschalk, and Wise, 1991). We believe that this last process does not qualify as motor learning per se, but it is discussed because cortical motor areas have been implicated in mediating changes in stimulus-response couplings. Similarly, classical conditioning as another form of stimulus-response coupling may also be included in discussions of cortical role(s) in learning, because under appropriate conditions this form of learning leads to changes that can be observed within MI.

Although several findings indicate participation of motor cortical areas in the acquisition of new behaviors, the exact role of each cortical area and the neural mechanisms underlying the three previously mentioned forms of skill learning remain unclear. Here, we review the evidence from experiments using various techniques that suggest a role for MI in the types of learning just described. We then discuss the evidence that a cellular architecture exists within the motor cortex to support these sorts of learning-related phenomena. Finally, we discuss the formidable body of data showing cellular and representational plasticity within the motor cortex. We define *plasticity* as any enduring change in motor cortical properties (e.g., in the strength of internal connections, representation pattern, or neuronal properties either morphological or functional). We will argue that motor cortical areas contain abundant neural machinery to support reorganization and contain several useful mechanisms for it to play a central role in learning.

In the context of this review, it is necessary to define the term *motor cortex*. This term is applied broadly to include frontal and parietal cortical regions contributing to attentional, preparatory, mnemonic, executive, and regulatory aspects of voluntary actions (Kalaska and Crammond, 1992). Anatomical, neurophysiological, and behavioral findings in nonhuman primates (primarily macaque monkeys) have provided evidence for a sizable number of motor areas in the frontal and parietal cortex (e.g., Pandya and Vignolo, 1971; Mountcastle, Lynch, Georgopoulos, Sakata, and Acuna, 1975; Matelli, Camarda, Glickstein, and Rizzolatti, 1986; Gentilucci et al., 1988; Kalaska, Cohen,

Prud'homme, and Hyde, 1990; Luppino, Matelli, and Rizzolatti, 1990; Dum and Strick, 1991; di Pellegrino and Wise, 1991; Shima et al., 1991). In the monkey, this parcellation most often typically distinguishes MI (Brodmann area 4) and a number of nonprimary areas, (such as the premotor [PMA] and supplementary motor [SMA] areas). Dynamic modifications in this larger cortical network, which itself has a profusion of anatomical interconnections, may contribute to the impressive behavioral flexibility of mammals. However, for expediency we will discuss nearly exclusively the role of the MI in motor learning.

ROLE OF THE MOTOR CORTEX IN LEARNING

There currently exists a diverse collection of studies using lesion, electrophysiological, imaging, and stimulation techniques suggesting that the motor cortex is involved in all three forms of learning defined earlier.

Adaptation

Though adaptation processes have traditionally been ascribed to the cerebellum, there is some evidence to suggest a role for MI in adaptation. For example, when Martin and Ghez (1993) blocked neuronal activity with injections of muscimol into cat MI, the animals could not learn to correct aberrant limb trajectories caused by the inactivation. Similarly, removal of the primary somatic sensory cortex (SI), which disrupts somatic sensory input to MI, also interferes with capabilities to correct movement errors, according to Asanuma and Mackel (1989). These experimenters interpreted this result as indicating particular importance for the SI input to MI to mediate motor learning. An alternative view of the SI (and the MI) lesion study might be that disrupting the integrity of motor cortical circuits simply prevents learning by modifying one of myriad processes needed for adaptation, while not definitively placing MI as *the* structure required for motor adaptation. Further, cats with SI ablations can eventually learn to make correct movements, which shows that other pathways are available for learning motor adjustments. Grafton et al. (1992), using positron emission tomography (PET) imaging, found relative cerebral blood flow (CBF) increases in the human MI (and SMA) during the early phases of learning a pursuit rotor task, suggestive of a role for these motor areas in motor learning (see also chapters 11 and 13). Rather than being a sign of involvement in learning, these changes might be attributed to increased number of movements during adaptation to the task.

Skill Learning

Several different tasks have been used to evaluate a motor cortical role in skill learning. Most of the tasks employed the learning of finger movement sequences and most recently, experimenters used a method that can distinguish the implicit and explicit forms of motor learning (Nissen and Bullemer, 1987). In one study of particular interest, Pascual-Leone, Grafman, and Hallett (1994; see also chapter 13) used transcranial magnetic stimulation (albeit a relatively crude method) to map muscle territories in cortex. Cortical muscle representations "expanded" during sequence acquisition but before the subjects had explicit knowledge of the sequence, then it retracted when subjects acquired knowledge of the sequential skill. Brain imaging studies have also reported plasticity of cortical representations with sequence learning, though in contrast to the Pascual-Leone et al. (1994) result, the overall effect appears an increased size of representation in MI after the learning of finger sequences (Karni et al., 1994; Grafton, Hazelton, and Ivry, 1995). A possible reason for the differences in the stimulation and brain imaging studies is not immediately apparent, though they may be related to differences in the time of evaluation; stimulation maps were obtained during a no-movement condition, between practice sessions, whereas movement representations using vascular imaging were obtained *during* performance of the new movement. It is noteworthy, though currently unexplained, that other human functional imaging studies using motor "learning" tasks have reported changes in the nonprimary motor cortex, but not in MI (Lang et al., 1988; Seitz and Roland, 1992; cf. Schlaug, Knorr, and Seitz, 1994).

An experiment examining a type of motor skill learning different from sequential learning used electrical stimulation through individual microwires chronically implanted in MI of monkeys to evaluate whether the functional coupling of MI to muscles changed with learning (Suner, Gutman, Gaal, Sanes, and Donoghue, 1993). Muscle activation patterns following MI intracortical stimulation were evaluated after learning a conditioned wrist *flexion* movement, then after learning a conditioned wrist *extension* over a period of weeks, and again when the monkeys returned to performing in a wrist flexion task. In this task, the monkeys moved against a spring load to align a position-feedback cursor with a narrow, (4 to 8-degree) visual target presented on a video monitor. We consider this to be a form of skill learning because precision alignment of the hand had to be achieved within a brief reaction time (both speed and accuracy had to be improved). MI stimulation while the monkey waited to perform the movements indicated that the muscle field and the magnitude of muscle responses related to individual cortical sites varied with training. At some cortical sites, the type of shift correlated with the particular task. For example, activation of wrist flexor muscles from a site decreased during the wrist extension task and then returned to previously observed levels on resumption of the wrist flexion task. A similar result has been reported by Milleken, Nudo, Grenda, Jenkins, and Merzenich (1992). Changes in MI discharge have been reported during learning of a new movement amplitude in an elbow flexion task (Burnod, Maton, and Calvet, 1983; Maton, Burnod, and Calvet, 1983), although kinematic changes may have contributed to these learning-related discharge modifications.

"Nonmotor" Learning

Several studies have reported a role for motor cortex in conditional associations, thereby suggesting that cortical motor areas may participate in both nonmotor and motor learning. Conditional associations are considered nonmotor because the tasks used in these experiments typically require the coupling of an auditory or visual cue to a movement already within the motor repertoire of the subject. In a series of studies, Gemba and Sasaki (1984; 1987; 1988) found that sensory-cued evoked potentials (EPs) recorded from MI become more prominent when a monkey learned to move in response to a "go" cue. Whether performance changes contributed significantly to the prominence of the EP is not fully evident in these experiments. Tests also have detected neurons that develop cue responses when a monkey learned to associate an arbitrary visual cue with an already learned arm movement (Mitz et al., 1991), although the majority of these neurons were found in PMA and not in MI. A predominant role for PMA in this type of conditional association is further supported by Germain and Lamarre's (1993) finding that the percentage of cue-responsive cells in a tone-conditioning task increased in PMA but not in MI, when pre- and postlearning populations were compared (see also chapter 12). Nevertheless, this work provides some of the most direct evidence for the development of new properties of motor cortex neurons during the learning of a new behavior, even though a new motor action was not learned. Some forms of classical conditioning may produce changes that in certain ways resemble those observed for the conditional associations described above, in that formerly irrelevant stimuli come to elicit a response in MI neurons after acquisition of a particular form of conditioned rapid eye blink (Woody, 1986). Further, this particular form of conditioning is blocked following MI lesions (Woody, Yarowsky, Owens, Black, and Crow, 1974), suggesting that the changes occurring in MI neurons are germane to the conditioning process.

Collectively these studies suggest that motor cortex is linked to processes involved in several different forms of learning and is therefore likely capable of plastic reorganization of its functional properties. Additional data concerning the plasticity of motor cortex representation patterns support the view that motor cortex is both modifiable and involved in learning. In a series of experiments, we have demonstrated that MI representations in the rat undergo rapid reorganization following peripheral nerve lesions (see Sanes and Donoghue, 1992 for a review of these and related studies). Using electrical stimulation mapping, we found that it is possible to elicit movements of the forelimb from the former MI whisker representation within hours of a transection of the peripheral motor nerve to the whiskers. This change in adult rats occurs abruptly and persists over time so that the whisker area becomes occupied by new somatic representations. The capability to shift control from one set of muscles to another seems well-suited for motor learning.

These indications for motor cortical involvement in learning prompted us to examine whether motor cortex itself can support these sorts of changes. As we discuss further, it appears that motor cortex contains both a substrate and mechanisms to restructure its organization to permit the formation of new sensorimotor associations required for forms of motor or nonmotor learning that have been linked to it.

CONNECTIONAL SUBSTRATES FOR MOTOR LEARNING

Although activity-driven changes have been evaluated largely within the motor cortex, many of the changes measured in it may instead reflect changes at any of a number of central nervous system (CNS) sites (e.g., Iriki, Pavlides, and Asanuma, 1990; Ito and Oda, 1994). In this section, we demonstrate that MI contains a substrate to permit a flexible organization: the connectional arrangement of extrinsic and intrinsic fiber pathways. Such other sites as the subcortical targets of motor cortical efferent pathways or the cerebellum are also likely to participate in motor learning; these sites are discussed elsewhere (see chapters 8 and 15).

Motor Cortical Circuitry

Typical of most cortical areas, MI receives inputs from subcortical and cortical areas, and there is a complex pattern of internal connectivity. Details of MI input-output organization have been reviewed previously (Wise and Donoghue, 1986; Jones, 1987; Darian-Smith, Darian, Burman, and Ratcliffe, 1993; Darian-Smith and Darian, 1993; Donoghue and Sanes, 1994; Miyashita, Keller, and Asanuma, 1994). Therefore, only a select set of the connections most relevant to the present discussion will be briefly reviewed. Figure 17.1 summarizes extrinsic and intrinsic connections potentially important for a motor cortical role in learning. Extrinsic pathways typically enter the cortex vertically. Among the extrinsic connections of MI, the thalamic pathway, including information from the cerebellum and basal ganglia, forms one of the most significant inputs. Fibers from the ventrolateral thalamic complex (VL) project most prominently to one of the middle cortical layers (layer III), forming bands that extend in the rostrocaudal dimension (Shinoda, Kakei, Futami, and Wannier, 1993). From a variety of modalities, these fibers transmit information that can be used for the generation of movement-related signals in MI (Thach, 1987; Butler, Horne, and Rawson, 1992; Forlano, Horne, Butler, and Finkelstein, 1993). Also entering through a vertical trajectory are corticocortical connections that arise from adjacent frontal areas and from the parietal lobe (Asanuma and Mackel, 1989; Andersen, Asanuma, Essick, and Siegel, 1990; Darian Smith et al., 1993; Darian-Smith and Darian, 1993). The projection from parietal somatic sensory areas forms one of major corticocortical projections to MI and likely represents a principal route via which somatic sensory information reaches MI (DeFelipe, Conley, and Jones,

Sites of activity dependent plasticity in motor cortex

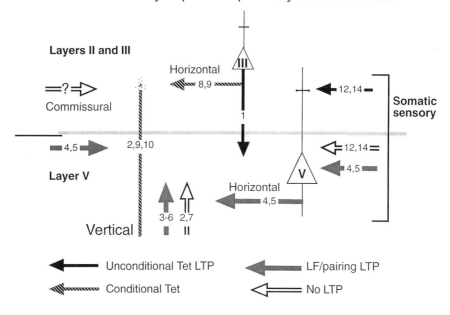

Figure 17.1 Schematic summary of major extrinsic and intrinsic MI pathways that undergo activity-dependent modification. The arrow style indicates the type of induction mechanisms currently identified at each site: Tet, tetanized; LTP, long-term potentiation; LF, low-frequency. Note that inhibitory local circuit neurons have been left out of this diagram. *Somatic sensory* refers to input from the primary somatic sensory cortex. Numbers indicate the appropriate references: 1, Kimura et al., 1994; 2, Asanuma and Mackel, 1989; 3, Baranyi and Feher, 1978; 4, Baranyi and Feher, 1981a; 5, Baranyi and Feher, 1981b; 6, Baranyi et al., 1991; 7, Castro-Alamancos et al., 1995; 8, Hess and Donoghue, 1994; 9, Hess et al., 1996; 10, Iriki et al., 1990; 11, Iriki et al., 1991; 12, Keller, Iriki, and Asanuma, 1990; 13, Sakamoto et al., 1987.

1986; Asanuma and Mackel, 1989; Porter and Sakamoto, 1988; Mackel, Iriki, Jorum, and Asanuma, 1991).

The *intrinsic* fiber systems of the motor cortex can be categorized as two types: vertical and horizontal. One prominent vertical intrinsic system descends radially from the pyramidal cells of the superficial layers (layers II and III) to layer V, but little is known about how this projection shapes the properties of layer V neurons, which are the source of descending MI pathways. Horizontally directed fibers form a diffuse but extensive intrinsic pathway within MI.[1] The pathway arises from pyramidal cells and projects across MI for long distances, forming connections along its route. Anatomical evidence in monkeys indicates that horizontal fibers branch extensively within the MI arm area to reach nearly all parts of this subdivision of the somatic motor representation (Huntley and Jones, 1991). Interestingly, the fibers appear to avoid adjacent representations insofar as fiber labeling diminishes abruptly at the arm-face border, even when a tracer injection is placed relatively close to this border. A similar trend has been suggested for the cat and rat MI (Aroniadou and Keller, 1993; Keller, 1993a, b) except that retrograde tracer injections (Keller, 1993a; Miyashita et al., 1994) and intracellular dye labeling of MI pyramidal neurons (Landry, Labelle, and Deschenes, 1980; Donoghue and Kitai, 1981; Landry, Wilson, and Kitai, 1984; Jacobs, 1993) suggest that horizontal connections more extensively interconnect different somatic subdivisions in the rat compared with the monkey MI. Recent electrophysiological studies in rats have demonstrated that horizontal projections exert excitatory influences over distances of at least 1.25 mm, comprising a considerable extent of MI's width (Aroniadou and Keller, 1993; Hess and Donoghue, 1994; Jacobs, Hess, Connors, and Donoghue, 1995). Field potential recordings, current source density (CSD) analysis, and intracellular recordings demonstrate two prominent horizontal pathways: across layers II and III and across layer V.[2] In addition, there is also a relatively strong projection from layer V to III (Hess, Jacobs, and Donoghue, 1994) that, although oblique in its trajectory, will be grouped with horizontal connections here because it serves to distribute information horizontally across MI. Thus, the horizontal fiber plexus forms a broadly distributed system that could serve to interconnect spatially distributed groups of neurons in MI; in the monkey, at least, these horizontal connections tie together MI neurons related to a major body part (e.g., the arm) but do not seem to interconnect together representations of different body parts.

Electrophysiological studies have demonstrated that horizontal pathways, similar to the other major extrinsic and intrinsic pathways, exert excitatory effects while using glutamate or a closely related amino acid as their transmitter (Hess et al., 1994). Each of these horizontal pathways also appears to have a small component linked to the activation of N-methyl-D-aspartate (NMDA) receptors (Aroniadou and Teyler, 1991; Hess et al., 1994). This suggests that synaptic modification is likely to occur at these sites because NMDA is associated with synaptic modification (Malenka and Nicoll, 1993). In addition to terminations on pyramidal neurons, horizontal fibers also terminate on nonpyramidal, presumably GABAergic, inhibitory neurons (Jones, 1993; Keller and Asanuma, 1993). In contrast to the widely dispersed and excitatory projections of pyramidal cells in MI, activation of nonpyramidal cells provides intracortical inhibition (Thomson and Deuchars, 1994) that exerts its effects locally, but see Kang, Kaneko, Ohishi, Endo, and Araki (1994), who suggest that some inhibitory neurons may distribute their influence up to 1.2 mm away. In MI, the role of the local inhibitory connections has not been identified, but we will argue that it is suited ideally to be a substrate to support reorganization of motor representations.

A Model of Intrinsic Connectivity in MI

The pattern of horizontal connectivity, with long-range excitation and shorter-range inhibition, led us to propose a simple model of MI's intrinsic connections that may form a basis for restructuring of cortical circuitry. Figure 17.2 depicts excitatory coupling of pyramidal cells in two functionally different

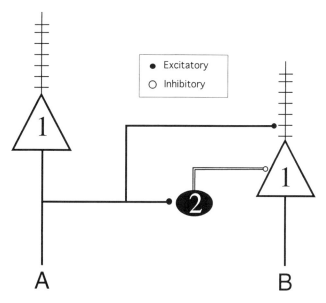

Figure 17.2 Simple model of circuit arrangement of excitatory and inhibitory elements involved in intrinsic horizontal interactions in MI. Pyramidal neurons (1) typically have long-ranging collaterals that form excitatory synapses on GABAergic inhibitory neurons (2) and on other pyramidal neurons. The inhibitory cells provide a disynaptic, feed-forward inhibition to the target pyramidal cell. The experimental data indicate that this arrangement typically prevents strong interactions among neighboring pyramidal neurons unless inhibition is reduced or the efficacy of the pyramidal cell connection is increased (as might occur with LTP). Note that increase in the coupling strength between the pyramidal cells could lead to coactivation so that target muscles A and B would be activated together, as shown experimentally in Jacobs and Donoghue (1991).

representations via a horizontally directed pyramidal cell axon collateral. This collateral additionally terminates on a local inhibitory neuron near the target pyramidal cell that can provide local feed-forward inhibition through this disynaptic connection (Hendry, Houser, Jones, and Vaughn, 1983). This connectional pattern could exist among any of the three described horizontal pathways (layers III–III, V–V, or V–III), although this generality requires additional experimental verification. A prediction of this model is that blockade of inhibition would strengthen the coupling between the two prototypic pyramidal cells. Such an arrangement could allow effectively for increased coupling of cells located in two separate MI regions. This model led us to hypothesize that a change in coupling would produce new motor output architectures. The hypothesis was explicitly tested in vivo in the rat MI using the GABA$_A$ receptor antagonist bicuculline to block feed-forward inhibition and reveal extant excitatory horizontal connections between representations (Jacobs and Donoghue, 1991). Focal application of bicuculline at a site in the forelimb representation made it possible to evoke forelimb movements by stimulation within the vibrissa area, presumably by unmasking the horizontal excitatory collateral depicted in figure 17.2. The changes transiently induced in MI by this pharmacological manipulation resembled that which occurs after nerve lesions (Sanes and Donoghue, 1992). This result supports the hypothesis that changes in the coupling strength of pyramidal cells through existing horizontal connections can permit the expression of one of a variety of possible MI output maps. Using cortical slice preparations, it has been possible to demonstrate more directly the masking of horizontal excitatory connections by feed-forward inhibition. Focal application of bicuculline revealed the expression of a considerably larger excitatory horizontal response, either in field potentials or in intracellularly recorded synaptic responses, than is present when inhibition is intact (Hess et al., 1994). Intracellular recordings indicate that monosynaptic excitatory connections are being uncovered, although polysynaptic components likely also contribute to the observed changes.

These observations suggest that intrinsic horizontal connections form an important part of a substrate for motor cortex plasticity. The remaining extrinsic and intrinsic fibers must also play a role, but it is less clear how their organization might participate in restructuring MI organization. It seems reasonable to assume that these pathways could carry the external cues to initiate or promote plastic changes. We will introduce some evidence in the next section that suggests that interactions among extrinsic and intrinsic fibers are important for remodeling MI organization.

MECHANISMS AVAILABLE IN MI FOR REORGANIZATION

In addition to MI containing a substrate for restructuring its organization, long-lasting shifts in MI organization would require that inherent mechanisms exist to implement and sustain such changes. Three important candidate mechanisms are considered on the basis of recent experimental evidence. Each of the three mechanisms has been detected in MI and has been implicated to some extent in the potential for MI to be a site of motor learning. The first is activity-dependent synaptic plasticity, which will be emphasized in this review. By this mechanism, long-term change in efficacy occurs in those synapses that have been recently active and able to drive (depolarize) their postsynaptic targets. This characterization generally fits into the category of Hebbian-type synaptic modification. The phenomenon LTP (Lømo and Bliss, 1973) has been documented extensively at a growing number of sites throughout the nervous system. It has appeal as a model for learning because LTP typically results in long-lasting modifications specific to active junctions, without producing global changes in the target neuron. There are several reasons to believe that motor cortical plasticity may occur by such activity-dependent mechanisms as LTP. Motor maps can be altered by electrical stimulation in MI (Nudo, Jenkins, and Merzenich, 1990), shifts in limb position (Sanes, Wang, and Donoghue, 1992), or repeated limb movement

(Humphrey, Qiu, Clavel, and O'Donoghue, 1990). Furthermore, blockade of NMDA receptors linked to activity-dependent plasticity, appears to prevent movement-initiated reorganization of MI (Qui, Donoghue, and Humphrey, 1990). A second mechanism available within MI for learning involves generalized excitability changes in postsynaptic neurons; a third is growth of new connections. The last two mechanisms have been discussed elsewhere and will be addressed only briefly in this chapter.

Activity-Driven Synaptic Modification

It is now very well documented that many excitatory, glutamatergic synapses undergo activity-dependent modulation in their efficacy. Whether the change in efficacy is an increase or a decrease seems to depend on the temporal pattern of the stimulation. High-frequency stimulation (HFS) using trains either in bursts or in a sustained fashion can produce a persistent change in synaptic efficacy. By contrast, low-frequency stimulation (LFS) at approximately 1 Hz produces weakening of synaptic strength in the stimulated pathway (see Bear and Kirkwood, 1993; Bear and Malenka, 1994; Malenka, 1994), namely, LTD.

Two general forms of LTP induction have been described: unconditional and conditional. They are introduced here because they may serve to differentiate distinct sets of conditions that must be fulfilled for synaptic modification to occur. *Unconditional* LTP occurs when stimulation of an afferent fiber pathway induces modification without other experimental manipulations. *Conditional* LTP requires an additional component, such as stimulation of additional afferent fiber pathways or the reduction of inhibition by applied pharmacological agents, such as the $GABA_A$ blocker bicuculline. This difference does not require fundamentally different synaptic properties; a less effective activation of the postsynaptic cell could prevent sufficient depolarization for modification to occur, and thereby necessitate an additional condition for LTP induction. The finding that no level of stimulation is ever adequate to induce LTP in some pathways without adding other factors indicates that real differences in the ability to induce LTP exist. We suggest that the specific arrangement of excitatory and inhibitory connections in the cortex plays an important role in dissociating conditionally from unconditionally induced LTP. However, as a cautionary note it must be added that many experiments on LTP are frequently carried out in brain slices. In slice preparations, cells sit at considerably hyperpolarized membrane potentials, which may affect conditions for LTP induction in addition to circuit architecture.

Pairing is a third method for LTP induction in which changes in input effectiveness are induced by stimulation (usually low frequency) of that afferent, paired with depolarization of the target neuron in a specific temporal relationship (e.g., Baranyi, Szente, and Woody, 1991). Depolarization is achieved either by passing current directly through an intracellular recording electrode or by antidromic activation of the cell under study. Although repetitive stimulation and pairing paradigms seem to be quite similar forms of conditional activation, in that they require two factors to induce LTP, there are distinct differences in the sites where one or the other form of potentiation can be induced at various points within motor cortical circuitry, as will be discussed further. Nevertheless, it is not clear that these two forms of induction are mutually exclusive or that the presence of two forms indicates that they necessarily operate by unique mechanisms. Two important features common to the set of activity driven forms of plasticity—unconditional, conditional, and pairing—are that synaptic modifications occur locally and that they are restricted to the activated synapses. This property has made LTP such an attractive model for learning.

SITES OF SYNAPTIC PLASTICITY IN MI

As noted earlier, figure 17.1 provides a synopsis of the experimental data concerning sites of synaptic plasticity in the major MI pathways. Although many cortical areas have been examined for plastic changes, it is noteworthy that individual circuits within MI have probably received the most experimental investigation of any other single neocortical field (see figure 17.1). It seems that activity-driven modification occurs at every possible synaptic junction, and this appears to be correct as a first approximation. Synapses formed by extrinsic and intrinsic fiber systems are modifiable. The presence of malleability at numerous MI sites is one important component of the argument that MI circuits contain all the essential elements for occurrence of learning.

Different arrows in figure 17.1 denote sites where conditional, unconditional, and pairing forms of modification have been identified. It appears that even for a single pathway, the forms of modification may vary, as for example the extrinsic projections from SI (labeled Somatic Sensory in figure 17.1) or the VL (labeled Vertical in figure 17.1). The corticocortical projection from SI to the superficial layers of MI shows unconditional potentiation (Sakamoto, Porter, and Asanuma, 1987; Iriki, Pavlides, Keller, and Asanuma, 1991), suggesting that the effectiveness of incoming sensory activation of layer II and III neurons would often be modified. By contrast, the same parameters of stimulation that evoke strengthening of this input to the superficial layers fail to modify connections within layer V. However, this pathway to the deep layers appears to be modifiable using a pairing paradigm (Baranyi and Feher, 1981a,b).[3]

A second example of mixed rules for LTP induction occurs in the VL projection. Vertical ascending projections within MI in general do not readily undergo unconditional LTP. Attempts at LTP induction in vivo in cats (Baranyi and Feher, 1978; Iriki et al., 1991) and in rat cortical slices (Castro-Alamancos, Donoghue, and Connors, 1995) are generally unsuccessful when vertical pathways are tetanized alone.[4] However, conditional or pairing paradigms can induce plastic modifications in vertical projections. Conditional potentiation of the vertical projection to the superficial layers occurs in both cats (VL stimulation in vivo; Iriki et al., 1991) and rats (vertical stimulation in slice; Hess, Aizenman, and Donoghue, 1995). In both species, LTP occurred when the vertical pathway was stimulated in conjunction with activation of a corticocortical pathway, either the intrinsic horizontal projection across the superficial MI layers or the cortical input from SI. By contrast, concurrent SI and VL stimulation using tetanizing stimulation failed to modify synaptic strength in the deep layers (Iriki et al., 1991). These connections are capable of modification under some conditions because pairing can successfully potentiate VL synapses onto layer V neurons (Baranyi and Feher, 1978, 1981a, b). These findings suggest that extrinsic inputs to the superficial layers may more readily modify compared to terminations in the deeper layers, even though all of these projections are capable of modification, should the appropriate conditions be met.

Local projections within MI also show differential abilities to undergo modification. Recently, it was demonstrated that the descending vertical connection from layer II and III to layer V undergoes unconditional LTP (Kimura, Caria, Melis, and Asanuma, 1994). This suggests that restructuring within the superficial layers may be readily imposed upon output neurons of the deep layers. Apart from this intrinsic connection, the remainder seem to require additional conditions to modify their efficacy. The intrinsic horizontal connections of the superficial layers undergo only conditional modification (Hess and Donoghue, 1994; Hess et al., 1995). Ordinarily, tetanizing stimulation produces no change in the effectiveness of these pathways in slice preparations, but a long-lasting increase in the effectiveness of the pathway is evident if inhibition is transiently reduced by pharmacological agents placed at the recording site during the tetanizing stimulation (figure 17.3). Previously we noted that blockade of inhibition unmasked horizontal excitatory connections (Jacobs and Donoghue, 1991; Hess and Donoghue, 1994) which may permit sufficient depolarization for LTP induction. This finding indicates that inhibitory circuits are critically placed to regulate interactions among pyramidal cells distributed across MI, both dynamically (for brief epochs) and over the long term, through LTP (or LTD). The data further indicate that any manipulation that influences the amount of inhibition in cortex may regulate the ability for these connections to modify. Whether inhibitory synaptic strength can be modified in these circuits is not clear, but considerable evidence suggests that mechanisms exist to effect such changes (McCarren and Alger, 1985; see also Sanes and Donoghue, 1992; Jones, 1993). LTP also can be induced in the intrinsic horizontal pathways of the superficial layers of MI if the vertical projection is co-tetanized with the horizontal projections (Hess et al., 1995; see also figure 17.4). The mechanism by which this paradigm permits horizontal (as well as vertical) changes is not known, although a

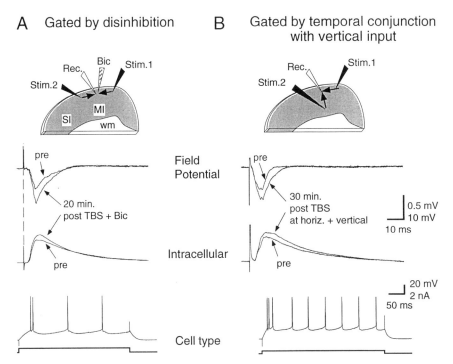

A Gated by disinhibition

B Gated by temporal conjunction with vertical input

Field Potential

Intracellular

Cell type

0.5 mV
10 mV
10 ms

20 mV
2 nA
50 ms

Figure 17.3 Two means of conditional LTP induction in the horizontal connections of MI (rat cortex, slice preparations). Columns A and B show typical configurations of stimulating, recording, and drug-application pipettes. Below, field potential and intracellular responses of the horizontal pathways are shown pre- and posttetanization. Bottom traces show intracellular responses to a depolarizing current pulse. Cells have discharge characteristics of layer III pyramidal neurons. Intracellular recordings made near (~ 100-μm) field potential recording electrodes (Rec.). A. LTP may be induced by the action of horizontal fibers alone but only when inhibition is pharmacologically reduced. B. LTP may also occur when there is close temporal conjunction of activity of vertical and horizontal pathways achieved by conjoint stimulation of electrodes (Stim. 1 and Stim. 2). TBS, Theta burst stimulation; bic, bicuculline.

convergence of inputs on common inhibitory interneurons could explain this interaction (see Hess et al., 1995). This hypothesis would further implicate inhibitory neurons in plasticity and suggests that temporal conjunction of activity in ascending thalamic pathways and the horizontal pathways may be a critical factor for restructuring horizontal interactions in the cortex. It remains speculative whether such patterns occur during learning, but this idea seems to be amenable to experimental testing.

So far, we have discussed only mechanisms that produce strengthening of synapses. A unidirectional mechanism could rapidly encounter ceiling or saturation effects. However, LTD provides a mechanism by which synapses may be weakened. Among all of the MI pathways the potential for *decreases* in synaptic strength has been investigated only for the intrinsic horizontal connections of the superficial layers (Hess and Donoghue, 1995; see also figure 17.4). LTD has been induced by low-frequency stimulation (2 Hz for 10 min)

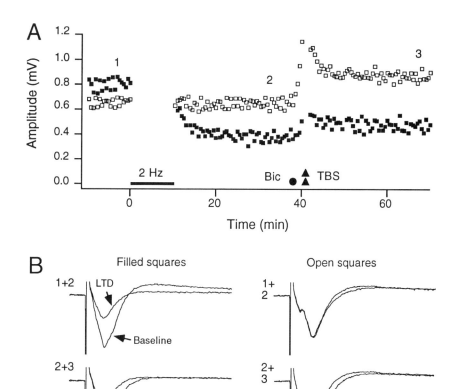

Figure 17.4 Horizontal connections of the superficial cortical layers show decreases and increases in synaptic efficacy dependent on stimulation frequency. A. Plot of field potential amplitude changes associated with low- (2-Hz) and high-frequency (theta burst) [TBS] stimulation of horizontal connections. Low-frequency stimulation of one horizontal pathway 500 μm from recording sites (filled squares) produced a weakening of the stimulated horizontal connection but no change in a control pathway (open squares, same recording site, but separate stimulation site). Subsequent high-frequency stimulation of both pathways simultaneously (during transient, local GABA blockade) increased the efficacy of both pathways. Note that the control pathway shows no heterosynaptic depression and that the depressed pathway can recover efficacy after LTD is induced. B. Examples of field potentials recorded in this experiment comparing waveforms before and after low-frequency stimulation for depressed (filled squares, 1 + 2) and control (open squares, 1 + 2) pathways and for these pathways after high-frequency stimulation (2 + 3). Numbers refer to points on graph in A from which potentials were selected. Bic, bicuculline. (Reprinted from Hess and Donoghue 1996.)

of the horizontal pathways within layers II and III. Note that depressed horizontal pathways retained the ability to increase synaptic strength at levels comparable to control unstimulated inputs because this shows that LTD did not result simply from transmission failure. These experiments point out another temporal dimension to synaptic strength modification: The frequency or pattern of activation of an input can determine whether a particular synapse increases or decreases its strength.

SUMMARY OF SITES OF SYNAPTIC MODIFICATION IN MI

The list of sites within MI circuits where synapses may modify is long and complex. However, certain principles seem to emerge. First, all excitatory synaptic connections within MI that have been tested appear capable of activity-dependent modification, though the rules for modifying each connection may vary. Second, it seems much easier to modify inputs directed toward superficial layers than those directed toward deeper cortical layers. Although the reasons for these laminar differences remain uncertain, it may be significant that certain markers for synaptic plasticity, such as the enrichment of calcium/calmodulin-dependent protein kinase II (Jacobs, Neve, and Donoghue, 1990), appear to be enriched in superficial cortical layers (cf. Huntley, Vickers, Janssen, Brose, and Heinemann, 1994). Third, the thalamic pathway seems particularly refractory to change, though the resistance seems to be peculiar to MI. Last, beyond a general ability for cortical excitatory synapses to modify, spatial and temporal factors appear to determine whether change will occur. In this context, spatial factors refer to the unique circuit architecture for each pathway. Increased knowledge of the organization of these circuits is required to determine how such factors as feed-forward inhibition can regulate the potential for synaptic plasticity.

Conditioning-Related Changes in Neuronal Excitability

LTP-like phenomena are not the only cortical mechanisms available for introducing change in motor cortical circuits. Work from Woody et al. has provided extensive data demonstrating that MI neurons can be conditioned to an auditory stimulus during classic conditoning of a short-latency eyeblink response. The mechanism for this change differs significantly from the LTP induction discussed above. Conditioning-induced sensory response increases appear to result from a long-lasting postsynaptic excitability increase that occurs during learning (Brons and Woody, 1980; Woody, 1986; Baranyi et al., 1991). Lesion studies further suggest that this learning depends on MI (Woody et al., 1974), which is required if MI is the site of learning in this paradigm. A postsynaptic excitability change of this sort would appear to be less specific than LTP because the effectiveness of every input to the neuron would be affected. Woody has made the interesting observation that stimulation of the hypothalamic-basal forebrain region dramatically reduces the number of training trials required for conditioning by one to two orders of magnitude (Kim, Woody, and Berthier, 1983; Aou, Oomura, Woody, and Nishino, 1988). This effect appears to work through the release of acetylcholine (Woody, 1986; Woody and Gruen, 1987), a transmitter of the basal forebrain projection to the cortex that can increase the excitability of motor cortical neurons (Matsumura, Sawaguchi, and Kubota, 1990) and appears to be tied closely to the conditioning-related modification of MI neurons. Thus it will be important to consider the interaction of modulatory inputs with more specific MI inputs during learning because neuromodulators may provide yet another "gating factor" that will determine the rules for modification at a particular site within MI circuitry. It is interesting to speculate that mechanisms regulating global excitability may be critical in providing the necessary depolarization of postsynaptic neurons (as in the pairing-type of conditioning described previously) so that more specific LTP-like mechanisms may be engaged more effectively during learning.

Morphological Changes as a Mechanism for Plasticity

The mechanisms described thus far rely on changes in the efficacy of existing synapses. A further possibility is that new synapses are formed or inactive ones are removed. It is generally held that overt morphologic restructuring of cortical connections ends early in postnatal development. However, Greenough, Larson, and Withers (1985) and Withers and Greenough (1989) reported that dendritic branches of MI neurons increase in number with motor training. This observation is consistent with the formation of new synapses, but there has been no direct demonstration of newly formed synaptic junctions. A recent report from Darian-Smith and Gilbert (1994) in visual cortex has provided additional evidence by showing that there is an increase in the number of axonal collaterals of horizontal pathways into a functionally reorganized area of the cortex. In MI, it has also been reported that electrical stimulation of the thalamus can increase synaptic density in MI (Keller, Arissian, and Asanuma, 1992). Another intriguing observation is that layer V neurons in normal rat MI are particularly enriched in messenger RNA for GAP-43, a growth-associated protein (Jacobs and Donoghue, 1991). It is not known whether this expression signals ongoing connectional restructuring for this cell class. The extent to which morphologic reorganization operates in learning is still poorly understood, but it remains an important consideration when considering plasticity of the adult cortex.

CONCLUSIONS

The evidence linking MI to various types of motor and nonmotor learning is not conclusive, but all the available evidence is sufficiently convincing to warrant further intensive investigation to understand its place among the set of neural structures that might participate in learning. Studies will be difficult to design because of the limitations in separating motor performance from learning functions when observing neural activity patterns, or because of the imprecision in precisely defining what is meant by learning. Nevertheless, the evidence is fairly compelling that MI contains the neural machinery required to participate in conditional associations, because of the apparent relative ease of generating LTP in the somatic sensory input to MI and the likelihood of similar inputs from other sensory modalities. In addition, the plasticity of horizontal connections may serve to restructure cortical neuronal assemblies, which could provide new connectional substrates necessary for skill learning. Our view is that sectors of the motor cortex, such as the MI arm area, function as a distributed neural network and not as a collection of independent controllers; we suggest that a large population of broadly distributed neurons contribute at any one time to ongoing motor processes (see Donoghue and Sanes, 1994) and for motor skill learning or for forming new conditional associations. The plasticity mechanisms we have identified also could participate in adaptation but, by our definition, it is not entirely clear that this occurs. However, the present definitions of these terms are sufficiently loose, and the data are sufficiently incomplete to make it difficult to draw any firm conclusion about the forms of learning that engage MI neurons.

The substrates and mechanisms we have described are not unique to MI. This machinery appears available throughout the neocortex, though it will be necessary to determine whether the rules for modification vary from area to area across cortex. However, these experiments suggest that each cortical area is continually reshaped as a result of its use. The precise form of this reshaping will be regulated by input-output organization, the availability of mechanisms for activity-dependent synaptic modification, the influence of neuromodulatory inputs, and the arrangement of intrinsic circuitry. The presently available data lead us to conclude that MI provides an adaptive, dynamic network able to provide immense flexibility to the motor system that can be used to reshape the skeletal motor system when the individual is confronted with novel situations requiring new behavioral responses.

ACKNOWLEDGMENTS

This research was supported by grants from the National Institute of Neurological Disorders and Stroke (NS 22517 and NS25074), the National Institute on Aging (AG 10634), the Whitehall Foundation, and the Charles E. Culpeper Foundation.

NOTES

1. For a review of what these fibers might do in visual cortex, where they have been most studied, see, for example, Gilbert, Hirsch, and Wiesel (1990); Hirsch and Gilbert (1991); and McGuire, Gilbert, Rivlin, and Wiesel (1991).

2. Because CSD analysis indicates solely the location of activated synapses and not their targets, it should be noted that the responses recorded from layers II and III may result from activation of synapses on dendrites of cells belonging to those layers as well as neurons in deeper layers. Similarly, responses recorded from layer V may contain components resulting from activation of layer V and layer VI cells.

3. A significant difference in these two studies is that Baranyi and Feher (1981a) stimulated peripheral nerves, whereas Asanuma stimulated the SI to MI pathway directly.

4. Studies in cats directly stimulated VL. Studies in rats have employed only slice preparations in which stimulation is applied in the deep layers or white matter. In this way, activation involves VL fibers but would also include a number of other fiber systems.

REFERENCES

Adams JA (1987). Historical review and appraisal of research on learning, retention, and transfer of human motor skills. Psychol Bull 101:41–74.

Andersen RA, Asanuma C, Essick G, Siegel RM (1990). Corticocortical connections of anatomically and physiologically defined subdivisions within the inferior parietal lobule. J Comp Neurol 296:65–113.

Aou S, Oomura Y, Woody CD, Nishino H (1988). Effects of behaviorally rewarding hypothalamic electrical stimulation on intracellularly recorded neuronal activity in the motor cortex of awake monkeys. Brain Res 439:31–38.

Aroniadou VA, Keller A (1993). The patterns and synaptic properties of horizontal intracortical connections in the rat motor cortex. J Neurophysiol 70:1553–1569.

Aroniadou VA, Teyler TJ (1991). The role of NMDA receptors in long-term potentiation (LTP) and depression (LTD) in rat visual cortex. Brain Res 562:136–143.

Asanuma H, Mackel R (1989). Direct and indirect sensory input pathways to the motor cortex: Its structure and function in relation to learning of motor skills. Jpn J Physiol 39:1–19.

Atkeson CG (1989). Learning arm kinematics and dynamics. Annu Rev Neurosci 12:157–183.

Baranyi A, Feher O (1978). Conditioned changes of synaptic transmission in the motor cortex of the cat. Exp Brain Res 33:283–298.

Baranyi A, Feher O (1981a). Long-term facilitation of excitatory synaptic transmission in single motor cortical neurones of the cat produced by repetitive pairing of synaptic potentials and action potentials following intracellular stimulation. Neurosci Lett 23:303–308.

Baranyi A, Feher O (1981b). Intracellular studies on cortical synaptic plasticity. Conditioning effect of antidromic activation on test-EPSPs. Exp Brain Res 41:124–134.

Baranyi A, Szente MB, Woody CD (1991). Properties of associative long-lasting potentiation induced by cellular conditioning in the motor cortex of conscious cats. Neuroscience 42:321–334.

Bear MF, Kirkwood A (1993). Neocortical long-term potentiation. Curr Opin Neurobiol 3:197–202.

Bear MF, Malenka RC (1994). Synaptic plasticity: LTP and LTD. Curr Opin Neurobiol 4:389–399.

Brons J, Woody C (1989). Long-term changes in excitability of cortical neuron after Pavlovian conditioning and excitation. J Neurophysiol 44:605–615.

Burnod Y, Maton B, Calvet J (1982). Short-term changes in cell activity of areas 4 and 5 during operant conditioning. Exp Neurol 78:227–240.

Butler EG, Horne MK, Rawson JA (1992). Sensory characteristics of monkey thalamic and motor cortex neurones. J Physiol (Lond) 445:1–24.

Castro-Alamancos MA, Donoghue JP, Connors BW (1995). Different forms of synaptic plasticity in somatosensory and motor areas of the neocortex. J Neurosci 15:5324–5333.

Darian-Smith C, Darian SI (1993). Thalamic projections to areas 3a, 3b, and 4 in the sensorimotor cortex of the mature and infant macaque monkey. J Comp Neurol 335:173–199.

Darian-Smith C, Darian SI, Burman K, Ratcliffe N (1993). Ipsilateral cortical projections to areas 3a, 3b, and 4 in the macaque monkey. J Comp Neurol 335:200–213.

Darian-Smith C, Gilbert CD (1994). Axonal sprouting accompanies functional reorganization in adult cat striate cortex. Nature 368:737–740.

DeFelipe J, Conley M, Jones EG (1986). Long-range focal collateralization of axons arising from cortico-cortical cells in monkey sensory-motor cortex. J Neurosci 6:3749–3765.

di Pellegrino G, Wise SP (1991). A neurophysiological comparison of three distinct regions of the primate frontal lobe. Brain 114:951–978.

Donoghue JP, Kitai ST (1981). A collateral pathway to the neostriatum from corticofugal neurons of the rat sensory-motor cortex: An intracellular HRP study. J Comp Neurol 201:1–13.

Donoghue JP, Sanes JN (1994). Motor areas of the cerebral cortex. J Clin Neurophysiol 11:382–396.

Dugas C, Marteniuk RG (1989). Strategy and learning effects on perturbed movements: An electromyographic and kinematic study. Behav Brain Res 35:181–193.

Dum RP, Strick PL (1991). The origin of corticospinal projections from the premotor areas in the frontal lobe. J Neurosci 11:667–689.

Fitts PM (1954). The information capacity of the human motor system in controlling the amplitude of movement. J Exp Psychol 67:381–391.

Forlano LM, Horne MK, Butler EG, Finkelstein D (1993). Neural activity in the monkey anterior ventrolateral thalamus during trained, ballistic movements. J Neurophysiol 70:2276–2288.

Gemba H, Sasaki KT (1984). Studies on cortical field potentials recorded during learning processes of visually initiated hand movements in monkeys. Exp Brain Res 55:28–32.

Gemba H, Sasaki K (1987). Cortical field potentials associated with audio-initiated hand movements in the monkey. Exp Brain Res 65:649–657.

Gemba H, Sasaki KT (1988). Changes in cortical field potentials associated with learning processes of audio-initiated hand movements in monkeys. Exp Brain Res 70:43–49.

Gentilucci M, Fogassi L, Luppino G, Matelli M, Camarda R, Rizzolatti G (1988). Functional organization of inferior area 6 in the macaque monkey: I. Somatotopy and the control of proximal movements. Exp Brain Res 71:475–490.

Germain L, Lamarre Y (1993). Neuronal activity in the motor and premotor cortices before and after learning the associations between auditory stimuli and motor responses. Brain Res 611:175–179.

Gilbert CD, Hirsch JA, Wiesel TN (1990). Lateral interactions in visual cortex. Cold Spring Harb Symp Quant Biol 55:663–677.

Gordon AM, Casabona A, Soechting JF (1994). The learning of novel finger movement sequences. J Neurophysiol 72:1596–1610.

Grafton ST, Hazeltine E, Ivry R (1995). Functional mapping of sequence learning in normal humans. J Cog Neurosci 7:497–510.

Grafton ST, Mazziotta JC, Presty S, Friston KJ, Frackowiak RS, Phelps ME (1992). Functional anatomy of human procedural learning determined with regional cerebral blood flow and PET. J Neurosci 12:2542–2548.

Greenough WT, Larson JR, Withers GS (1985). Effects of unilateral and bilateral training in a reaching task on dendritic branching of neurons in the rat motor-sensory forelimb cortex. Behav Neural Biol 44:301–314.

Halsband U, Freund H-J (1990). Premotor cortex and conditional motor learning in man. Brain 113:207–222.

Hendry SH, Houser CR, Jones EG, Vaughn JE (1983). Synaptic organization of immunocyto-chemically identified GABA neurons in the monkey sensory-motor cortex. J Neurocytol 12: 639–660.

Hess G, Aizenman CD, Donoghue JP (1996). Gating of long-term potentiation in layer II/III horizontal connections in rat motor cortex (in press).

Hess G, Donoghue JP (1994). Long-term potentiation of horizontal connections provides a mechanism to reorganize cortical motor maps. J Neurophysiol 71:2543–2547.

Hess G, Jacobs KM, Donoghue JP (1994). N-methyl-D-aspartate receptor-mediated component of field potentials evoked in horizontal pathways of rat motor cortex. Neuroscience 61:225–235.

Hess G, Donoghue JP (1996). Long-term depression of horizontal connections in rat motor cortex (in press).

Hirsch JA, Gilbert CD (1991). Synaptic physiology of horizontal connections in the cat's visual cortex. J Neurosci 11:1800–1809.

Humphrey DR, Qiu XO, Clavel P, O'Donoghue DL (1990). Changes in forelimb motor repre-sentation in rodent cortex induced by passive movements. Soc Neurosci Abstr 16:422.

Huntley GW, Jones EG (1991). Relationship of intrinsic connections to forelimb movement representations in monkey motor cortex: A correlative anatomic and physiological study. J Neurophysiol 66:390–413.

Huntley GW, Vickers JC, Janssen W, Brose N, Heinemann SF (1994). Distribution and synaptic localiztion of immunocytochemically identified NMDA receptor subunit proteins in sensory-motor and visual cortices of monkey and human. J Neurosci 14:3603–3619.

Iriki A, Keller A, Pavlides C, Asanuma H (1990). Long-lasting facilitation of pyramidal tract input to spinal interneurons. Neuroreport 1:157–160.

Iriki A, Pavlides C, Keller A, Asanuma H (1991). Long-term potentiation of thalamic input to the motor cortex induced by coactivation of thalamocortical and corticocortical afferents. J Neurophysiol 65:1435–1441.

Ito M, Oda Y (1994). Electrophysiological evidence for formation of new corticorubral syn-apses associated with classical conditioning in the cat. Exp Brain Res 99:277–288.

Jacobs KM (1993). The Functional Architecture of Neocortical Circuitry. Unpublished doctoral dissertation, Brown University, Providence.

Jacobs K, Donoghue J (1991). Reshaping the cortical map by unmasking latent intracortical connections. Science 251:944–947.

Jacobs KM, Hess G, Connors BW, Donoghue JP (1996). Intracortical vertical and horizontal response patterns produced by layer V stimulation in rat motor cortex in vitro (submitted for publication).

Jacobs KM, Neve RL, Donoghue JP (1990). Adult rat neocortex contains a laminar-specific distribution of both calcium/calmodulin-dependent protein kinase II and GAP-43 mRNA. Soc Neurosci Abstr 16:43.

Jaric S, Corcos DM, Gottlieb GL, Ilic DB, Latash ML (1994). The effects of practice on movement distance and final position reproduction: Implications for the equilibrium-point control of movements. Exp Brain Res 100:353–359.

Jones EG (1987). Ascending inputs to, and internal organization of, cortical motor areas. Ciba Found Symp 132:21–39.

Jones EG (1993). GABAergic neurons and their role in cortical plasticity in primates. Cereb Cortex 3:361–372.

Kalaska JF, Cohen DAD, Prud'homme M, Hyde ML (1990). Parietal area 5 neuronal activity encodes movement kinematics, not movement dynamics. Exp Brain Res 80:351–364.

Kalaska JF, Crammond DJ (1992). Cerebral cortical mechanisms of reaching movements. Science 255:1517–1523.

Kang Y, Kaneko T, Ohishi H, Endo K, Araki T (1994). Spatiotemporally differential inhibition of pyramidal cells in the cat motor cortex. J Neurophysiol 71:280–293.

Karni A, Meyer G, Jezzard P, Adams MG, Turner R, Ungerleider L (1995). Functional MRI evidence for adult motorcortex plasticity during motor skill learning. Nature 377:155–158.

Keller A (1993a). Intrinsic synaptic organization of the motor cortex. Cereb Cortex 3:430–441.

Keller A (1993b). Intrinsic connections between representation zones in the cat motor cortex. Neuroreport 4:515–518.

Keller A, Arissian K, Asanuma H (1992). Synaptic proliferation in the motor cortex of adult cats after long-term thalamic stimulation. J Neurophysiol 68:295–308.

Keller A, Asanuma H (1993). Synaptic relationships involving local axon collaterals of pyramidal neurons in the cat motor cortex. J Comp Neurol 336:229–242.

Keller A, Iriki A, Asanuma H (1990). Identification of neurons producing LTP in the cat motor cortex: Intracellular recordings and labelling. J Comp Neurol 300:47–60.

Kim EH, Woody CD, Berthier NE (1983). Rapid acquisition of conditioned eye blink responses in cats following pairing of an auditory CS with glabella tap US and hypothalamic stimulation. J Neurophysiol 49:767–779.

Kimura A, Caria MA, Melis F, Asanuma H (1994). Long-term potentiation within the cat motor cortex. Neuroreport 5:2372–2376.

Landry P, Labelle A, De henes M (1980). Intracortical distribution of axonal collaterals of pyramidal tract cells in the cat motor cortex. Brain Res 191:327–336.

Landry P, Wilson CJ, Kitai ST (1984). Morphological and electrophysiological characteristics of pyramidal tract neurons in the rat. Exp Brain Res 57:177–190.

Lang W, Lang M, Podreka I, Steiner M, Uhl F, Suess E, Muller C (1988). DC-potential shifts and regional cerebral blood flow reveal frontal cortex involvement in human visuomotor learning. Exp Brain Res 71:353–364.

Lisberger SG (1988). The neural basis for motor learning in the vestibulo-ocular reflex in monkeys. Trends Neurosci 11:147–152.

Lømo T, Bliss TVP (1973). Long-lasting potentiation of synaptic transmission in the dentate area of the anesthisized rabbit following stimulation of the perforant path. J Physiol (Lond) 232:331–356.

Luppino G, Matelli M, Rizzolatti G (1990). Cortico-cortical connections of two electrophysiologically identified arm representations in the mesial agranular frontal cortex. Exp Brain Res 82:214–218.

Mackel R, Iriki A, Jorum E, Asanuma H (1991). Neurons of the pretectal area convey spinal input to the motor thalamus of the cat. Exp Brain Res 84:12–24.

Malenka RC (1994). Synaptic plasticity in the hippocampus: LTP and LTD. Cell 78:535–538.

Malenka RC, Nicoll RA (1993). NMDA-receptor-dependent synaptic plasticity: Multiple forms and mechanisms. Trends Neurosci 16:521–527.

Martin JH, Ghez C (1993). Differential impairments in reaching and grasping produced by local inactivation within the forelimb representation of the motor cortex in the cat. Exp Brain Res 94:429–443.

Matelli M, Camarda R, Glickstein M, Rizzolatti G (1986). Afferent and efferent projections of the inferior area 6 in the macaque monkey. J Comp Neurol 251:281–298.

Maton B, Burnod Y, Calvet J (1983). Evolution of myoelectrical and precentral cell activities during learning of a new amplitude of movement. Brain Res 267:241–248.

Matsumura M, Sawaguchi T, Kubota K (1990). Modulation of neuronal activities by iontophoretically applied catecholamines and acetylcholine in the primate motor cortex during a visual reaction-time task. Neurosci Res NY. 8:138–145.

McCarren M, Alger BE (1985). Use-dependent depression of IPSPs in rat hippocampal pyramidal cells in vitro. J Neurophysiol 53:557–571.

McGuire BA, Gilbert CD, Rivlin PK, Wiesel TN (1991). Targets of horizontal connections in macaque primary visual cortex. J Comp Neurol 305:370–392.

Milliken G, Nudo R, Grenda R, Jenkins WM, Merzenich MM (1992). Expansion of distal forelimb representations in primary motor cortex of adult squirrel monkeys following motor training. Soc Neurosci Abstr 18:214.

Mitz AR, Godschalk M, Wise SP (1991). Learning-dependent neuronal activity in the premotor cortex: activity during the acquisition of conditional motor associations. J Neurosci 11:1855–1872.

Miyashita E, Keller A, Asanuma H (1994). Input-output organization of the rat vibrissal motor cortex. Exp Brain Res 99:223–232.

Mountcastle VB, Lynch JC, Georgopoulos A, Sakata H, Acuna C (1975). Posterior parietal association cortex of the monkey: Command functions for operations within extrapersonal space. J Neurophysiol 38:871–908.

Nissen MJ, Bullemer P (1987). Attentional requirements of learning: Evidence from performance measures. Cogn Psychol 19:1–33.

Nudo RJ, Jenkins WM, Merzenich MM (1990). Repetitive microstimulation alters the cortical representation of movements in adult rats. Somatosens Mot Res 7:463–483.

Pandya DN, Vignolo L (1971). Intra- and interhemispheric projections of the precentral, premotor and arcuate areas in the rhesus monkeys. Brain Res 26:217–223.

Pascual-Leone A, Grafman J, Hallett M (1994). Modulation of cortical motor outptut maps during development of implicit and explicit knowledge. Science 263:1287–1289.

Pew RW (1966). Acquisition of hierarchical control over the temporal organization of a skill. J Exp Psychol 71:764–771.

Porter LL, Sakamoto K (1988). Organization and synaptic relationships of the projection from the primary sensory to the primary motor cortex in the cat. J Comp Neurol 271:387–396.

Qiu XQ, O'Donoghue DL, Humphrey DR (1990). NMDA antagonist (MK-801) blocks plasticity of motor cortex maps induced by passive limb movement. Soc Neurosci Abstr 16:422.

Sakamoto T, Porter LL, Asanuma H (1987). Long-lasting potentiation of synaptic potentials in the motor cortex produced by stimulation of the sensory cortex in the cat: A basis of motor learning. Brain Res 413:360–364.

Sanes J, Donoghue J (1992). Organization and adaptability of muscle represenations in primary motor cortex. Exp Brain Res Suppl 22:103–127.

Sanes JN, Wang J, Donoghue JP (1992). Immediate and delayed changes of rat motor cortical output representation with new forelimb configurations. Cereb Cortex 2:141–152.

Schlaug G, Knorr U, Seitz R (1994). Inter-subject variability of cerebral activations in acquiring a motor skill: A study with positron emission tomography. Exp Brain Res 98:523–534.

Schmidt RA (1976). The schema as a solution to some persistent problems in motor learning theory. In GE Stelmach (ed), Motor Control. New York: Academic, pp 41–65.

Seitz RJ, Roland PE (1992). Learning of sequential finger movements in man: A combined kinematic and positron emission tomography (PET) study. Eur J Neurosci 4:154–165.

Shima K, Aya K, Mushiake H, Inase M, Aizawa H, Tanji J (1991). Two movement-related foci in the primate cingulate cortex observed in signal-triggered and self-paced forelimb movements. J Neurophysiol 65:188–202.

Shinoda Y, Kakei S, Futami T, Wannier T (1993). Thalamocortical organization in the cerebello-thalamo-cortical system. Cereb Cortex 3:421–429.

Suner S, Gutman D, Gaal G, Sanes J, Donoghue JP (1993). Reorganization of monkey motor cortex related to motor skill learning. Soc Neurosci Abstr 19:775.

Thach WT (1987). Cerebellar inputs to motor cortex. Ciba Found Symp 132:201–220.

Thomson AM, Deuchars J (1994). Temporal and spatial properties of local circuits in neocortex. Trends Neurosci 17:119–126.

Wise SP, Donoghue JP (1986). The motor cortex of rodents. In EG Jones, A Peters (eds). The Cerebral Cortex: The Functional Areas of the Cerebral Cortex. New York: Plenum, vol 5, pp 243–270.

Withers GS, Greenough WT (1989). Reach training selectively alters dendritic branching in subpopulations of layer II-III pyramids in rat motor-somatosensory forelimb cortex. Neuropsychologia 27:61–69.

Woody CD (1986). Understanding the cellular basis of memory and learning. Annu Rev Psychol 37:433–493.

Woody CD, Gruen E (1987). Acetylcholine reduces net outward currents measured in vivo with single electrode voltage clamp techniques in neurons of the motor cortex of cats. Brain Res 424:193–198.

Woody C, Yarowsky P, Owens J, Black CP, Crow T (1974). Effect of lesions of cortical motor areas on acquisition of conditioned eye blink in the cat. J Neurophysiol 37:385–394.

18 Neuronal Mechanisms Subserving the Acquisition of New Skilled Movements in Mammals

Hiroshi Asanuma

Understanding the neural basis of learning and memory, especially, the mechanisms underlying consciousness, is of concern to neuroscientists. However, our knowledge about such mechanisms remains fragmentary because of the diversity of the problem. On the other hand, studying the mechanisms of motor learning is much simpler because it does not necessitate consciousness or language, making experimental approaches easier. In both cases, it is assumed that learned skills are stored in selected circuits in the central nervous system. Determining how these circuits are created has been the purpose of our experiments.

The type of motor learning we are interested in is acquisition of new skilled movements, such as a baseball player hitting a home run. We must ask first what is meant by a skilled movement. A skilled movement consists of a series of movement patterns which are called movement segments (Adams, 1984). Each segment consists of simultaneous contraction of a group of muscles. In the early stages of investigation, ethologists thought that these movement segments were inborn and that skilled movements were accomplished by retrieval of existing segments (as seen in fighting, nest building, etc.) (Lorenz, 1970). However, experimental psychologists soon recognized that not all the segments are inborn and that skilled movements have to be acquired by learning new movement segments. Therefore, it seems reasonable to propose that one of the important processes of motor learning is the creation of new movement segments that are necessary for new movements. A question then arises: What is the actual location of these circuits. Many sites in the central nervous system can be considered but because of its large size and unique structure, we would speculate that this learning is processed by reorganization of the motor cortex (see also chapter 17).

The motor cortex consists of cortical efferent zones (Asanuma, 1981; Asanuma, 1989). Each zone is innervated by the projection from the ventrolateral nucleus (VL) of the thalamus and part of the the somatosensory cortex (area 2). The innervation from the VL is diffuse, each neuron in the VL innervating many efferent zones located in a wide area of the motor cortex (Strick, 1973). On the other hand, the projection from area 2 to the motor cortex is specific, and each sensory column is thought to innervate a few efferent zones (Porter and Sakamoto, 1988). This organization suggests that the input from area 2 to the motor cortex serves as a teacher in learning new motor skills. We have started experiments by examining whether intracortical microstimulation (ICMS) of the sensory cortex can produce long-term potentiation (LTP) in the motor cortex. It was found that tetanic ICMS in area 2 could produce LTP at their terminals in the motor cortex (Sakamoto, Porter, and Asanuma, 1987; see also chapter 17). The results can be interpreted in the following way: In learning a new motor skill, repeated practice of a particular movement is necessary. During that time, the sensory input related to the contraction of the target muscles ascends to the sensory cortex and activates related sensory columns, which then transfers the input to the motor cortex to produce LTP at their terminals. This LTP increases the efficiency of synaptic transmission in selected groups of corticocortical projection. When the VL input is combined with this corticocortical input, it activates (by summation) a selected group of efferent zones. This interpretation agrees with the experience that, in the beginning of motor learning, movement is hectic, producing contraction of unnecessary muscles. As practice continues, these unnecessary contractions are eliminated, and only necessary muscles contract.

According to this interpretation, execution of skilled movement always necessitates feedback information from the periphery. However, we know that after the completion of learning, the feedback becomes unnecessary. A typical example of this phenomenon is seen in a pianist (see chapter 16). The movement of the finger is too fast for the feedback input to participate; therefore there must be other mechanisms participating in learning new motor skills. In spite of our extensive attempts, tetanic stimulation of the VL never produced LTP at their terminals (Sakamoto et al., 1987). However, when VL stimulation was combined with area 2 stimulation, associative LTP could be produced at the VL terminals (Iriki, Pavlides, Keller, and Asanuma, 1989; see chapter 17). The result indicates that after sufficient practice, the efficiency of a selected portion of VL terminals becomes enhanced, and activation of a selected group of efferent zones can be accomplished by the same command signal coming through the VL.

Altogether, the results may indicate the following: In the early stages of learning, the somatosensory cortex is necessary to create new movement segments but, after establishing the new segments, input from area 2 becomes unnecessary. To examine whether this is the case, we trained monkeys with and without the sensory cortex (Pavlides, Miyashita, and Asanuma, 1993). The hand area of the sensory cortex of one hemisphere was removed prior to the behavioral experiments. It has been reported that removal of the somatosensory cortex produces unnoticeable motor deficits (Asanuma and Arissian, 1984; Travis and Woolsey, 1956). After recovery from the surgery, the monkeys were trained to catch a food pellet falling through a semicircular tube as shown in figure 18.1A. The speed of the food pellet was controlled by changing the angle of the tube. The task that the monkey had to learn was to swing the hand and, at an appropriate time to grab the food. Neither hand

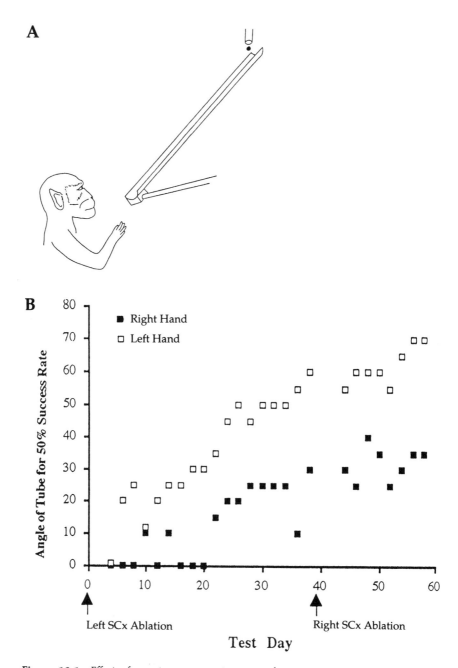

Figure 18.1 Effect of somatosensory cortex removal on motor activity. A. A macaque monkey faced a semicylindrical tube held by a bar attached at the bottom. Tube angle was adjusted by rotating the bar. The task was to catch a spherical food pellet dropped to the tube from a dispenser after a tone signal. The monkey caught the falling food by swinging its arm. B. Learning curves for food-catching task. Ordinate: angle of the tube at which the monkey could catch the food pellet in 50 percent of the trials. Abscissa: days after the first operation that removed left somatosensory cortex. The second operation; which removed the remaining (right) somatosensory cortex; did not eliminate the previously learned skill. (Modified from Pavlides et al., 1993.)

Neuronal Mechanisms for Acquisition of Skilled Movements

had difficulty in swinging and reaching the falling target or in grabbing stationary food. As training progressed, the hand contralateral to the lesion could not combine the two movements. As a result, the learning of the new skill was severely retarded (as shown by the filled squares in figure 18.1B). After completion of the training, the remaining sensory cortex was removed. As shown, the already-acquired motor skill did not disappear (open squares of figure 18.1). The results support the hypothesis that the projection from the sensory cortex to the motor cortex is significant in learning new motor skills.

REFERENCES

Adams JA (1984). Learning of movement sequences. Psychol Bull 96:3–28.

Asanuma H (1981). The pyramidal tract. In VB Brooks (ed), Handbook of Physiology, Section 1: The Nervous System, Bethesda: American Physiological Society. pp 703–733.

Asanuma H (1989). The Motor Cortex. New York: Raven Press.

Asanuma H, Arissian K (1984). Experiments on functional role of peripheral input to motor cortex during voluntary movements in the monkey. J Neurophysiol 52:212–227.

Iriki A, Pavlides C, Keller A, Asanuma H (1989). Long-term potentiation in the motor cortex. Science 245:1385–1387.

Lorenz K (1970). Studies in Animal and Human Behavior. Cambridge, MA: Harvard University Press.

Pavlides C, Miyashita E, Asanuma H (1993). Projection from the sensory to the motor cortex is important in learning motor skills in the monkey. J Neurophysiol 70:733–741.

Porter LL, Sakamoto K (1988). Organization and synaptic relationship of the projection from the primary sensory to the primary motor cortex in the cat. J Comp Neurol 271:387–396.

Sakamoto T, Porter LL, Asanuma H (1987). Long-lasting potentiation of synaptic potentials in the motor cortex produced by stimulation of the sensory cortex in the cat: A basis of motor learning. Brain Res 413:360–364.

Strick PL (1973). Light microscopic analysis of the cortical projection of the thalamic ventro-lateral nucleus in the cat. Brain Res 55:1–24.

Travis AM, Woolsey CN (1956). Motor performance of monkeys after bilateral partial and total cerebral decortications. Am J Phys Med 35:273–289.

19 Motor Learning: Toward Understanding Acquired Representations

George E. Stelmach

It goes without saying that motor skill improves with practice. With training or practice, we expect improvement, and this improvement is assumed to be ubiquitous, though there are limits in the scope and extent. An enormous research effort has been devoted to the behavioral phenomena associated with recording performance changes as individuals acquire a new or novel form of voluntary motor behavior (see Adams, 1987, for review). This chapter discusses recent conceptions of human motor learning that have implications on how the acquisition processes should be characterized.

These emerging conceptions contrast in a major way from much of the earlier work on motor learning. During the early period, considerable effort was spent on describing the benefits of practice by documenting the rate and magnitude of changes in performance resulting from practice. For the most part, this research dealt with the law of practice, which almost always was demonstrated by plotting the logarithm of task performance time against the logarithm of the trial number (Newell and Rosenbloom, 1981). Such plots typically yielded a straight line. According to Newell and Rosenbloom, this relationship is often referred to as the *power law of practice*. This empirical law has been around for a long time; it was apparently discovered first by Snoddy (1926) in a study on mirror tracing, a skill that involves intimate and continuous coordination of the perceptual and motor systems. Its ubiquity is widely recognized, as it occupied a major position in early books on human performance (e.g., Fitts and Posner, 1967; Welford, 1968).

Current research in motor learning is focused more on what is learned than on how a motor skill can be learned best. Throughout this chapter, a prevalent theme will be the elucidation of the limits of making inferences about motor learning from performance curves. As will be shown, motor performance is a less-than-perfect indicator of motor learning. The use of transfer tests will be introduced as a method to clarify performance and learning differences. As the chapter proceeds, an attempt will be made to examine the nature of the movement representation acquired during practice. Again, the use of transfer tests will be demonstrated. Two questions focus the emerging debate: As skills are learned, how are they acquired, and once a motor skill has been acquired, what is the nature of its underlying memory representation? We will demonstrate that emerging transfer paradigms hold promise for understanding how motor actions are neurally coded and represented.

MOTOR LEARNING DEFINED

Over the years, motor learning has been defined in several ways by various authors (see chapter 6). In general, these definitions share certain distinct characteristics. First, learning is a process of acquiring the capability for producing skilled action. As stated by Schmidt (1991b), learning is a set of underlying events, occurrences, or changes that take place when practice enables an individual to improve motor control and coordination. Second, learning occurs as a direct result of practice or training. Third, learning cannot be observed directly, as the processes leading to changes in behavior are internal and are usually not available for direct examination. At best in an experimental paradigm, learning must be inferred on the basis of changes in motor performance. Fourth, learning is assumed to produce relatively permanent changes in motor control. This latter restriction is needed to rule out temporary effects due to motivation, excitation, and arousal.

By combining the foregoing features, it is possible to offer the following global definition: *Motor learning* is defined as a change in the capability of an individual to perform a skill that must be inferred from a relatively permanent improvement in performance as a result of practice (Stelmach, 1982; Schmidt 1991b). In many ways, understanding motor skill learning is more difficult than associative learning or vestibuloocular reflex adaptation because: (1) The control parameters of voluntary movements have highly nonlinear dynamics with multiple degrees of freedom, (2) many neural networks and pathways are organized in a hierarchical manner, and (3) volition participates in the highest level of control (Kawato, 1989).

EARLIER RESEARCH IN MOTOR LEARNING

Much of the earlier analysis of motor skill learning concentrated on methods of learning rather than on conceptualization of what is learned. During that period, one of researchers' major goals was to understand which independent variables are involved in the optimization of learning, which are involved in degrading learning, and which are neutral or have no effect (Keele, 1986). Though such information may be important for the development of descriptive theories of learning, it does not contribute to the more basic questions of how learning takes place and what is acquired with practice (Schmidt, 1991a).

During the aforementioned period, methods of learning were prominent. For example, it has been shown by many that motor skills are best learned with distributed practice schedules (see Keele, 1986; Adams, 1987). During practice, short, frequent rests benefit performance more than massed practice does; hence, experiments that dealt with massed versus distributed practice

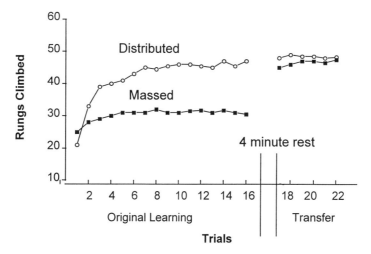

Figure 19.1 The effects of distributed and massed practice on Bachman ladder test performance. Transfer testing reveals that not all of the difference between the two groups is due to learning; most was due to temporary fatigue arising from massed practice. Adapted from Stelmach, 1969.

focused on the amount of rest imposed between trials of a fixed length. In a 1969 study, Stelmach addressed the issue of the effects of massed practice on the learning of a novel motor task. He used sixteen 30-second trials on a Bachman ladder task (in which the subject had to climb a free-standing ladder, attempting to maximize the number of rungs climbed in a 30-s trial). The distributed-practice condition had 30-s rests between trials, whereas a massed group had no rest between trials.

The results of this study are presented in figure 19.1, where the number of rungs climbed is plotted against trials for the massed and distributed groups. Both groups began practice at essentially the same initial level, but the massed group's rate of improvement did not approach that of the distributed. By the end of the acquisition trials, there was a clear advantage for the distributed group. The difference between groups was 67 percent in favor of the distributed group.

Which group learned more? The obvious answer is that it was the distributed group, based on the performance curve data during original learning. However, this conclusion is based on the assumption that the performance curves reflect the amount learned. As is shown in the transfer part of the data in figure 19.1, that interpretation is not correct. That is, when both groups are given a four-minute rest interval and are retested, the massed group's performance jumps dramatically during transfer; now the group differences are no longer apparent. The massed group's performance was temporarily impaired due to the frequency of training, thus it should be apparent that transfer tests can play a useful role in motor learning research. If solely the performance curves during original learning were available, it is obvious that the incorrect conclusion would have been made from these data. The major point made by these data is that performance curves do not always reflect the amount learned; therefore, it is difficult to infer the amount learned without transfer tests (Schmidt, 1991b; Stelmach, 1969).

TRANSFER PARADIGMS

Transfer designs are critical to the study of motor learning, as they provide a way for various independent variables to be studied with respect to their effects on motor learning. The essential feature of such paradigms is that after practice, all groups transfer to some common level of an independent variable. These designs make it possible to categorize variables into two types: performance variables and learning variables. A *performance variable* is one that affects performance but not learning, and a *learning variable* is one that influences performance in a relatively permanent way.

Random Versus Blocked Practice

An experiment by Shea and Morgan (1979) provides a further illustration of how the performance curve during acquisition can be misleading and does not reveal the amount learned. They compared random and blocked types of practice on a complex arm sequencing task. The tasks required rapid, multiple-component arm movements, where the subjects attempted to minimize the time taken to complete the sequence. Blocked practice involved sequential trials of three arm sequences in which subjects were required to practice each task pattern repeatedly before moving on to the next pattern. In contrast, random practice involved the same number of trials on the three separate tasks, but the order was randomized so that a given task was never practiced on successive trials. After an original practice phase, retention tests were given after 10 min and after 10 days. These retention tests were given under either random or blocked conditions so that half the subjects in the blocked or random condition were switched to the opposite practice pattern.

The results are reported in figure 19.2. During the original learning phase, there was a substantial advantage for the subjects who practiced under blocked conditions, particularly during the initial stages of practice. With practice, the random group improved at a fast rate until they were almost as good as the blocked group. However, amount of learning during the transfer tests revealed a completely different story. There was a strong advantage in retention for those subjects who practiced under random conditions during original learning. What is surprising is that, even though the random group subjects performed at a much lower rate during acquisition, they performed substantially better compared to the blocked group during the retention tests (Schmidt, 1991a). Moreover, these results (which may appear to be counterintuitive) indicate that regardless of whether the retention test was itself random or blocked, it was always more effective to have practiced under random conditions. As pointed out by Schmidt and Bjork (1992), "[R]emark-

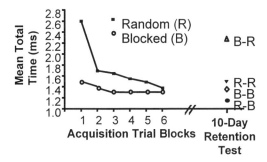

Figure 19.2 Performance on movement speed tasks under random (R) and blocked (B) conditions in acquisition and after 10 days. The first letter indicates the acquisition condition, and the second represents the retention condition. Adapted from Shea and Morgan, 1979.

ably, this was the case even though the random condition was detrimental to performance during original learning." This phenomenon has been observed by others (Baddéley and Longmann, 1978; Lee and Magill, 1983; Goode and Magill, 1986).

How are such results explained? According to Schmidt and Bjork (1992), the condition that produced the best retention performance appeared to have a characteristic that provided added difficulty for the learner during the acquisition phase. They suggest that random practice serves to keep the performance from generating a stable "set" for a particular task and forces the learner to retrieve and organize a different motor plan in every trial. Therefore, the speculation is that this type of practice may enrich the nature of the learned representation which translates into better retention.

Feedback During Original Learning

Variation of feedback is one of the most robust variables influencing the performance curve during acquisition. It has been shown repeatedly that the accuracy, frequency, and latency in which feedback is provided can influence performance during acquisition. A study by Schmidt, Young, Swinner and Shapiro (1989) suggests that, as with random and blocked designs, the frequency of knowledge of results (KR) differentially affects performance as it is compared to learning. In this experiment, subjects had to learn a relatively complex arm movement in which they were to produce two reversals in direction so that action time was as close as possible to a defined goal. In one condition, feedback about the movement-time error was given after each trial. In other conditions, the feedback was delayed and given in a summary form in every 5 or 15 trials. The summary form of feedback provided was identical in content to that given in every trial except that it covered a spectrum of trials. Subjects in each of these three feedback conditions performed six blocks of acquisition practice and then were retested after 2 days. The retention transfer task consisted of practice without any feedback.

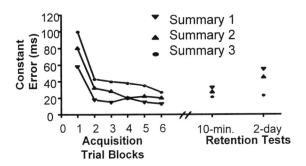

Figure 19.3 Mean errors in a movement-patterning task for three different summary-feedback lengths in acquisition and on no-feedback retention tests given after 10 min or 2 days. Conditions: Summary 1, feedback every trial; Summary 2, every 5 trials; Summary 3, every 15 trials. Adapted from Schmidt et al., 1989.

The results of the experiment are seen in figure 19.3. During the original learning, subjects in the feedback on every trial condition performed more accurately throughout practice than the other two groups. From the data, it is apparent that delaying the feedback and giving it only in every 5 or 15 trials reduced performance throughout acquisition trials. This reduction was apparent in slowing the rate of improvement and the final level of performance achieved during the acquisition trials. However, a different view is obtained if one inspects the transfer retention tests. The most effective retention performance was generated by the 15-trial summary KR group. According to Schmidt and Bjork (1992), these data seem to contradict the notion that frequent feedback translates into optimal learning. Schmidt et al. have shown similar effects in other studies over the years (Winstein and Schmidt, 1990; Schmidt, 1991a). How are these data explained? One hypothesis is that frequent feedback tends to become part of the task so that performance is disrupted in retention when feedback is not provided. In addition, some have speculated that frequent feedback could block information-processing activities that are important during the acquisition. Such processing of response-produced feedback leads to less effective error-detection capabilities. Finally, frequent feedback makes performance too variable during practice, inhibiting the capability to learn a stabilized representation that can be retained.

Modularity

Keele, Cohen, and Ivry (1990) analyzed the modularity of learning a motor sequence using a key-pressing task, their primary question being whether a learned sequence of key presses is independent of the effector system that executes the sequence. To answer this question, a transfer test placed response targets at one of three horizontal locations on a monitor and required the subjects to press keys that corresponded to the positions of the visual signals. As each key was pressed, the visual signals disappeared, and 200 msec later another appeared. There were two acquisition situations: First,

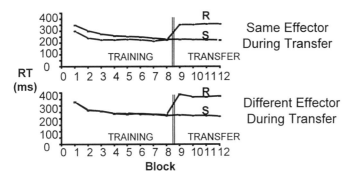

Figure 19.4 Reaction time to visual signals at three screen locations; location is fixed in blocks 1 to 18. R, random during transfer; S, sequence during transfer; RT, reaction time. Adapted from Keele et al., 1990.

signals appeared at random with the restriction of no immediate repetition, and second, signals appeared in a particular order of five elements (e.g., 31231) before repeating. In this condition, the five-sequence combination of stimuli and responses was repeated for 20 cycles totalling 100 trials. Thus the difference between conditions was that the repetitive sequence condition permitted the subjects to learn the five-element pattern though the random condition did not. The expectation was that with practice, the subjects would learn to produce faster reaction times to the predictable sequence, and no such benefit would be in the random condition.

During the original training phase, subjects in both conditions practiced a sequence of eight blocks of 100 trials per block. During this training phase, half the subjects responded with three fingers on the three keys. The other half of the subjects hit the keys with their index finger by moving their arms back and forth over the keys (Keele et al., 1990). The primary difference was that some subjects used finger responses and the others used arm movements to execute the sequence.

In a subsequent phase, blocks 9 to 12 were transfer trials. For these trials, half the subjects kept the same effectors as before, but the other half changed from fingers to arms or from arms to fingers. Moreover, half of each of these groups continued the identical sequence as in original training, whereas the other half received signals at random (Keele et al., 1990). The reaction time data for these task conditions are shown in figure 19.4.

During transfer, the group that maintained the sequence continued to perform at the original learning rate, but reaction times of the group that shifted to the random condition produced considerably slower response latencies. This difference in reaction times between the two groups indicates the degree of sequence learning.

The primary issue is what happens to the performance of the groups that changed effectors from original training to transfer. As can be seen in figure 19.4, the results indicated that there is no difference in performance between groups, regardless of maintaining the same effector or switching. The advantage of sequence-maintenance trials over random targets is the same regardless of whether the effectors change. These results suggest that a sequence acquired in the course of performance with a particular muscle effector system is completely independent of that effector system (Keele et al., 1990).

Other studies also provide examples that the acquired behavior can be exported to a different muscle system. Pew (1974) had subjects track an apparently random movement of a moving target. Unknown to the subjects, one segment of the moving spot was the same across trials, and tracking during that segment exhibited greater than normal improvement. Quite surprisingly, the improvement transferred to a mirror-image display, which required a totally different movement sequence. Moreover, an experiment by Rosenbloom (1977) showed that fatigue that accrues during training with a strenuous arm-cranking movement and is pattern-specific during acquisition, transfers to muscles in a previously unused arm.

In many ways, these foregoing experiments are similar to the example provided by Bernstein (1967) first addressing the extent to which the representation of a sequence of action is separable from and able to be interfaced with difficult effector systems (Keele et al., 1990). Bernstein showed that handwriting samples from the hand, arm, mouth, and foot can illustrate a number of similarities. The similarity of spatial configurations across effectors suggests that the sequence representation is independent of the muscular systems that execute them (Castiello and Stelmach, 1993). The Bernstein example is primarily heuristic as it does not provide precise information on how the acquired representation specifies the temporal and spatial aspects of the handwriting.

As Keele (1986) points out, these observations do not mean that no learning occurs at a motoric level. However, these data do suggest some division between the motor level and the representation level (MacKay, 1982; Keele et al., 1990; Castiello and Stelmach, 1993). Keele suggests that the representation level contains the temporal and sequencing information. If learning is to occur, the muscle level must learn how to accept the representation level commands and to move in a coordinated fashion specified by the motor output.

Generalized Representations

It is a common procedure in motor learning research to provide practice in rather restrictive conditions to enhance performance improvements (Schmidt, 1991b). Many experiments have demonstrated that by keeping the stimulus and response conditions constant and repetitive, very substantial performance improvements occur with rather small amounts of practice (Keele, 1986; Schmidt and Bjork, 1992). What kind of learning do such practice regimens yield? To answer this question, one may employ again a transfer design; such a design permits one to address whether the learning acquired during practice

Table 19.1 Design for an Experiment on Variability in Practice

Group	Original Practice Phase 300 trials; Day 1	Transfer Test Phase Immediate, Day 1	Delayed, Day 2
Constant			
Subgroup a	15 cm only	50 cm	50 cm
Subgroup b	35 cm only	50 cm	50 cm
Subgroup c	60 cm only	50 cm	50 cm
Subgroup d	65 cm only	50 cm	50 cm
Variable	15, 35, 60, and 65 cm in random order	50 cm	50 cm

Source: Adapted from Stelmach and McCracken, 1977.

is generalizable. In other words, does the learned motor pattern transfer to novel situations?

There have been a number of experiments that have addressed this issue. McCracken and Stelmach (1977) did one such study illustrating that variability of practice produces a more modular representation compared to fixed practice. The researchers had subjects move their right arm from a starting key to knock over a barrier, with a goal of producing the movement in a 200-ms time period (from initiation to barrier contact). In essence, this was a ballistic aiming task, requiring a controlled-force output to propel the arm to the target in the required time. In variable practice, the distance to each barrier was changed in different conditions (15, 35, 60, and 65 cm). While keeping the time goal of 200 ms constant over practice, the subjects received 300 practice trials presented in a random order so that each distance was practiced equally (see table 19.1). This condition was contrasted with a constant practice condition which consisted of four subgroups, wherein subjects practiced only one movement distance for the 300 trials. In the transfer test phase, both groups transferred to a novel (50-cm) distance, both immediately after training and 2 days later. In this way, the experiment examined the effect of varied versus constant practice on the capability to perform a similar but new action.

The results from the McCracken and Stelmach (1977) study are shown in figure 19.5 wherein the absolute errors are plotted for the trials during the acquisition phase and for the trials at immediate transfer. As might be expected, during the original training the constant group performed with less error than the variable group. The critical comparison that yields information about the nature of the learned representation is the immediate transfer test in which subjects are required to produce a novel movement (Schmidt and Bjork, 1992). In figure 19.5, it can be seen that the variable-practice group performs with less error. From this finding, it appeared that the variability in practice (during original practice) allowed the subjects to learn the task more effectively, permitting them to perform the new version of the task

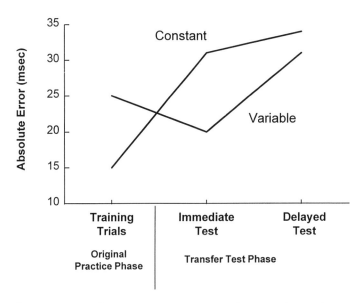

Figure 19.5 Performance in a movement-production task as a function of variability in practice during final acquisition and transfer trials. Adapted from McCracken and Stelmach, 1977.

with less error. The results suggest that variable practice created a learned motor representation that was different from the one obtained from constant practice.

Similar results have been reported by others using different tasks, such as throwing objects at targets of different distances (Kerr and Booth, 1978; Wulf, 1991) and propelling objects to targets at different distances (Kelso and Norman, 1977). These variability-of-practice studies suggest that practicing similar movement patterns containing different force-amplitudes or durations to achieve a task goal can heighten the learned motor representation and improve retention and transfer capabilities (Schmidt, 1991a). The data from these foregoing studies are used often as support for a type of motor learning that promotes the development of response schemata.

Summary

Though motor learning research has existed for many years, for the most part it has not addressed what individuals learn, how they learn, and how the learning is transferred into performance. Transfer tests are one step toward answering such questions. As seen in the foregoing examples, transfer tests permit inspection of what part of the motor learning can be transferred to different task conditions. Substantial positive transfer implies that fundamental parts of the acquired motor pattern are scalable and consist of invariant properties of the learned representation. These data then address one of the basic questions in motor learning research: whether learning involves acquiring a specific pattern or a more general pattern. This controversy in turn centers on another question: whether the acquired representation consists of abstract rules or parameters, or whether it is instance- or example-based. The suggestion of a rule-based schema theory provides a knowledge representation protocol that is in some ways similar to the notion of frames as used in artificial intelligence, but it is distinguished by its special attention to perception structures and distributed motor control (Arbib, 1991). The transfer data reviewed in this chapter seem to suggest that the learned or acquired representation may be abstract in nature, which permits the subjects to transfer (scale) the learned motor control pattern to novel movement patterns. Such data add to the growing evidence that over practice, a generalized abstract representation is formed permitting movements that share invariant features. This representation also permits scaling of the movement pattern to preserved relative timing (size and speed).

TASK CONSTRAINTS AND MOTOR LEARNING

This chapter began with the suggestion that practice leads to improvements in performance. Ensuing sections then described factors that influence the nature of these improvements. It was shown that these improvements in performance are imperfect reflections of learning. Moreover, it was demonstrated through transfer tests that the conditions of practice often determine the nature of the learned representation. This section will continue this theme, but the emphasis will switch to how individuals cope with alterations to well-learned movement patterns.

The task chosen for study is prehensile movements for reaching and grasping objects of different sizes. Such movements are well-learned and are used daily, so this skill is a good medium in which to study the characteristics of learned representations. Jeannerod (1981) provided some evidence that movements of reaching toward and grasping an object involve parallel-acting components, each of which is under independent control. One component, the reach, carries the hand over the requisite distance and is sensitive to the location of the object. While the hand is being transported, independent grasping mechanisms are thought to shape the hand to conform to the size and shape of the object.

At issue in these experiments is whether these tasks can provide further evidence on how the motor system adapts to task variations that are not part of the normal routine. Such variations share many of the common principles of transfer tests, wherein subjects are required to make novel motor responses. Such variations provide an opportunity to examine how the motor system adapts on-line and to determine how the motor system preserves relative timing. By analyzing the kinematics of a movement (e.g., displacement, velocity, and acceleration), investigators are able to generate logical hypotheses about the underlying movement representation (Jeannerod, 1984). When one creates an altered state (initial position or trajectory formation), kinematics can provide insight into how the acquired representative parameters modify the motor output for novel movement patterns. An essential feature of abstract representation is its capability to produce scalable properties of the acquired motor behavior. Such scalability suggests that relative timing reflecting spatial and temporal organization is an essential feature of generalized (abstract) motor programs.

Grasping with an Altered Aperture

Past studies have examined the coupling of the reach and grasp components during prehensile movements. Many such studies have supported the view that these components reflect the output of two parallel, though temporarily coupled, motor program representations. An essential characteristic of prehensile movement is its ability to accommodate objects of varying sizes and shapes in a multitude of locations. To accomplish such actions requires each component to be controlled by a learned generalized representation capable of incorporating such information as the initial hand and arm configurations in addition to the characteristics of the object (location, size, shape, etc.). To execute an accurate prehensile movement, the central nervous system needs a good memorial representation of the reach and grasp pattern required. Introducing novel movement conditions is one way to exploit that representation in attempting to understand its invariant features.

In a recent experiment, Saling, Mescheriakov, Molokanova, Stelmach, and Berger (in press) studied the nature of learned representations that guide prehensile movements. At issue was how the learned pattern, which has such robust kinematic features under normal conditions, responds to altered initial hand postures. The data from this experiment suggested that the representation may be abstract in nature, as the grip aperture was able to reorganize itself during wrist transport without influencing transport. Moreover, as the reach progressed toward the object, both the transport and the manipulation components became codependent, and the relative timing was well-preserved.

In this experiment, subjects reached for and grasped two different size objects located on a table. The targets were two objects of different diameter, one 22 mm in diameter, the other 67 mm in diameter. The subjects grasped the small object with a precision grip (thumb opposite index finger) and the large object with a whole-hand grip (thumb opposite all fingers). After 10 trials of reaching and grasping one of the two objects under normal conditions, the subjects were instructed to extend the aperture fully, thumb and fingers maximally apart prior to the reach. The subject continued this style of reaching and grasping for 10 trials. This procedure was followed for each object size. Under normal conditions, the grip aperture is closed with the fingers in a slightly flexed position and in contact with the thumb. The primary question was how the acquired representation responds to the altered hand posture.

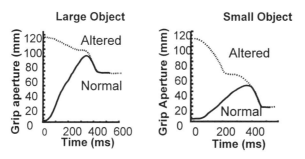

Figure 19.6 The effects of object size and altered grasp on grip aperture in a reaching task. From Saling et al., in press.

Figure 19.6 reports the kinematics of the grip for both the normal and altered conditions for both object sizes. The most striking feature of these data is that in the condition with the fingers and thumb maximally apart, the aperture does not continuously close until it makes contact with the object. It either hesitates momentarily (as seen in the figure) or slightly reopens before closure on the object. This pattern was true for either the small or the large object. These data indicate that some form of reorganization is occurring during the reach. Moreover, as can be seen in the figure, this reorganization is related to object size. The changes to the grip aperture are much larger when grasping the smaller object. When the closing and opening velocities were analyzed, it was found that both were sensitive to object size. Data from the main part of the study also showed that this grip reorganization did not affect the relative timing between the two components, the time to peak aperture and movement duration remaining invariant.

These data suggest that the learned representation for prehensile movements is quite adaptable with generalized features. That is, the representation is capable of accommodating the altered thumb-fingers posture without distorting the relationship between two components of the prehensile action. This interpretation is similar to the conclusion reached by Stelmach, Castiello, and Jeannerod (1994) that the memorial representation for prehensile acts contains scalable attributes that preserve relative timing. The scalable features appear to permit the aperture some flexibility during the early phase of the transport. In fact, the data suggest that the grip can operate independently from the transport component prior to reaching maximum grip aperture.

Grasping with Altered Trajectories

The previous experiment showed that by introducing a transfer-like condition (an altered initial hand posture prior to the reach), the learned representation demonstrated remarkable adaptability. The resultant data also suggested that the flexibility was organized somewhat separately, as the grip did all the accommodation. To achieve the task goal, the grip aperture reorganized itself independently from the transport component.

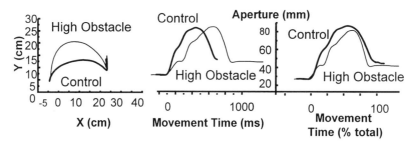

Figure 19.7 Effects of obstacle on reach-to-grasp movements. The trajectory is affected (left panel) by the obstacle, producing alterations in the grip (center panel); the right panel demonstrates that movement scaling exists across conditions. From M Saling, J Alberts, GE Stelmach, and JR Bloedel, unpublished data.

The experiment raised a related question: Do required changes to the trajectory also produce corresponding changes to the grip? M Saling, J Alberts, GE Stelmach, and JR Bloedel (unpublished data) used a paradigm requiring subjects to grasp an object 30 cm directly in front. After control trials without obstacle, the subjects had to reach for the object over obstacles placed in front of the object (about halfway between the starting position and the object). The two obstacles (10 cm and 13 cm in height) rested on the table. Reaching for the object required subjects to add vertical height to the hand transport to avoid contact with the obstacles. In this way, the experiment specifically altered the formation and execution of the trajectory of the transport component. The primary question was whether changes to the transport component produce corresponding changes to the aperture.

The data from this experiment are reported in figure 19.7. As can be seen in the left-hand graph, placing the obstacles in the path of the wrist definitely altered the trajectory of the hand. As can be seen, there is much more movement in the vertical plane when the obstacle is present.

In the center graph in figure 19.7, the aperture size is plotted for a typical subject as a function of movement time for the control and obstacle conditions. It can be seen that when the obstacle is present, the opening of the aperture is delayed and the closing is prolonged. These data suggest that the grip aperture is tightly coupled to the transport component. Moreover, the data also suggest that the grip aperture gets its primary information from the wrist. In the right-hand graph in figure 19.7, grip aperture is plotted as a function of percent of movement time. In contrast to the absolute difference previously reported for the same variables, when expressed on a relative time basis, the opening and closing of the aperture is nearly identical for the control and high-obstacle conditions. This finding is similar to the altered-grasp data also showing that the relative timing is preserved. It appears that the learned representation that guides prehensile acts has the ability to alter absolute time parameters for both the transport and grip components, yet preserves the relative timing between them.

These two prehension experiments offer yet another view of the nature of the representations that guide motor action. We may ask what has been acquired through many years of daily practice in performing prehensile actions. This highly practical skill was introduced to a transfer-like situation where the kinematics of two components can be examined in a novel state. These data offer a seminal look at which features are preserved and suggest both that learners have acquired the ability to produce a prehensile movement task that contains invariant relative timing features and that this capability is manifested in scalable parameters. Moreover, the altered grasping experiment found that the grip aperture reorganization occurred without influencing the transport of the wrist. These results are consistent with the postulate that the grip reorganizes itself during the transport to preserve the relative timing between the transport and grip components.

CONCLUSIONS

In this chapter, an attempt has been made to document how motor learning research has changed over the years. Early research was focused primarily on determining the optimal conditions of practice and how improvement in performance could be precisely documented. During most of this research period, the debate focused on rates of learning and retention curves. Recently, learning research has begun to address more fundamental questions, such as what is acquired through practice. Through the use of transfer tests, these experiments are addressing questions aimed at understanding the nature of the motor representation acquired through pratice. Such research has led to the view that the acquired representation contains invariant features that permit scaling of the movement pattern to preserve relative timing. The renewal of interest in motor learning, due in part to the availability of new recording techniques for movement, has drawn attention to determining what aspects of movement control change through extended practice. As stated by Jeannerod (1990), a complete kinematic description of how control changes with practice can be regarded as a reasonable description of how the neural commands also have changed. A major advantage of this analytical approach over the traditional task-oriented approach is that research is focused on identifying the features contained in the acquired representation. Of course, a full understanding of motor learning can come about only if behavioral work is integrated with biomechanics and neurophysiology.

ACKNOWLEDGMENTS

I thank Marian Saling for discussing the sections that dealt with prehension and Rachael Seidler for preparing the graphs contained in this chapter. Financial assistance from the Flinn Foundation and the National Institute of Neurological Diseases and Stroke (NS17421 and NS13312) helped in the preparation of this manuscript.

REFERENCES

Adams JA (1987). Historical review and appraisal of research on the learning retention and transfer of human motor skills. Psychol Bull 101:41–74.

Arbib M (1991). Programs, schemas, and neural networks for control of hand movements. In M Jeannerod (ed), Attention and Performance XIII. Hillsdale, NJ: Lawrence Erlbaum Associates, pp 111–138.

Baddeley AD, Longman DJA (1978). The influence of length and frequency of training session on the rate of learning to type. Ergonomics 21:627–635.

Bernstein N (1967). The Coordination and Regulation of Movement. Oxford: Pergamon.

Castiello U, Stelmach GE (1993). Generalized representation of handwriting: Evidence of effector independence. Acta Psychol (Amst) 31:395–402.

Fitts PM, Posner MI (1967). Human Performance. Belmont, CA: Brooks/Cole.

Goode S, Magill RA (1986). The contextual interference effects in learning three badminton serves. Res Q Exerc Sport 57:308–314.

Jeannerod M (1981). Intersegmental coordination during reaching at natural visual objects. In J Long, A Baddeley (eds), Attention and Performance. Hillsdale, NJ: Lawrence Erlbaum Associates, pp 153–168.

Jeannerod M (1984). The timing of natural prehension movements. J Mot Behav 16:235–254.

Jeannerod M (1990). The Neural and Behavioral Organization of Goal-Directed Movements. Oxford: Oxford Science.

Kawato M (1989). Adaptation and learning in control of voluntary movement by the central nervous system. Adv Robot 3:229–249.

Keele SW (1986). Motor control. In K Boff, L Kaufman, J Thomas (eds), Handbook of Perception and Human Performance: II. Cognitive Processes and Performance. New York: Wiley, pp 1–60.

Keele SW, Cohen A, Ivry R (1990). Motor programs: Concepts and issues. In M Jeannerod (ed), Attention and Performance XIII. Hillsdale, NJ: Lawrence Erlbaum Associates, pp 77–111.

Kelso JAS, Norman PE (1977). Motor schema formation in children. Devel Psych 14:153–156.

Kerr R, Booth B (1978). Specific and varied practice of motor skill. Percept Mot Skills 46:395–401.

Lee TD (1988). Transfer-appropriate processing: A framework for conceptualizing practice effects in motor learning. In OG Meijer, K Roth (eds), Complex Motor Behaviour: The Motor-Action Controversy. Amsterdam: Elsevier, pp 201–215.

Lee TD, Magill RA (1983). The locus of contextual interference in motor skill acquisition. J Exp Psychol Learn Mem Cogn 9:730–746.

McCracken HD, Stelmach GE (1977). A test of schema theory of discrete motor learning. J Mot Behav 9:193–201.

MacKay DG (1982). A theory of the representation and enactment of intentions. In D Magill (ed), Memory and Control in Motor Behavior. Amsterdam: North Holland.

Newell A, Rosenbloom (1981). Mechanisms of skill acquisition and the law of practice. In JR Anderson (ed), Cognitive Skills and Their Acquisition. Hillsdale, NJ: Lawrence Erlbaum Associates, pp 1–54.

Pew RW (1974). Levels of analysis in motor control. Brain Res 71:393–400.

Rosenbloom DA (1977). Selective adaptation of "command neurons" in the human motor system. Neuropsychologia 15:81–91.

Sailing M, Mecheriakov S, Molokarova E, Stelmoch GE, Berger M (in press). Exp Brain Res.

Schmidt RA (1991a). Frequent augmented feedback can degrade learning: Evidence and interpretations. In GE Stelmach, J Requin (eds), Tutorials in Motor Neuroscience. Dordrecht, The Netherlands: Kluwer, pp 59–75.

Schmidt RA (1991b). Motor Learning and Performance: From Principles to Practice. Champaign, IL: Human Kinetics.

Schmidt RA, Bjork RA (1992). New conceptions of practice: Common principles in three paradigms suggest new concepts for training. Psych Sci 3:207–217.

Schmidt RA, Young DE, Swinner S, Shapiro DC (1989). Summary knowledge of results for skill acquisition: Support for the guidance hypothesis. J Exp Psychol 15:352–359.

Shea JB, Morgan RL (1979). Contextual interference effects on the acquisition, retention, and transfer of a motor skill. J Exp Psychol Hum Learn Mem 5:179–187.

Snoddy GS (1926). Learning and stability. J Appl Psychol 10:1–36.

Stelmach GE (1969). Efficiency of motor learning as a function of inter-trial rest. Res Q Exerc Sport 40:192–200.

Stelmach GE (1982). Motor control and motor learning: The closed-loop perspective. In JA Kelso (ed), Human Motor Behavior: An Introduction. Hillsdale, NJ: Lawrence Erlbaum Associates, pp 93–116.

Stelmach GE, Castiello U, Jeannerod M (1994). Orienting the finger opposition space during prehension movements. J Mot Behav 26:178–186.

Welford AT (1968). Fundamentals of Skill. London: Methuen.

Winstein CJ, Schmidt RA (1990). Reduced frequency of knowledge of results enhances motor skill learning. J Exp Psychol Learn Mem Cogn 16:677–691.

Wulf G (1991). The effect of type of practice on motor learning in children. Appl Cogn Psych 5:123–134.

20 Learning Internal Models of the Motor Apparatus

Mitsuo Kawato

The problem of controlling goal-directed limb movements can be partitioned conceptually into a set of information-processing subprocesses: trajectory planning, coordinate transformation from extracorporal space to intrinsic body coordinates, and motor command generation. These subprocesses are required for translating the spatial characteristics of the target or goal of the movement into an appropriate pattern of muscle activation. Over the past decade, computational studies of motor control have become much more advanced as a result of concentrating on these three computational problems. These studies demonstrated that each of the three problems is computationally difficult in the sense that the solution cannot be determined uniquely. This computational difficulty, often referred to as *ill-posedness*, necessitates both forward and inverse models of the motor apparatus (Kawato, 1992). Here we will concentrate only on the motor command–generation problem.

Fast and coordinated arm movements should be executed under feedforward control because biological feedback loops (in particular those via the periphery) are slow and have small gains. Flash (1987) explained slight curvatures observed in point-to-point paths in front of the body by combining the minimum-jerk model (Flash and Hogan, 1985) with the virtual-trajectory control hypothesis (Bizzi, Accornero, Chapple, and Hogan, 1984; Hogan, 1984). The minimum-jerk model determines a unique trajectory by minimizing the time integral of the squared jerk (rate of change of acceleration) taken from the hand position represented in Cartesian space. The *virtual trajectory* is defined as "a time-varying position"; each position at a given moment is an equilibrium position determined by the viscoelastic property of the limb when motor commands at that moment are maintained for an indefinite time interval. In the virtual-trajectory control hypothesis, necessary joint torques are generated as a product of the limb's mechanical stiffness and of the difference between the actual and the virtual trajectory. It was also advocated that with this mechanism, the brain does not need to solve the inverse dynamics problem (computational problem of transforming the desired trajectory into the necessary motor commands, equivalent to the foregoing motor command–generation problem; details of this argument will be given in the next section) and does not need to possess internal inverse models to solve the problem.

In the work of Flash (1987), the virtual (not the real) trajectory, was assumed to be planned as the minimum-jerk trajectory. Although the virtual trajectory is straight, the real trajectory is slightly curved because of imperfect control by the virtual trajectory control. However, the stiffness values assumed in Flash's simulation (1987) are controversial. Bennett, Hollerbach, Xu, and Hunter (1992), Gomi, Koike, and Kawato (1992), Bennett (1993), and Gomi and Kawato (1996) found that dynamic stiffness during movement was much less than was assumed by Flash (1987).

Subsequently, based on the measured values of stiffness during movement, Katayama and Kawato (1993) showed that to reproduce roughly straight hand paths, the virtual trajectory must be dramatically curved. The differences between Flash's and Katayama's simulations can be understood readily if one recalls that the required joint torques are generated as the product both of mechanical stiffness and of the difference between the virtual and real trajectories under the virtual-trajectory control hypothesis. If such physical parameters as moment of inertia, mass, and link length are given, and the desired hand trajectory is fixed, the required joint torques can be determined uniquely from the inverse dynamics equation (see figure 20.1C). When the stiffness is large, the difference between the virtual and real trajectories is small but if the stiffness is small, this difference becomes large. Human multijoint hand paths are roughly straight for point-to-point movements. Consequently in Flash's simulation, where a relatively high stiffness was assumed, the virtual trajectory could be close to the real trajectory (i.e., it could be a simple straight trajectory). However, in Katayama's simulation, where a relatively low stiffness was assumed, the virtual trajectory was very different from the real trajectory. Conversely, if the virtual trajectory is planned as the minimum-jerk trajectory, the real trajectories are overly curved and do not get close enough to the target point when using the dynamic stiffness values measured during movement (Katayama and Kawato, 1993).

Thus if we consider the low mechanical stiffness values recently measured during movement (Bennett et al., 1992; Gomi et al., 1992; Gomi and Kawato, 1996), it would seem difficult to reproduce slightly curved hand paths by combining the virtual-trajectory control hypothesis with the minimum-jerk model. Planning the necessary complicated shapes of the virtual trajectory is computationally as difficult as solving the inverse dynamics problem, and actually is mathematically equivalent to it. Thus we believe that the most radical version of the virtual-trajectory control hypothesis (which posits that the brain does not solve the inverse dynamics problem) can be refuted on the basis of the stiffness measurements and simulation studies noted above. This situation necessitates the use of internal, neural models such as an inverse dynamics model for feed-forward control (Kawato, Gomi, Katayama, and Koike, 1993).

INTERNAL MODELS AND THE CEREBELLUM

The internal models in the brain must be acquired through motor learning so as to accommodate the changes that occur with the growth of such controlled objects as hands, legs, and torso and also the unpredictable variability of their dynamic properties because of injury, disease, or aging.

Where in the brain are internal models of the motor apparatus likely to be stored? First, the locus should exhibit a remarkable adaptive capability essential for acquisition and continuous updating of internal models of the motor apparatus. A number of physiological studies have suggested important functional roles of the cerebellum in motor learning and remarkable synaptic plasticity in the cerebellar cortex (Ito, 1984, 1989). Second, such biological objects of motor control as arms, speech articulators, and the torso possess many degrees of freedom and complicated nonlinear dynamics. Correspondingly, neural internal models should receive a broad range of sensory inputs and possess a capacity high enough to approximate complex dynamics. Extensive sensory signals carried by mossy fiber inputs and an enormous number of granule cells in the cerebellar cortex seem to fulfill the preceding prerequisites for internal models. Furthermore, both the recurrent and feedforward networks in the cerebellar cortex achieved by different kinds of inhibitory interneurons can provide temporal and spatial filtering and some nonlinear transformations on the mossy fiber inputs to finally feed an enormously rich set of synaptic inputs to Purkinje cells. Finally, the cerebellar symptoms usually classified as the *triad* of hypotonia—hypermetria, and intention tremor—could be understood as degraded performance when control is forced to rely solely on negative feedback control after internal models are destroyed or cannot be updated. This is because precise, fast, and coordinated movements can be executed if accurate internal models of the motor apparatus can be used, whereas pure feedback controllers with long feedback delays and small gains can attain only poor performance in these computations and usually lead to oscillatory instability for forced fast movements.

Miall, Weir, Wolpert, and Stein (1993) classified into several classes many theories regarding cerebellar role in the control of visually guided movements (such as coordination by Flourens, comparators by Holmes, gain controllers, associative learning, etc.), and they suggested that the most complete class of theories involves the cerebellum in forming an internal model of the motor system, as these theories can encompass all alternative theories while fitting many of the known facts of cerebellar organization. This "internal model" class of theories requires theories that call for the cerebellum to be an adaptive system capable of learning and of updating a model as the behavior of the motor system changes. These theories also require that the cerebellum store relevant parameters of the motor system, as these parameters form part of the description of the motor system behavior. Another requirement is timing capabilities; the motor system is dynamic, so a useful model will also need dynamic (i.e., time-dependent behavior). These theories also account for the connectivity of the cerebellum at a reasonable level of detail and can account for many of the symptoms of cerebellar disorder (Miall et al., 1993). How might internal models be acquired in the cerebellum through motor learning?

INTERNAL MODELS OF MOTOR APPARATUS

Controlled objects in biological movement can generally be described as *multivariable nonlinear dynamical systems* (figure 20.1C) whose inputs are muscle tensions, joint torques, or firing rates of nerve fibers to innervate muscles, and whose outputs are muscle lengths, joint angles, or the position of the hand in Cartesian coordinates. Thus, the direction of information flow in the controlled objects is from the motor commands to the movement trajectory. Following robotics jargon, we can say that this information flow direction is *forward*, and the opposite direction is *inverse*. Accordingly, internal models of the motor system can be divided into two types: forward models and inverse models (figure 20.1C). By *forward model* we mean a neural representation of the transformation from motor commands to the resultant behavior of the controlled object. In other words, a forward model is just a simple model (emulator, predictor, simulator) of the controlled object and can be used as its substitute. If the actual motor command given to the motor apparatus is also fed to the forward models as its input (i.e., as corollary discharge or efference copy), its output predicts the produced trajectory. The neural computation time (say 30 ms) for this prediction is expected to be much shorter than the external visual or proprioceptive feedback delay (say 100–200 ms). Thus if a forward model is used in the internal feedback loop, feedback control performance is improved significantly because large external feedback delays can be avoided (Ito, 1970). However, it is well-known in control theory that high gains cannot be set even for this internal feedback control because feedback delays are unavoidable.

On the other hand, more sophisticated, satisfactory, and fast feed-forward control can be achieved through an inverse model of the controlled object (Albus, 1975; Kawato, Furukawa, and Suzuki, 1987; Atkeson, 1989). By *inverse model* we mean a neural representation of the transformation from the desired movement of the controlled object to the motor commands required to attain these movement goals. Because the inverse model possesses input-output transfer characteristics that are the inverse of those of the controlled object, the cascade of the two systems gives an approximate identity function (i.e., the output is equivalent to the input for any input) (figure 20.1A). Stated otherwise, if a desired trajectory is given to the inverse model, at the end of the cascade the produced trajectory is fairly close to the desired trajectory. Thus accurate inverse models could be used as ideal feed-forward controllers. The training of inverse models is therefore crucial to the performance in feed-forward control.

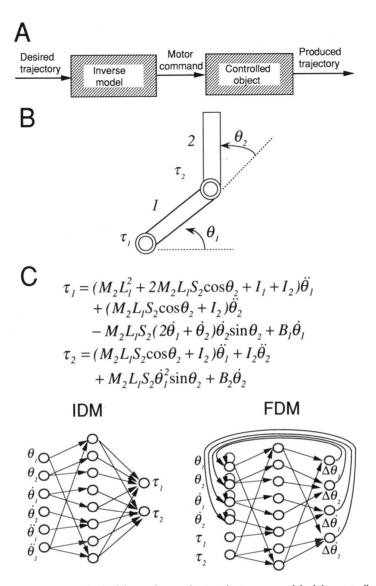

Figure 20.1 A. Feed-forward control using the inverse model of the controlled object. B. A two-link manipulator as an example of the controlled object. C. Different hardware and representational implementations of the inverse dynamics model (IDM) and the forward dynamics model (FDM). M_1, M_2, L_1, L_2, S_1, S_2, I_1, I_2, B_1, and B_2 are the mass, length, center of mass, moment of inertia, and viscosity coefficient of the first and the second links and joints, respectively.

　　Learning Internal Models of the Motor Apparatus

Though the inverse dynamics model of a controlled object is defined uniquely from a computational viewpoint, many different representations and hardware implementations are possible even for the same inverse dynamics model. This can be explained by using a simple example of a two-link, two-joint robotic manipulator (figure 20.1B) (a simple model of the human forearm and upper arm constrained in the horizontal plane at the shoulder level). θ_1, θ_2, τ_1, and τ_2 are the shoulder joint angle, the elbow joint angle, the shoulder joint torque, and the elbow joint torque, respectively (figure 20.1B). The Lagrangean equations of motion are shown in figure 20.1C, and relate the joint torques on the left to the joint angular accelerations, velocities, and positions on the right. M_1, M_2, L_1, L_2, S_1, S_2, I_1, I_2, B_1, and B_2 are the mass, length, center of mass, inertia moment, and viscosity coefficient of the first and the second links and joints, respectively. These equations can be viewed in two different ways. If we regard the left side, the joint *torque* as the input, and the right side the *output*, each equation gives the forward model of the manipulator (i.e., the equation predicts the movement from the motor command or torque). If we take the view that the right side defines the desired trajectory as an input and the left side computes the necessary torque as an output, the equation defines the inverse dynamics model (i.e., the equation calculates necessary torques to achieve the desired movement trajectory). The equations look complicated, but note that equations for robots with 6 or 7 degrees of freedom (the human arm has at least 7 degrees of freedom) are far more complicated and lengthy. If we print out the equations using some mathematical formula–handling software, the thickness of the printed sheets will be like a pile of newspapers received over a 1-week period. Thus biological researchers do not think that such inverse dynamics or forward dynamics equations are represented in the brain. This may be one of the motivations for developing the virtual-trajectory control hypothesis.

However, recent developments of artificial neural networks have demonstrated that the same inverse and forward models can be achieved easily by artificial neural networks with very simple structures (as shown in figure 20.1C). The simplest neural network structure for the inverse (left) and the forward (right) dynamics models are shown. The network for the inverse dynamics model is a feed-forward three-layer neural network model, whereas that for the forward model is a three-layer recurrent-type neural network model. Six neurons in the input layer of the inverse dynamics neural network represent positions, velocities, and accelerations of the two joints ($2 \times 3 = 6$), and the two output neurons represent torques of the two joints. Neurons in the second (hidden, intermediate) layer are necessary to approximate nonlinear transformations appearing in the Lagrangean equation. Synaptic weights between the first and the second layers, and between the second and the third layers, must be chosen carefully so that the input-output characteristic of the network well approximates that of the Lagrangean equation. It is mathematically shown that the approximation error goes to zero as the number of neurons in the second layer increases, as long as the synaptic weight values are optimally selected. Synaptic weights can be set by using some automatic learning method such as the Widrow-Hoff rule or the backpropagation-learning rule.

Because the network structures are very simple, it would not be surprising if biological neural networks with more complicated structures somehow implement inverse and forward dynamics models of a controlled object (i.e., a motor apparatus). One striking advantage of the neural network implementations of internal models is that pure and simple representations can be used but are not at all necessary. In the brain, it is difficult to imagine that any single neuron represents only the joint angle, joint angular velocity, joint angular acceleration, or joint torque. Even if the firing frequency of a single neuron is related to the muscle length, muscle spindle output, or motor neuron firing, it is more likely that a single-neuron firing frequency is a combination of temporally filtered and nonlinearly transformed sensory or motor variables.

If the input and output of the internal models are represented in this biological yet complicated manner, it is almost impossible to write down model equations (e.g., figure 20.1C) using those representations. Instead, neural networks can implement internal models with the same ease as in the pure representation of their inputs and outputs only if we can determine appropriate synaptic weights between neurons as previously explained.

Consequently, we believe that it would not be surprising if the brain acquires both the inverse and forward models based on some synaptic plasticity rules in the form of feed-forward and recurrent neural networks and uses them to solve various motor control problems including the motor command–generation problem.

SUPERVISED LEARNING FOR ACQUISITION OF INTERNAL MODELS

How can an internal inverse model be acquired? If a computational "teacher" can provide the correct motor commands, motor learning can be done in the framework of what is known as the *Widrow-Hoff rule*, consistent with biologically demonstrable heterosynaptic plasticity processes. However, in the context of motor learning it is unrealistic to assume the existence of a teacher with access to the correct motor commands prior to the learning of the movement pattern itself. It is more realistic to assume that a teacher has access only to the movement trajectory desired for the controlled object. For example, parents teach their children the correct pronunciation of words by providing speech samples in acoustic space but cannot directly communicate the neuronal firing patterns that activate articulator muscles. Correspondingly, a biologically plausible teacher for a neural network would have direct access not to the correct pattern of articulatory commands but rather to the desired "higher level" trajectory and the resultant discrepancy or error between the desired and currently produced trajectories. To train the inverse model, such trajectory errors must be converted first to motor command coordinates.

In the feedback-error learning approach (Kawato et al., 1987; figure 20.2A), the summation of the feedback motor command and the feed-forward command generated by the inverse model is fed to the controlled object, and the feedback controller transforms trajectory errors into motor command errors. The inverse model is trained during motor control while using the feedback motor command as the error signal. In this scheme, the feedback controller plays the role of a linear approximator of the inverse model of the controlled object, and converts trajectory errors into motor command errors. The feedforward controller does not mimic the feedback controller but acquires a fully nonlinear inverse model by trying to reduce the feedback motor command.

As explained in the previous section using figure 20.1C, the inverse dynamics model can be achieved by a simple, three-layer, feed-forward neural network model. Figure 20.2B shows the combination of the feedback-error learning scheme and the implementation of the inverse dynamics model by the three-layer network. This approach was applied to the control of robots possessing kinematic or dynamic redundancy and a 300-ms feedback loop delay (Kawato, 1990; Katayama and Kawato, 1991). Controlled objects used in experiments were a 6-degree-of-freedom PUMA robot, a 5-degree-of-freedom Bridgestone rubbertuator (artificial muscles made by pneumatic rubber actuators) SoftArm, and an automobile. The artificial network architecture that was used is shown in figure 20.3 which shows all the different degrees of freedom. Because of the feedback delay, the produced trajectory was compared with an earlier desired trajectory in the feedback controller. Though this seems quite difficult, the feedback-error learning was successful in these situations.

LONG-TERM DEPRESSION AND FEEDBACK-ERROR LEARNING

Marr (1969) and Albus (1971) proposed a detailed cerebellar model that can form associative memories between particular patterns on parallel fiber inputs and Purkinje cell outputs. The basic idea is that the parallel fiber–Purkinje cell synapses can be modified by input from climbing fibers. In perceptron models, the efficacy of a parallel fiber–Purkinje cell synapse is assumed to change when there exists a parallel fiber and climbing fiber input conjunction. The presence of the putative heterosynaptic plasticity of Purkinje cells was demonstrated as a long-term depression (LTD; Ito, 1989). An associative LTD found in Purkinje cells can be modeled as a heterosynaptic plasticity rule: The rate of change of the synaptic efficacy of a single parallel fiber synapse is proportional to the negative product of the firing rate of that synapse's input and the increment of the climbing fiber firing rate from its spontaneous level:

$$T \, dw_i/dt = -x_i(F - F_{\text{spont}}) \tag{1}$$

A

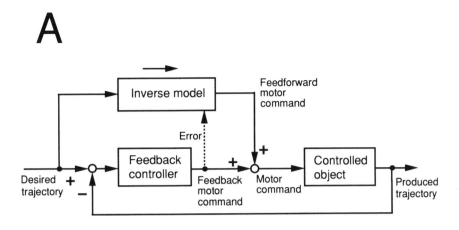

B

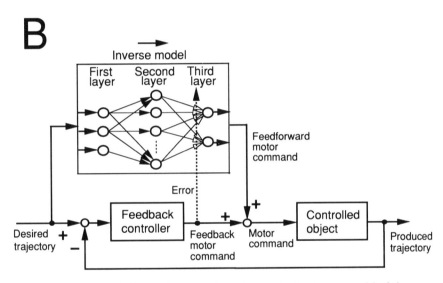

Figure 20.2 A. Feedback-error learning scheme to acquire the inverse model of the controlled object. B. The same learning scheme while using a three-layer feed-forward neural network model as the inverse dynamics model.

where T is a time constant; w_i is the synaptic weight of the ith parallel fiber–Purkinje cell synapse; x_i is the firing frequency of the ith parallel fiber–Purkinje cell synapse; F is the firing frequency of the climbing fiber input; and F_{spont} is its spontaneous level. This single rule reproduces both the LTD and long-term potentiation (LTP) found in Purkinje cells (Sakurai, 1987). When the climbing fiber and the parallel fiber are simultaneously stimulated, the parallel fiber synaptic efficacy decreases (LTD). In contrast, the parallel fiber synaptic efficacy increases (LTP) when only the parallel fiber is stimulated

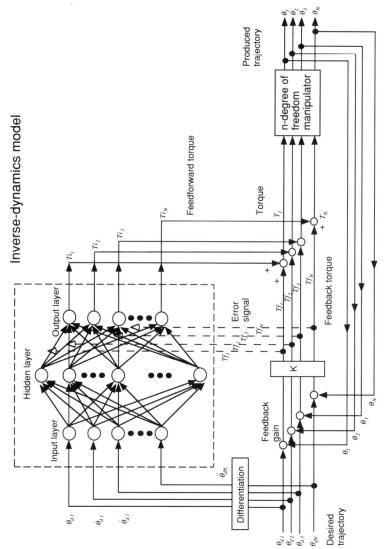

Figure 20.3 Detailed hardware structure of the artificial neural network model used in control experiments with different robotic manipulators.

(i.e., the climbing fiber firing frequency is lower than its spontaneous level) (Sakurai, 1987).

It can be shown that the previously mentioned learning rule can implement the feedback-error learning only if the climbing fiber input represents the feedback motor command (i.e., the error signal in the motor command space).

Marr (1982) pointed out that the brain must be understood at the following different levels: (1) computational theory (what is the goal of the computation?); (2) representation and algorithm (how can this computational theory be implemented?); and (3) hardware implementation. Though early-day cerebellar models (Marr, 1969; Albus, 1971) were epoch-making in proposing heterosynaptic plasticity as a basis of motor learning at the hardware level, Marr (1982) criticized these models because they could not provide a clear understanding at the first two levels mentioned previously. We proposed models that addressed these levels (introduced in this chapter). For example, in the feedback-error learning model, the cerebellum is postulated to acquire inverse models of controlled objects by using the heterosynaptic plasticity, whereas the climbing fiber inputs represent error signals in the motor command space.

We do not believe that the climbing fiber response is a random signal. The most important prerequisite for feedback-error learning is that the climbing fiber system convey the motor command errors in terms of both direction and amplitude. Support for this assumption was first reported by Simpson and Alley (1974) in experiments involving the flocculus of rabbits during vestibuloocular reflex (VOR). By accumulating spikes of climbing fibers for several tens of seconds, they showed that the firing frequency approximately codes the amplitude of the retinal slip velocity and is lower than the spontaneous level when the direction of image motion on the retina is opposite to the optimal direction. This observation in rabbits also was found in monkeys (Watanabe, 1985; Stone and Lisberger, 1990). The "learning" of information conveyed by these low-frequency climbing fibers could be accomplished over the relatively long time (1 hr) provided during LTD. Here, LTD computationally constitutes a biological spike-correlation accumulator.

MODEL OF SENSORIMOTOR LEARNING IN THE CEREBELLUM

We proposed a coherent model of cerebellar motor learning based on the feedback-error learning scheme (Kawato and Gomi, 1992a,b). The premotor network and the network-calculating climbing fiber activities in figure 20.4 correspond to the feedback controller of figure 20.3. The cerebellar cortex in figure 20.4 corresponds to the inverse dynamics model in figure 20.3. The climbing fiber inputs in figure 20.4 convey motor command errors (i.e., the feedback motor command in figure 20.3). The motor neurons, muscles, and the motor apparatus in figure 20.4 correspond to the controlled object in figure 20.3. The parallel fiber inputs are assumed to carry the desired motor pattern information and also the current state of the motor apparatus. We

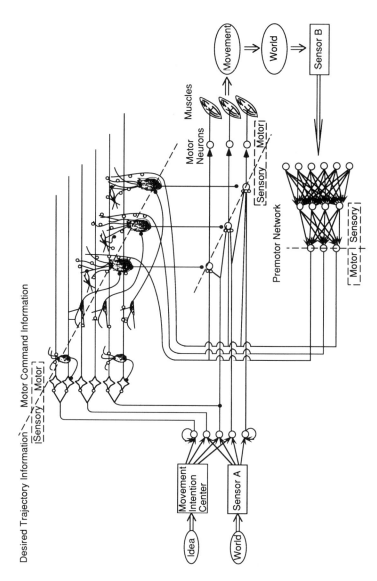

Figure 20.4 Cerebellar learning model motivated from the feedback-error learning scheme.

assume that climbing fiber responses represent motor commands generated by some of the premotor networks (i.e., networks that are upstream of the motor neurons and include feedback controllers at the spinal, brainstem, and cerebral levels (including the motor cortex). We do not assume necessarily that every premotor network literally compares a desired trajectory with an actual trajectory. However, it is required that the premotor network calculate the motor error in motor command coordinates, which vanishes (at the spontaneous firing level) when the resultant movement is desirable.

Based on the LTD in Purkinje cells, each longitudinal microzone in the cerebellar cortex with a 200-μm width and more than 50 mm long, in conjunction with a small portion of the deep cerebellar nucleus connected to the microzone, learns to execute predictive and coordinative control of different types of movements. This is achieved by a closed-loop and a one-to-one anatomical correspondence among each premotor network, a small region in the inferior olive, and a microzone of the cerebellar cortex. If one premotor network is regulated by one microzone of the cerebellar cortex, the latter must receive climbing fiber inputs from the specific part of the inferior olive that receives inputs from the earlier part of the same premotor network. With this anatomical organization, the cerebellar microzone is trained by feedback-error, which represents a copy of the motor-error command generated by the corresponding premotor network. Ultimately, each microzone acquires an inverse model of a specific controlled object and complements the relatively crude feedback control provided by the premotor networks. Thus the activity of the corresponding earlier part of the premotor network decreases as cerebellar learning proceeds, if it works in the feedback control mode. However, the latter half of the premotor circuit is quite active. If the premotor network constitutes a part of the feed-forward controller, as in the case of VOR, the premotor network activity does not decrease to zero. Moreover, it must be noted that other premotor networks not connected to the cerebellum may be active even after learning.

Two of the most important differences between the engineering (figure 20.3) and biological (figure 20.4) implementations of feedback-error learning by multilayer neural networks are their representations of inputs and outputs and how the intermediate layer representations are prepared.

In engineering implementations, the inputs to the three-layer network giving the inverse dynamics model are position, velocity, and acceleration of the desired trajectory for each degree of freedom. The outputs are feed-forward torque for each degree of freedom. On the other hand, though the inputs to the cerebellar cortex (mossy fibers) certainly convey information about the desired trajectory, they by no means represent pure positions, velocities, or accelerations. Based on what we know best about the mossy fiber inputs (ocular following responses for the ventral paraflocculus and the VORs for the flocculus), they represent complicated combinations of nonlinearly transformed desired velocity and acceleration.

In engineering implementations, the synaptic weights from the input layer to the hidden layer are learned by using the backpropagation learning rule. This cannot be expected in biological implementations; instead, a large number of granule cells and different kinds of inhibitory interneurons in the cerebellar cortex provide a rich class of temporally filtered and nonlinearly transformed signals from the mossy fiber inputs. It is not surprising if synapses on granule cells and the inhibitory interneurons are also plastic, but we expect that their synaptic plasticity is not supervised by the climbing fiber signals. In fact, Kano, Rexhausen, Dressen, and Konnerth (1992) found the LTP of synapses on Purkinje cells from inhibitory interneurons after occurrences of conjunctions of climbing fibers and inhibitory synaptic inputs. This makes perfect sense in the framework of feedback-error learning and can still be represented by Equation 1.

Our model in the simplest form (figure 20.2A) is quite restrictive in that not only does each microzone complement the relatively crude feedback control provided by the premotor networks, but it does so in time to provide a complete inverse model. This is the case only when the premotor network constitutes a feedback controller and there exists no fixed feed-forward pathway other than that via the cerebellar microzone. In most biological cases, the combination of the cerebellar cortex and the feed-forward part of the premotor network achieves the inverse dynamics model (figure 20.4).

Many researchers believe that the cerebellum modulates motor pattern generators or provides a correction to the premotor networks, rather than causing the activity of those premotor networks to go to zero. In response to this alternative view, we emphasize that what goes to zero is only the activity of premotor networks that work in feedback control and send their corollary discharges to the inferior olive. It might be that our inverse-model theory is appropriate to the most basic and (perhaps) phylogenetically older functions of the cerebellum but is not sufficiently comprehensive to cover all the functions of the cerebellum. Even in that case, our hope is that our simple inverse-dynamics theory will establish guidelines for more complicated and diverse computational functions of the cerebellum during motor learning.

Despite the crude nature of the signals from the premotor feedback networks, the premotor commands are the only source of motor coordinate information for training the cerebellum. There are two reasons why a relatively crude premotor command can serve as training information for the correct cerebellar command: First, the premotor command is not a teaching signal but rather an error signal. Second, though the premotor command is faulty, it at least roughly indicates the directions and magnitudes of cerebellar command modifications. This latter point is controversial because the range of firing frequencies of the climbing fibers is unusually low; hence it has seemed difficult to understand how climbing fiber activity could convey directional or amplitude information. By contrast, the apparent all-or-nothing firing characteristics of climbing fibers may be useful for somatic event detection, providing information to the Purkinje cells about the occurrence of undesirable movements (penalty signals). However, because the LTD has a time-constant of approximately 1 hr, even a low firing frequency can be integrated to give analog information. If the firing frequency is lower than the spontaneous level, it can give direction (negative) information. In the feedback-error learning framework, the climbing fibers must be able to convey amplitude as well as directional information regarding the error. This prerequisite is supported in the vestibulocerebellum (Simpson and Alley, 1974), but the problem is still open for other regions.

Despite the foregoing arguments, doubt may still remain regarding the effectiveness of Equation 1 because averaging loses the information content provided by specific parallel fiber contexts. In other words, it seems difficult for long-term averaging of climbing fiber activities to be used to modify those mossy fibers acting during a narrow time window, as seems to be required for any of the current theories on the role of the cerebellum in motor control. This concern is quite reasonable, but actually it is not the problem it is taken to be. One of the most remarkable aspects of our feedback-error learning model is that the correct feed-forward motor command, which has a high-frequency component, is learned from a smeared low-frequency feedback motor command because the latter signal is not a teaching signal but an error signal. This characteristic was demonstrated both by a number of practical applications in robotics and by mathematical analysis. Because Equation 1 calculates the product of two terms, even if the error term is of a low frequency, the learned feed-forward command can be of a frequency high enough for coordinated movement if the input term (from parallel fibers) is of a sufficiently high frequency. A simple (and thus perhaps unrealistic) example of this situation—where high-frequency motor command can be learned from low-frequency error signal—might be an assumed climbing fiber firing frequency of 5 pulses per second for 300 ms (low frequency) which is larger than its spontaneous value, say 1 pulse per second. During this time window of 300 ms, a set of parallel fibers is supposed to fire at high frequencies only during 10 ms (high frequency). Then, from Equation 1, synaptic weights of only this set of parallel fiber synapses are depressed. After learning, if the same input pattern is given on the whole set of parallel fibers, the Purkinje cell firing is suppressed and modified only during the preceding 10 ms (high frequency). By generalizing this simple case, we can expect that a precise inverse model with a high-frequency component can be learned even from an error signal provided by an approximate and low-frequency inverse model.

INVERSE DYNAMICS ENCODING OF OCULAR FOLLOWING EYE MOVEMENTS BY THE VENTRAL PARAFLOCCULUS

Recently, Shidara, Kawano, Gomi, and Kawato (1993) examined an inverse-dynamics representation of the firing pattern of ventral paraflocculus Purkinje cells during the ocular following response in monkeys. Movements of the visual scene evoke tracking movements of the eyes, termed *ocular following*.

When an observer's head turns, the eyes counterrotate in the head under the influence of the VOR, but because this reflex is not perfect, some disturbance of gaze (and hence also of the retinal image) often occurs. By working to stabilize the eye with respect to the environment, ocular following helps to compensate for the observer's own movements.

Simple-spike activity of a Purkinje cell in the left ventral paraflocculus was recorded together with the ocular following response from 50 to 200 presentations of a 20 °/s to 160 °/s downward or ipsilateral test ramp of a large-field random dot pattern. The responses were aligned with stimulus onset. The ensemble's average spike response over the trials—eye acceleration, eye velocity, eye position, and stimulus velocity—were calculated. The temporal pattern of the ensemble's mean firing frequency of cells was reconstructed as a linear weighted superposition of the position, velocity, and acceleration of the actual eye movement according to the following equation:

$$f(t - \Delta) = M \cdot \ddot{\theta}(t) + B \cdot \dot{\theta}(t) + K \cdot \theta(t) + f_{\text{spont}} \tag{2}$$

Here, $f(t)$, $\theta(t)$, $\dot{\theta}(t)$, $\ddot{\theta}(t)$, Δ, and f_{spont} are the firing frequency at time t, the eye position, velocity, acceleration at time t, the time delay, and the spontaneous firing level, respectively. The four coefficients and the time delay were estimated to minimize the squared error between the average and reconstructed firing frequencies.

Shidara et al. (1993) found that the cell firing frequency is fairly well reproduced by this expression: Square of the correlation coefficient was larger than 0.7 for more than 80 percent of the neurons studied (19 of 23). These authors used the parameters of the 19 well-fitted Purkinje cells for the statistical analysis that follows. The mean ratio of acceleration coefficient to velocity coefficient (M/B) of the Purkinje cells was 72.1, which was close to that of the motoneurons: 67.39. On the other hand, whereas the mean ratio of acceleration coefficient to position coefficient ($M/K = -294.5$) of the Purkinje cells was of a similar size, it was different from, and had the sign reverse of, that of the motoneurons: 344.8. These results indicate that the activity of the Purkinje cells encodes not the static but the dynamic part of the motor command for the required eye movement.

It was found that for more than half (13 of 21) of examined Purkinje cells, a single set of parameter values can reconstruct firing frequencies at different stimulus speeds (10, 20, 40, 80, and 160 °/s) (Gomi et al., 1994). As further evidence, figure 20.5 shows that a single set of parameter values can reconstruct firing frequencies for the five different stimulus speeds in the preferred direction (down for this Purkinje cell) and for the five different stimulus speeds in the antipreferred direction (up).

Figure 20.6 shows a current model of neural networks involved in the ocular following response.

For a satisfactory ocular following response, the desired trajectory information given by the ramp velocity profile must be converted into a motor command that produces the desired eye movement. Although this inverse dynamics problem could be solved at multiple sites in the brain, these results support the hypothesis that the cerebellum may be the major site of the inverse dynamics model for controlled movements. They do so for three reasons: (1) the Purkinje cell firing profiles were well-reconstructed by the inverse-dynamics representation; (2) though the ratio of acceleration and velocity coefficients of the Purkinje cells was very close to that of the motoneurons, that of mossy fiber inputs to them was only approximately half (i.e., though the outputs of the Purkinje cells could constitute the dynamic part of the final motor command, the inputs could not; and (3) the preferred directions of the Purkinje cells could be classified into only two groups, downward and ipsilateral, indicating that Purkinje cells encode coordinates suitable for generating the motor output, whereas the mossy fibers do not.

Thus the ventral paraflocculus constitutes a dynamic part of the inverse dynamics model of the eye plant, compensating only inertia and viscosity forces. This is similar to the separation of the full inverse dynamics model into an inverse statics model (which compensates only equilibrium posture maintenance) and an inverse dynamics model (which compensates only dynamic forces). We observed this separation in a previous application of our feedback-error learning neural network model (Katayama and Kawato, 1991), and it was successfully used for learning control of a robot arm with muscle-like pneumatic rubber actuators (i.e., rubbertuator SoftArm system). We found that the separation of static and dynamic components of the model was beneficial for stable and robust performance in learning and control, especially early in the learning phase.

CONCLUSION

Fast and well-coordinated movements by a motor apparatus with many degrees of freedom can be achieved only if the brain possesses and uses certain kinds of internal models of the motor apparatus. The cerebellum is one of the most plausible loci for the acquisition and storage of these internal models. We propose a cerebellar learning model based on a computationally developed feedback-error learning scheme. This computational model is supported by a reconstruction based on an inverse dynamics representation of firing frequencies of Purkinje cells during an ocular following response in the monkey ventral paraflocculus.

ACKNOWLEDGMENTS

I thank Dr. Yoh'ichi Tohkura of ATR Human Information Processing Research Laboratories for his continuing encouragement. Preparation of this manuscript was supported by a Human Frontier Science Project Grant to Mitsuo Kawato.

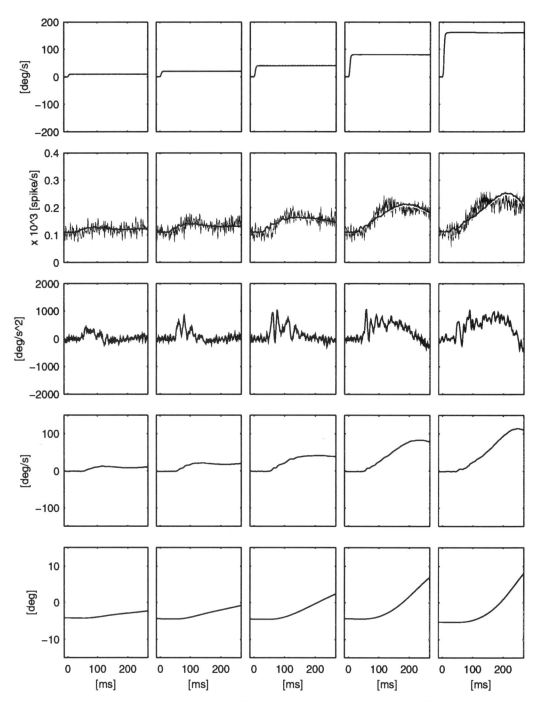

Figure 20.5 Reconstruction of firing frequencies of a single Purkinje cell under different-direction and different-speed visual stimuli. From top to bottom row: stimulus velocity patterns, observed single Purkinji cell firing frequency patterns (gray line), eye acceleration patterns, eye velocity patterns, and eye position patterns under five different stimulus velocities in the preferred (left 5 columns) and antipreferred (right 5 columns) directions. The reconstructed Purkinji cell firing frequency patterns by one set of parameter values are superimposed in the graphs in the second row (solid line).

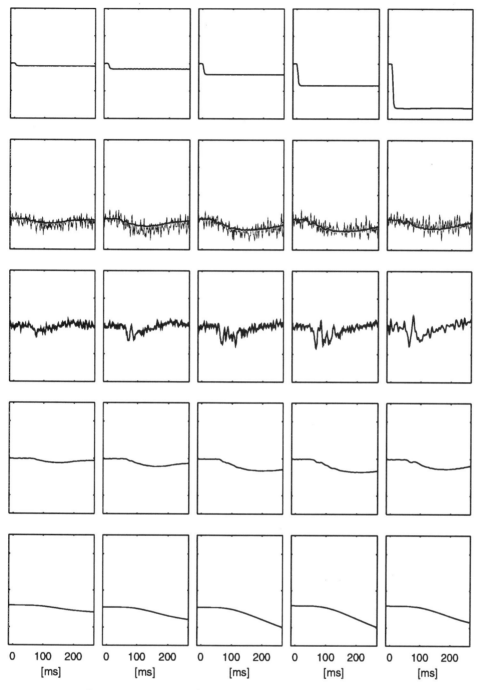

Figure 20.5 (continued)

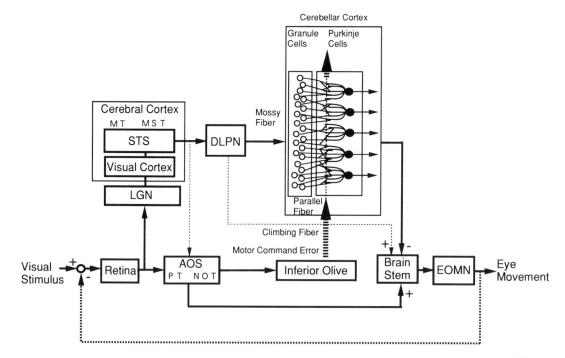

Figure 20.6 Schematic diagram of main neural pathways and neural networks responsible for control of ocular following responses in monkeys. STS, superior temporal sulcus; DLPN, dorsolateral pontine nucleus; AOS, accessory optic system; PT, pretectum; NOT, nucleus optic tract; and EOMN, extraocular motor neurons. Different brain regions are arranged so that the overall figure resembles the feedback-error learning model of the cerebellum shown in figure 20.4.

REFERENCES

Albus JS (1971). A theory of cerebellar functions. Math Biosci 10:25−61.

Albus JS (1975). A new approach to manipulator control: The cerebellar model articulation controller (CMAC). Trans ASME, J Dyn Syst Meas Cont 97:220−227.

Atkeson CG (1989). Learning arm kinematics and dynamics. Annu Rev Neurosci 12:157−183.

Bennett DJ (1993). Torques generated at the human elbow joint in response to constant position errors imposed during voluntary movements. Exp Brain Res 95:488−498.

Bennett DJ, Hollerbach JM, Xu Y, Hunter IW (1992). Time-varying stiffness of human elbow joint during cyclic voluntary movement. Exp Brain Res 88:433−442.

Bizzi E, Accornero N, Chapple W, Hogan N (1984). Posture control and trajectory formation during arm movement. J Neurosci 4:2738−2744.

Flash T (1987). The control of hand equilibrium trajectories in multi-joint arm movements. Biol Cybern 57:257−274.

Flash T, Hogan N (1985). The coordination of arm movements: An experimentally confirmed mathematical model. J Neurosci 5:1688−1703.

Gomi H, Kawato M (1996). Equilibrium-point control hypothesis examined by measured arm-stiffness during multi-joint movement. Science, in press.

Gomi H, Koike Y, Kawato M (1992). Human hand stiffness during discrete point-to-point multi-joint movement. Proc IEEE Eng Med Biol Soc 1628–1629.

Gomi H, Shidara M, Takemura A, Inoue Y, Kawano K, Kawato M (1994). Using an inverse dynamics representation to reconstruct temporal firing patterns of Purkinje cells in monkey ventral paraflocculus (ATR Tech Rep TR-H-086:1–36). Kyoto: ATR.

Hogan N (1984). An organizing principle for a class of voluntary movements. J Neurosci 4:2745–2754.

Ito M (1970). Neurophysiological aspects of the cerebellar motor control system. Int J Neurol 7:162–176.

Ito M (1984). The Cerebellum and Neural Control. New York: Raven Press.

Ito M (1989). Long-term depression. Annu Rev Neurosci 12:85–102.

Kano M, Rexhausen U, Dreessen J, Konnerth A (1992). Synaptic excitation produces a long-lasting rebound potentiation of inhibitory synaptic signals in cerebellar Purkinje cells. Nature 356:601–604.

Katayama M, Kawato M (1991). Learning trajectory and force control of an artifical muscle arm by parallel-hierarchical neural network model. In RP Lippmann, JE Moody, DS Touretzky (eds), Advances in Neural Information Processing Systems. San Mateo: Morgan Kaufmann, pp 436–442.

Katayama M, Kawato M (1993). Virtual trajectory and stiffness ellipse during multijoint arm movement predicted by neural inverse models. Biol Cybern 69:353–362.

Kawato M (1990). Computational schemes and neural network models for formation and control of multijoint arm trajectory. In T Miller, RS Sutton, PJ Werbos (eds), Neural Networks for Control. Cambridge, MA: MIT Press, pp 197–228.

Kawato M (1992). Optimization and learning in neural networks for formation and control of coordinated movement. In D Meyer, S Kornblum (eds), Attention and Performance: XIV. Synergies in Experimental Psychology, Artificial Intelligence, and Cognitive Neuroscience—A Silver Jubilee. Cambridge, MA: MIT Press, pp 821–849.

Kawato M, Furukawa K, Suzuki R (1987). A hierarchical neural-network model for control and learning of voluntary movement. Biol Cybern 57:169–185.

Kawato M, Gomi H (1992a). The cerebellum and VOR/OKR learning models. Trend Neurosci 15:445–453.

Kawato M, Gomi H (1992b). A computational model of four regions of the cerebellum based on feedback-error-learning. Biol Cybern 68:95–103.

Kawato M, Gomi H, Katayama M, Koike Y (1993). Supervised learning for coordinative motor control. In EB Baum (ed), Computational Learning and Cognition, SIAM Frontier Series. Philadelphia: Society for Industrial and Applied Mathematics, pp 126–161.

Marr D (1969). A theory of cerebellar cortex. J Physiol (Lond) 202:437–470.

Marr D (1982). Vision. New York: Freeman.

Miall RC, Weir DJ, Wolpert DM, Stein JF (1993). Is the cerebellum a Smith predictor? J Mot Behav 25:203–216.

Sakurai M (1987). Synaptic modification of parallel fiber-Purkinje cell transmission in *in vivo* guinea pig cerebellar slices. J Physiol (Lond) 394:463–480.

Shidara M, Kawano K, Gomi H, Kawato M (1993). Inverse-dynamics model eye movement control by Purkinje cells in the cerebellum. Nature 365:50–52.

Simpson JI, Alley KE (1974). Visual climbing fiber input to rabbit vestibulo-cerebellum: A source of direction-specific information. Brain Res 82:302–308.

Stone LS, Lisberger SG (1990). Visual responses of Purkinje cells in the cerebellar flocculus during smooth pursuit eye movements in monkeys. J Neurophysiol 63:1241–1261.

Watanabe E (1985). Role of the primate flocculus in adaptation of the vestibulo-ocular reflex. Neurosci Res 3:20–38.

Contributors

Hiroshi Asanuma
Rockefeller University
New York, New York

Robert Baker
Department of Physiology and
Neuroscience
New York University Medical
Center
New York, New York

James R. Bloedel
Division of Neurobiology
Barrow Neurological Institute
Phoenix, Arizona

Vlastislav Bracha
Division of Neurobiology
Barrow Neurological Institute
Phoenix, Arizona

John F. Disterhoft
Department of Cell and Molecular
Biology
Northwestern University Medical
School
Chicago, Illinois

John P. Donoghue
Department of Neuroscience
Brown University
Providence, Rhode Island

Timothy J. Ebner
Neurosurgery Department
University of Minnesota
Minneapolis, Minnesota

Kevin C. Engel
Department of Physiology
University of Minnesota
Minneapolis, Minnesota

Didier Flament
Neurosurgery Department
University of Minnesota
Minneapolis, Minnesota

Edwin Gilland
Department of Physiology and
Neuroscience
New York University Medical
Center
New York, New York

Andrew M. Gordon
Department of Physiology
University of Minnesota
Minneapolis, Minnesota

Mark Hallett
Medical Neurology Branch
National Institute of Neurological
Diseases and Stroke
Bethesda, Maryland

John A. Harvey
Department of Pharmacology
Medical College of Pennsylvania
Philadelphia, Pennsylvania

Grzegorz Hess
Department of Animal Physiology
Jagiellonian University
Krakow, Poland

Okihide Hikosaka
Department of Physiology
Juntendo University School of
Medicine
Tokyo, Japan

Fay B. Horak
R.S. Dow Neurological Sciences
Institute
Legacy Good Samaritan
Hospital
Portland, Oregon

Mitsuo Kawato
ATR Human Information Processing
Research Labs
Kyoto, Japan

Michelle A. Kronforst
Department of Cell and Molecular
Biology
Northwestern University Medical
School
Chicago, Illinois

Stephen G. Lisberger
Department of Physiology
University of California, San
Francisco
San Francisco, California

Matthew S. Milak
Division of Neurobiology
Barrow Neurological
Institute
Phoenix, Arizona

Shigehiro Miyachi
Department of Physiology
Juntendo University School of
Medicine
Tokyo, Japan

Kae Miyashita
Department of Physiology
Juntendo University School of
Medicine
Tokyo, Japan

James R. Moyer, Jr.
Department of Psychology
Yale University
New Haven, Connecticut

Alvaro Pascual-Leone
Departamento de Fisiologia
Universidad de Valencia
Valencia, Spain

Miya K. Rand
Department of Exercise Science and
Physical Education
Arizona State University
Tempe, Arizona

Jerome N. Sanes
Department of Neuroscience
Brown University
Providence, Rhode Island

Sharad J. Shanbhag
Neurosurgery Department
University of Minnesota
Minneapolis, Minnesota

Yury Shimansky
Division of Neurobiology
Barrow Neurological Institute
Phoenix, Arizona

John F. Soechting
Department of Physiology
University of Minnesota
Minneapolis, Minnesota

Joseph E. Steinmetz
Department of Psychology
Indiana University
Bloomington, Indiana

George E. Stelmach
Department of Exercise Science
and Physical Education
Arizona State University
Tempe, Arizona

W. Thomas Thach
Department of Neurology and
Neurological Surgery
Irene Walter Johnson Rehabilitation
Research Institute
Washington University School of
Medicine
St. Louis, Missouri

L. T. Thompson
Department of Cell and Molecular
Biology
Northwestern University Medical
School
Chicago, Illinois

Helge Topka
Department of Neurology
Universität Tübingen
Tübingen, Germany

Eddy A. Van der Zee
Department of Cell and Molecular
Biology
Northwestern University Medical
School
Chicago, Illinois

Craig Weiss
Department of Cell and Molecular
Biology
Northwestern University Medical
School
Chicago, Illinois

John P. Welsh
Department of Physiology and
Neuroscience
New York University Medical
Center
New York, New York

Steven P. Wise
Laboratory of Neurophysiology
National Institute of Mental Health
Poolesville, Maryland

Charles D. Woody
UCLA Medical Center
Los Angeles, California

Index